Men and Their Dogs

Christopher Blazina · Lori R. Kogan
Editors

Men and Their Dogs

A New Understanding of Man's Best Friend

Springer

Editors
Christopher Blazina
New Mexico State University
Las Cruces, NM
USA

Lori R. Kogan
Colorado State University
Fort Collins, CO
USA

ISBN 978-3-319-30095-5 ISBN 978-3-319-30097-9 (eBook)
DOI 10.1007/978-3-319-30097-9

Library of Congress Control Number: 2016933321

Printed on acid-free paper

This Springer imprint is published by Springer Nature
The registered company is Springer International Publishing AG Switzerland

Contents

Editors and Contributors

About the Editors

Christopher Blazina Ph.D. is a psychologist, professor, and author/editor of six books, and more than 50 publications. The books include: *The Cultural Myth of Masculinity; The Secret Lives of Men; An International Psychology of Men; The Psychology of the Human-Animal Bond; When Man Meets Dog*. His main area of research and clinical practice involves men's psychology, and most recently, how human–animal interaction especially impacts males across the life span. Dr. Blazina is currently a faculty member at New Mexico State University.

Lori R. Kogan Ph.D. is licensed psychologist and Associate Professor of Clinical Sciences for the College of Veterinary Medicine and Biomedical Sciences at Colorado State University. She is currently engaged in several research projects pertaining to the intersection of the human animal interactions, the human animal bond, and veterinary medicine. She is the editor of the Human–Animal Interaction Bulletin, an open-access, online publication supported by Division 17 (Counseling Psychology) of the American Psychological Association. She is also the founder/director of Pets Forever, an intergenerational service learning course and community program which functions in partnership with the Colorado State University Foundation to help low-income elderly and/or disabled pet owners. In addition, Dr. Kogan has years of experience providing individual and couples counseling to veterinary students, faculty and staff. She has published numerous journal articles, co-authored book chapters, and given invited presentations on topics related to human animal interactions in both psychology and veterinary medicine venues.

Contributors

Cynthia L. Bathurst Ph.D. is Co-founder, President and Executive Director of Safe Humane, a first-of-its kind organization founded on the concept that a humane community is a safer community. Safe Humane Chicago incorporates its mission to inspire positive relationships between people and animals into nontraditional programs that benefit youth, veterans, and at-risk animals through education, advocacy, outreach, and hands-on programs in communities challenged by crime and a lack of needed resources.

Dr. Bathurst earned a Bachelor of Science degree in Mathematics and Computer Science from the University of Alabama and a Ph.D. through the English Department at the University of Iowa. Her professional career started with more than 5 years of college-level teaching at Iowa and continued in Chicago with more than 25 years in contract mathematical analysis and consulting. During that time, she was led to community policing and organizing, prompted by crime and violence in Chicago and the need for safer, more humane neighborhoods. In 2009 the American Veterinary Medical Association awarded her their Humane Award, an award given to a non-veterinarian who has advanced animal well-being, shown exemplary dedication to the care of animals, and contributed to the community and society. In 2012 she became Safe Humane Chicago's Executive Director and continues working on taking Safe Humane concepts and programs to other cities. She has served on numerous public safety, community policing and animal welfare boards, and task forces and is currently Vice-Chair of Chicago's Commission on Animal Care and Control and an advisor to the National Canine Research Council.

Laura Bruneau Ph.D. is an Associate Professor of Counselor Education at Adams State University in Alamosa, Colorado. She completed her doctorate degree in Counselor Education and Supervision at Kent State University. Dr. Bruneau has published in several peer-reviewed counseling journals (e.g., Journal of Humanistic Counseling, Journal of Creativity in Mental Health, Journal of School Counseling). Her research interests include creativity in counseling, therapeutic reading, counseling theory, animal assisted therapy, and animal assisted education. She and her dog are a registered Pet Partners team. Since 2012, she has implemented a Reading Education Assistance Dog program at local elementary schools. This program helps struggling readers by providing a space for supervised, enjoyable reading practice. Dr. Bruneau is also a member of the Advisory Board Committee for the Center for Human Animal Interventions at Oakland University in Rochester, Michigan.

Dr. Cori Bussolari is a licensed psychologist and credentialed school psychologist. For most of her professional clinical career, Dr. Bussolari has worked with individuals and families coping with illness, death, or a significant life transition, In addition to her clinical work in private practice in San Francisco, Dr. Bussolari is an Associate Professor at the University of San Francisco in the Counseling Psychology Department. While Dr. Bussolari's current research involvement is in the area of pet loss and grief and she has always been immersed within the area of bereavement and trauma, especially in regards to positive and lifelong coping. Dr. Bussolari is an active consultant for schools, families, and community mental health clinics regarding issues related to illness, bereavement, or learning difficulties. She also facilitates the San Francisco SPCA Pet Loss Support Group.

Dr. Betty J. Carmack Professor Emerita in the School of Nursing at the University of San Francisco, has worked in the area of pet loss since 1982. She initiated and has led the monthly pet loss support groups at the SF/SPCA from 1982 to 2015. In addition to working with individuals grieving the death of their companion animals, she has worked with the staff of humane societies, veterinary hospitals, and animal care organizations vis-à-vis their specific grief and stress issues as these relate to their work with and care of animals. She is particularly interested in compassion fatigue. She has authored articles in both the professional and the lay literature, presented at numerous professional conferences, engaged in research related to pet loss, and mentored others who feel called to this work. She has conducted research on the lived experience of losing a companion animal as well as on the continuing connections people have after the death of a beloved animal. She is the author of the book Grieving the Death of a Pet. She continues to collaborate on research related to continuing bonds and pet loss. She has served on the Board of Trustees of Pet Unlimited in San Francisco and the Advisory Board of VET Street Outreach Services also in San Francisco. She was on the faculty of the Schools of Nursing at both the University of California, San Francisco and the University of San Francisco.

Teri L. Carper Ph.D. is a Staff Psychologist at the Orlando VAMC specializing in EBT for PTSD via Telehealth. She completed her undergraduate work at Boston University and earned her Ph.D. in 2010 from the University of Central Florida (UCF). Dr. Carper completed her Pre-doctoral internship at Boston Consortium for Clinical Psychology and her postdoctoral fellowship at the National Center for PTSD at Boston VA, where she also held the positions of Clinical Fellow in Psychiatry at Harvard Medical School and Teaching Fellow in Psychiatry at Boston University School of Medicine. Dr. Carper's clinical and research interests center around trauma trajectories and resiliency factors, and she is currently an Investigator on a grant examining the impact of human–animal interaction on extant PTSD treatments. In addition to her clinical responsibilities, Dr. Carper also serves on the Orlando VAMC Training Committee and is a certified LEAN/Six Sigma consultant for the mental health services. Dr. Carper's personal interests include animal rescue, distance running, skiing, spending time with family and friends, and most importantly, raising her daughter and son.

Robyn Denke B.A. is a graduate student in the Educational Psychology Department of the Neag School of Education at the University of Connecticut pursuing her Master of Arts in School Counseling. Passionate about social justice issues, Robyn's research interests include positive youth development, educational equity, and prevention and intervention programs for students.

Angela K. Fournier Ph.D., LP is a graduate of Virginia Tech with an MS and Ph.D. in Clinical Psychology. She is a licensed psychologist in Minnesota and Associate Professor at Bemidji State University. Dr. Fournier is an EAGALA- certified MH and co-facilitates EAP/L at Eagle Vista Ranch and Wellness Center in Bemidji, MN, providing group therapy services to women and at-risk youth in chemical dependency treatment. Her research focuses on the psychological outcomes of human–animal interaction. Recent works include development of a human–animal interaction scale and measuring outcomes of equine-assisted interventions.

Mary Harlinger is a Ph.D. candidate in Counseling Psychology. She values the importance of finding balance in life and this has recently focused on incorporating play into adult life. This has been applied to include the behavioral health applications for chronic illness and the use of canine companionship especially in consideration of gender differences.

Amy Johnson MA, MAT, LPC, TLS has been working in the field of Animal Assisted Interventions, both through practice and education, for over 10 years. She is the Director and Founder of Teacher's Pet: Dogs and Kids Learning Together, a nonprofit that pairs at-risk and court-adjudicated youth with hard-to-adopt shelter dogs for training and education. She is the Director of the Center for Human Animal Interventions and Director of the online Animal Assisted Therapy Certificate Program, both located at Oakland University in Rochester, Michigan. Most recently, she has received the University of Professional and Continuing Education (UPCEA) Central Region 2015 Celebration of Excellence Professional Educator Award for this program. Johnson is a licensed professional counselor with a certification in Trauma and Loss who specializes in working with adolescents in court-referred placement programs and juveniles charged with sexual offenses. She completed a national certification through the Council of Professional Dog Trainers. She has also served on the Curriculum Committee for Pet Partners continuing education.

Rachel Katz is a San Francisco-based spiritual director in private practice, writer, researcher and end-of-life care practitioner with the nationally acclaimed Zen Hospice Project. Her scope of expertise includes death/dying, the human/animal bond, grief/loss, spirituality, and chronic illness. Rachel leads workshops using creative modalities to explore one's relationship with death. Her writing has appeared in a variety of publications and blogs, including her own.

Dr. Michelle Lem is a 2001 graduate of the Ontario Veterinary College (OVC), and the Founder and Director of Community Veterinary Outreach, a veterinary-based registered charity that has provided pro bono preventive veterinary care for animals of the homeless and marginally housed in Ottawa since 2003. This program has been successfully reproduced in other communities. Community Veterinary Outreach programs also operate in Hamilton, Toronto and Kitchener-Waterloo, and Guelph, Ontario Canada.

Dr. Lem provided behavioral consultations for companion animals on a referral basis; was the contract veterinarian for Department of National Defence's military working dogs from 2009 to 2011; and has taught in the Veterinary Assistant and Technician programs at Algonquin College since 2004. In 2009, Dr. Lem received an OVC fellowship to pursue graduate research in the Department of Population Medicine, studying the effects of pet ownership on street-involved youth, receiving her MSc in 2012. Dr. Lem has served on the College of Veterinarians of Ontario's (CVO) Shelter Medicine Task Force and represented the CVO on Emergency Management Ontario's (EMO) committee for resourcing. Dr. Lem is an active member of the Canadian Veterinary Medical Association (CVMA) as a trained member of the Canadian Veterinary Reserve and serves on the CVMA's Animal Welfare Committee.

In 2011, Dr. Lem received the Ottawa Humane Society's Muriel Davies Award for her contribution to animal welfare in the Ottawa community. Her outreach work has been recognized at the Summit for Urban Animal Strategies, where she was awarded the Thought Leadership Scholarship and Individual Achievement Award in 2011, the Community Collaboration Award in 2013, the OVC Young Alumnus Award in 2014, and the CVMA's President's Award in 2015. In 2012, Dr. Lem was humbled to receive the Queen Elizabeth II Diamond Jubilee Medal for her service. In May 2013, Dr. Lem was elected as an Ashoka Fellow, one of only 49 Canadian Fellows and joining an international community of 3,000 leading social entrepreneurs in over 70 countries (www.ashoka.org).

Lisa Lunghofer Ph.D. is Founder and Executive Director of Making Good Work, LLC, which provides consulting services to nonprofits nationwide. Since 2009 she has worked with animal-related programs, including Safe Humane Chicago, helping them to create strategic plans, develop logic models, write grant proposals, build successful programs, develop evaluation plans, and track outcomes. Examples of her work include designing an education initiative, based on a public health model, to prevent animal cruelty in Philadelphia; writing grant proposals for programs that promote the human–animal bond; conducting strategic planning with animal and child welfare organizations; evaluating the effects of shelter dogs on veterans diagnosed with PTSD; and directing the Animals and Society Institute's Animal Abuse Prevention Program.

Dr. Lisa Lunghofer, Executive Director of Making Good Work, has 20 years of experience working successfully with public sector and nonprofit clients in the areas of child welfare, violence prevention, animal welfare, and the human–animal bond. Since 2009 she has served as a consultant to animal-related programs nationwide, including Safe Humane Chicago, helping them to develop program models, develop evaluation plans and identify and track outcomes. Prior to founding Making Good Work, Lisa led a variety of national evaluation projects for which she received grants from the Department of Health and Human Services' Administration for Children and Families, the National Institute of Justice and the Office of Juvenile Justice and Delinquency Prevention.

James M. O'Neil Ph.D. is Professor of Educational Psychology and Family Studies at the University of Connecticut and a licensed psychologist in private practice in South Windsor, Connecticut. In 1975, he received his doctorate from the Department of Counseling and Personnel Services at the University of Maryland. He is a fellow of the American Psychological Association in Divisions 17, 35, 43, 51, 52, and 56. He is one of the founding members of the Society for the Psychological Study of Men and Masculinity (SPSMM), Division 51 of the American Psychological Association. SPSMM named him Researcher of the Year in 1997 for his 20-year research program on men's gender role conflict. His research programs relate to men and masculinity, gender role conflict, psychology of men and women, and violence and victimization. He has published over 100 journal articles and books chapters and is the author of the Gender Role Conflict Scale (GRCS), a widely used measure of men's conflict with their gender roles. Over 300 studies have used the

GRCS with over 200 of the studies being published in psychological journals. He published (with Michele Harway) What Causes Men's Violence Against Women? in 1999 (Sage Publications) and his last book, Men's Gender Role Conflict: Psychological Costs, Consequences, and an Agenda for Change was published in November, 2014 by APA Books. In 1991, he was awarded a Fulbright Teaching Scholarship by the Council for International Exchange of Scholars, to lecture in the former Soviet Union. He lectured at Moscow State Pedagogical University from February to April, 1992, on topics such as psychological counseling, psychology of gender roles, and victimization. In 1995, he was awarded Teaching Fellow status by the University of Connecticut for his outstanding excellence and dedication to the university teaching profession. In August, 2008, he received the Distinguished Professional Service Award from Division 51 of the American Psychological Association for his 25-year research program on men's gender role conflict and his advocacy for teaching of the psychology of men in the United States. He has advocated professional activism with gender role and social justice issues throughout his 40 years as a counseling psychologist.

Wendy Packman JD, Ph.D. is a Professor of Psychology at Palo Alto University (PAU). She is the Director of the Joint JD-Ph.D. Program in Psychology and Law at PAU and Golden Gate University Law School. Dr. Packman has studied, presented, and written extensively on sibling bereavement and continuing bonds, the impact of a child's death on parents, and the psychological sequelae of pet loss. She is the primary investigator of an international cross-cultural study examining the use of continuing bonds following a pet's death.

Frederick C. Petty Ph.D., MD is Professor of Psychiatry in the College of Medicine at the University of Central Florida, and Supervisory Psychiatrist at the Orlando VA Medical Center.

Jessica Thomas Psy.D completed her doctoral coursework in Clinical Psychology with an emphasis on child and adolescent psychology at the Chicago School of Professional Psychology, Los Angeles. Her work with youth began in 2008 and continues to be fueled by her enthusiasm to encourage recovery and foster resilience in the youth many clinicians' struggle to work with. Since that time, she has been honored by both the city and the county of Los Angeles for 'Outstanding Community Dedication' and currently works for the Los Angeles County Department of Mental Health, in the Enhanced Specialized Foster Care Unit. Jessica is passionate about not only counseling trauma-affected youth but also seeking out more proactive interventions in an effort to prevent the escalation of those youth, into the criminal justice system. This impetus led to her involvement with the k9 Connection program, inspired her dissertation research on the use of human–animal interaction and continues to motivate her work toward certification as an Animal Assisted Therapy team with her rescue dog, Mr. Bentley Jackson.

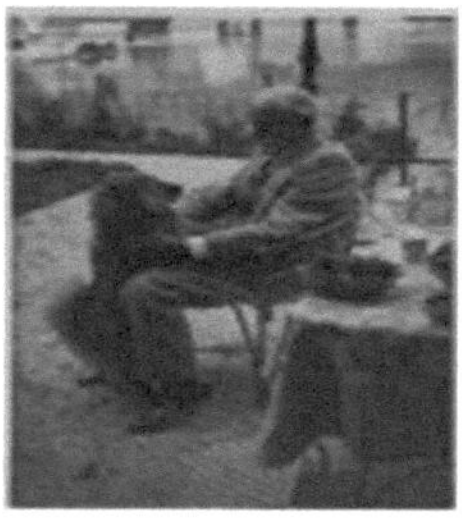

Freud and his dog Luna

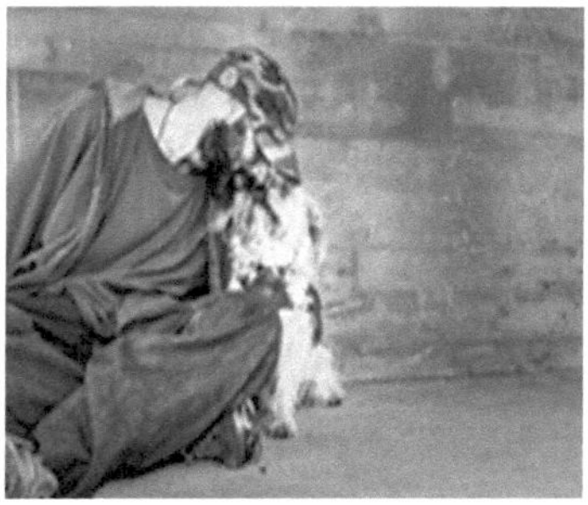

A homeless youth and his dog

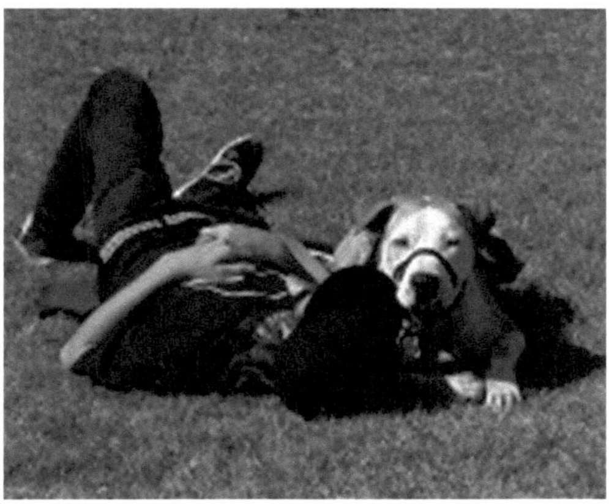

A youth participate in a dog trianing program

Chapter 1
An Introduction to Men and Their Dogs: A New Understanding of "Man's Best Friend"

Chris Blazina and Lori Kogan

From the time I (Chris Blazina) began my career as a psychologist, I knew it would be difficult to reach the men I sought to help. As a general rule, males in North America have very negative attitudes about seeking support. I might even go so far as to say the same men struggle with a "crisis of connection," which equates to a number of challenges, such as the difficulty in making and sustaining connections with others. It also involves mistaking self-reliance for total self-sufficiency and pressure to keep vulnerability firmly in check. A significant percentage of American men endorse some form of these traditional male norms or at least have familiarity with them. One troubling aspect of this prevalence is many men believe they are just fulfilling the requirements of mature masculinity. Through a string of iconic heroes and role models, Western culture teaches that adult males naturally transition into a state of self-imposed seclusion and emotional detachment. This is true even when surrounded by those who are interested and available. Needless to say, these acquired practices impact our relationships with companions, friends, and family. The net effect is that men are at risk and in need of innovative ways to help.

In an attempt to counter men's isolation, the bulk of my clinical and research work has focused on helping males develop more substantial relationships and skill sets. A reliable tie that breaks through the well-worn masculine persona that keeps others at bay is beneficial, but unfortunately also hard to come by. Steps toward a meaningful social network may begin in an unexpected way and involve

C. Blazina (✉)
Department. of Counseling and Educational Psychology, New Mexico State University, College of Education, MSC 3CEP, PO Box 30001, Las Cruces, NM 88003, USA
e-mail: cblazina@nmsu.edu

L. Kogan
Clinical Sciences Department, Colorado State University, College of Veterinary Medicine and Biomedical Sciences, 1601, Campus Delivery, Fort Collins, CO 80523, USA
e-mail: Lori.kogan@colostate.edu

C. Blazina and L.R. Kogan (eds.), *Men and Their Dogs*,
DOI 10.1007/978-3-319-30097-9_1

"man's best friend." While there are a number of reasons to be concerned about males in our culture, the bond with canine companions offers hope.

In this volume, we explore the rich, complex bond that men share with their dogs in hopes of generating a new psychological understanding of this unique relationship. We have deliberately chosen to use the phrase "animal companion" instead of "pet" to set the tone for the type of scientific inquires made within this text. While both terms can be used to express fondness and endearment, animal companion carries a distinct connotation. The existence of a special bond between man and dog may be for many readers, an a priori assumption. This supposition may be derived in part from studies conducted in North America that propose a high percentage of human counterparts, (some studies have found between 85 and 99 %—most of whom are female), define their dogs as being like a close friend or family member (e.g., Cain, 1983; Voith, 1985). How much these findings generalize to men, however, remains relatively unanswered. For example, to what degree do men share that same level of depth and connection toward their dogs? What is the role of male socialization across the life span and its impact on how males express their sentiments for animal companions? If masculinity does play a key role, can researchers and clinicians accurately identify and address the strength and type of bond shared? Our choice of terminology (animal companion) suggests the type of attachment men experience has a unique meaning in their lives, but this assumption is in need of further investigating.

The research examining males' experiences of attachment and loss regarding an animal companion is a work in progress, with much remaining unknown. Some studies suggests that males show lower levels of attachment (Kidd & Kidd, 1985), while others find no gender differences (Prato-Previde et al., 2006; Ramirez, 2006). Likewise, research suggests males report less grief upon losing their dogs (Brown, 2006). Yet, although male socialization is an important contextual variable, it is seldom included in the line of inquiry involving both Human–Animal Interaction (HAI) and attachment and loss. In many studies, males are assumed to be a single homogenous group uninfluenced by any other categories, characteristics, or life experiences. What is often implied is that a simple statistical mean or checking the demographic box of being male on a research questionnaire is all that is needed to explain the complete story of how men relate toward their dogs. It is our position in this book that attempting to understand HAI without also including an appreciation of context omits critical and necessary information for researchers and clinicians. In this case, one of the key contextual factors not only involves gender, but how males have been taught to enact the descriptive and prescriptive rules of Western cultural masculinity or traditional male gender roles.

Men and the Bond in Context

Researchers within the field of gender studies have argued that context is a viable avenue of exploration when studying gender roles (see Blazina, 2001; Blazina & Shen-Miller, 2010; Ennis, 2008; Falmagne, 2000; Liu, 2005; O'Neil, 2015;

Stewart & McDermott, 2004; Vacha-Hasse et al., 2010). Context allows for a more nuanced understanding of key characteristics by studying them in conjunction with other variables of interest. Context applied to the study of masculinity includes the culturally constructed ways men are taught and reinforced to enact traditional male roles at the cultural, familial, interpersonal, and intrapsychic levels. Various theorists and researchers have identified some of the limiting effects of constricted forms of traditional male gender roles (see: Blazina, 2001; Blazina & Shen-Miller, 2010; Levant, 1995; O'Neil, 1986, 2008, 2015; Pleck, 1981; Pollack, 1995; Vacha-Hasse et al., 2010; Wester, 2008). Traditional male roles can include overly restricted emotionality, homophobia, striving for skewed versions of success and power, and unsuccessful attempts to balance work and family demands. Men who feel constricted by traditional gender roles are adversely impacted by psychological distress and limited opportunities for intimacy (O'Neil, 1986, 2008, 2015). An abundance of research over the past 40 years supports the link between gender role confliction of men and psychological distress such as increases in depression, anxiety, substance usage, and interpersonal problems (O'Neil, 2008, 2015). We believe that the bond between man and dog has the potential to offset some of these challenges. However, to understand how this process occurs, it is crucial to place male socialization and the bond in context with other variables of interest.

When we pair masculinity with other factors such as age, emotional intelligence, relational skill sets, perceived emotional support, prior relationship success and failure, current life stress, history of trauma and loss, and attachment style and strength with humans and animal companions, a more nuanced understanding of the bond's role is obtained. For example, recent research has examined how psychoanalyst John Bowlby's (1969/1982) attachment figures' characteristics originally devised to describe the caregiver and child relationship (e.g., safe base, safe haven, proximity seeking, and distress at being apart), are also applicable to the human–animal bond (Kurdek, 2008, 2009; Sharkin & Knox, 2003).

An attachment figure represents someone to whom we have formed an emotional and psychological bond, and who is integral in supplying certain basic psychological experiences; someone to return to in times of distress who can act as an encouraging presence to help us explore the world and develop the various complexities of our personalities (Bowlby, 1969/1982, 1980). It has been argued that animal companions, specifically a dog, can serve for some as an attachment figure (Kurdek, 2008, 2009). Part of the research supporting this notion is how the presence of an animal companion has been shown to reduce levels of anxiety, depression, and loneliness (Zarski, 1984; Garrity et al., 1989) as well as ameliorate the effects of potentially stressful life-events (e.g., divorce and bereavement) (Folse et al., 1994) and enhance feelings of autonomy, competence and self-esteem (Beck & Katcher, 1996; Kidd & Kidd, 1985; Levinson, 1972; Robin & Ten Bensel, 1985; Triebenbacher, 1998). Animal companions can also encourage playfulness and provide laughter and entertainment to their human counterparts (Muschel, 1984). We argue that animal companions offer many men a respite from the strain of traditional male gender roles. The shared bond may also be one that prompts transformation in males' lives. This can involve change on many levels including rethinking dysfunctional gender roles/norms, healing psychological wounds, and maturation to becoming more relational persons able to build and sustaining connections with others. This short list of potential benefits is especially important for at risk populations.

Due to their cultural history and dynamics, many people do not instinctively consider men in Western culture as an at risk population. This may be especially true if the males in question are Caucasian, heterosexual, middleclass, and have been college educated. Instead, assumptions are made about these and others males of varying contextual backgrounds as having great privilege both at home and at work (e.g., less time child-rearing, better pay, and positions, etc.). Until fairly recently, these contextual dynamics of historical privilege were thought to play some role in shielding males from stress. Yet, males' that face masculine gender role strain in combination with other contextual factors are certainly in a tenuous position. When dynamics such as attachment-loss history, economic strife, societal injustice, lack of social support are interfaced with already present masculine role stress, the result is a cumulative challenge on mental health and well-being. Adding to the configuration are situation-specific stressors such as being a male with a history of incarceration, or that of having intense military service in war torn areas. Taken together, males' lives become a much more complex, nuanced narrative that is in need of understanding.

Finally, is the dilemma of males' reluctance to seek help. There is a prevailing trend for males of all races and ethnicities in North American to report negative attitudes toward seeking psychological and medical support services (Addis & Cohane, 2005). Many of these same men often seem to struggle with difficulty making and sustaining emotionally meaningful ties with others (Levant, 1995; Pleck, 1981). Those within Division 51 of the American Psychological Association, the Society for the Psychological Study of Men and Masculinity, argue that these circumstances are less likely the result of male biological hard-wiring but instead largely occur through the culturally conditioned ways men are socialized to think, feel, and act (see: Levant, 1995; O'Neil, 1986, 2008, 2015; Pleck, 1981). This socialization process often leaves men confused and in a double-bind (Good & Wood, 1995). Males often mistake self-reliance for total self-sufficiency and feel pressure to keep any types of vulnerability firmly in check. While they might potentially benefit from many types of social support, they simultaneously feel blocked from accessing them. These acquired perceptions and resultant behaviors often also have negative effects on significant others, friends, and family (O'Neil, 2008, 2013, 2015; Pollack, 1995). While some men may try to offset a lack of connection with various coping skills and stereotypical psychological defenses, there is no substitute for a real bond. Contemporary psychoanalytic perspectives such as Bowlby's Attachment theory (1969/1982) argue for the importance of making and sustaining emotional ties throughout the life span. Our relationships with others ultimately give our lives meaning and direction. This is where man's best friend can play a pivotal role.

To illustrate, a recent study asked devoted middle-aged dog owners to rate both their human and animal companions on attachment figure characteristics (Kurdek, 2009). The results revealed that 45 % of the participants gave their dogs the highest ratings on all four attachment figure features. The differences between human and canine companion relationships were especially notable in the area of the safe haven dimension (the bond as a source of comfort in stressful times). Respondents reported being more likely to turn to their animal companions in times of emotional distress than to their mothers, fathers, brothers, sisters, best friends, and children. There was also an important result reported regarding middle-aged men and attachment. While middle-aged males followed the general trend of the attachment figure findings, they were more likely to rely on their dogs when under stress than any other potential human supports. The only connection that rivaled the bond between man and dog on this soothing dimension was one's romantic significant other. These results lend support to the notion that in some contexts, dogs really are "man's best friend." This adage may be especially true for middle-aged men with a limited support system who are uncomfortable revealing personal matters to others. Unfortunately, dimensions of this state of relating can be all too familiar for many men across the life span.

Part of the challenge in helping males is uncovering the key factors that perpetuate the constricting nature of male socialization. It also includes finding innovative ways to neutralize those dynamics, renorm gender expectations, and/or overcome them. One tool in this process can be a better understanding of men's utilization of the HAI to meet connection needs and psychological closeness. While we cannot assume that all men have the same experiences in terms of how they construct or experience masculinity, we can more likely accept that male socialization is a variable of interest, impacting a wide number of areas including work, love, and even the perceptions of the human–animal bond. Approaching the wide range of men's experiences from a contextual framework allows for a clearer picture detailing how various themes interact to create a unique experience of human–animal relatedness. While the bond with animal companions should not be viewed as a panacea, it is nevertheless, an important connection that needs further study.

John Bowlby suggested at the core of attachment theory (1969/1982) that all mammalian animals are predisposed to make and sustain attachment bonds with others. Yet, much of the stringent socially constructed rules for masculinity can cause boys and men to feel that deep bonds with human companions go against the grain of what it means to be a man (see: Blazina, 2001, 2011; O'Neil, 1986, 2008; Pollack, 1995). It is also our position that HAI can produce a gender-neutral encounter where males feel, at least temporarily, freedom from constricting male roles. These moments can also be emotionally corrective, healing past emotional wounds, or at least, provide a respite from the various strains that can be prevalent in men's lives.

We cannot say that all men subscribe to the same definition of traditional conflicted masculinity or subsequently experience equal amounts of gender role strain. It still may be accurate to say most males are very aware of the old rules and in some situation-specific contexts are influenced by them. Traditional masculine socialization can result in a male's Achilles heel, a place of vulnerability that may be best summarized as not only a crisis of connection but also one that involves dealing with loss. Purported social networks are often smaller for men (Barbee et al., 1993) especially as they age, and become divorced or widowed (Doka & Martin, 2010). Research also suggest males are often less likely to receive support for their losses. These findings imply there may be fewer chances for connection but also when meaningful ties are established, they carry more of the burden of meeting essential psychological needs. The conundrum of male attachment also has very clear implications for issues of grief and loss. When would-be attachment figures make it successfully through what can seem to be a gauntlet of male emotional defenses are then lost, understandably many men are left in a difficult place.

We need to understand more how HAI may potentially offset some of attachment-loss challenges men experience and in doing so, inadvertently create other dynamics we are just beginning to understand. For instance, what are the male-dog dynamics that makes bonding in this dyad seem different, perhaps easier? Is it more than the gender-neutral space that is being created? When males walk, run, and play with their dogs, do they enter into a different sphere of relating, one not easily quantified but certainly emotionally significant? Perhaps this is a type of bond that helps males' counterbalance the attachment challenges found elsewhere that sometimes occur with human companions, friends, and family. Freud made mention of the unambivalent nature of dogs—"They love their friends and bite their enemies" (Roth, 2005). Being with a canine friend that offers such clarity may be a welcome relief for many men confused by the nature of relationship rules and proper protocol in other relational contexts with human companions. It may also enable males to act in a similar canine-inspired direct manner of healthy relating, being an impetus for revealing parts of themselves male socialization has taught to keep hidden. In either case, having established a meaningful bond with animal companion for upwards of 12–14 years, how does a man adjust to the loss? Does male socialization also prevent him from seeking support from others; instead, dealing with grief in a more private introspective way as argued by Doka and Martin (2010) when losing human companions?

Finally, does one's sense of masculinity affect the making of a *continued bond*, (see Klass, Silverman, & Nickman, 1996) a new way of establishing an attachment bond with an attachment figure or significant other that has been loss? Do males feel blocked from remaking the lost connection with animal companion, or do they just keep the process private, fearing others would not understand? If males have turned to an animal companion because that seems safe, can he also learn to call on the memory of his animal companion, thereby utilizing the continued bond even after the more tangible connection has been broken? Even with these dynamics, we expect there will be individual differences and variation among males in the ways each is approached.

Herzog (2007) suggested it is the within group differences among men (and women) that accounts for some of the potential gender confusion regarding attitudes toward the bond. Some research treats all men as if they have the same HA attitudes when clearly they do not. While our focus in this book is on those men who value and derive a psychological benefit from the bond, we do not gloss over the reality that other males use animals as a means of psychological control, harming them in various destructive ways. This can occur among perpetrators of animal and family abuse, violence, and neglect. By beginning to investigate the role of healthy connections with animal companions, it may also shed light on those who struggle and are extremely conflicted not only with HAI but all their attachment bonds.

There is also expected variability regarding male's willingness to report experiences and emotions surrounding their companion animals due to it being a potentially emotionally laden topic. Some males may deem this information as off-limits to discuss. To do otherwise may lead to the violation of stringent male roles regarding restricted emotionality and self-sufficiency. Again, this leads to erroneous conclusions regarding men and animal companions—chief among these men do not attach or grieve for their loss. We see these same potential influences beginning to shape behavior toward the bond at a young age. In one study examining boys and girls levels of attachment to their animal companions, as measured through the likelihood of expressing love to them, saying they were loved by them, and reporting missing them when apart, boys showed significantly lower levels than girls (Kidd & Kidd, 1985). The researchers concluded that male socialization may have influenced boys' willingness to report their actual feelings, because when examining the actual behaviors shown toward their animal companions, no gender differences were found.

It is suggested throughout this volume that some males who have experienced traditionally male gender socialization and the burden of other contextual dynamics, will turn to animal companions to meet important affiliation needs, especially in times of distress. This does not mean all males will follow this pattern nor do so in health ways. Much of the original basis for the man's best friend assumption is derived from limited empirical evidence or clinical case studies. Scenarios included instances from the formative years when a boy felt alone except for the presence of an animal friend; or as an adult, how the bond is experienced by some men as a reliable connection amid a series of life frustrations or relationship failures. In this book, various chapter topics attempt to shed additional light upon the bond between man and dog. It is argued that for many males, the HA bond takes on a different contextual meaning, one both nuanced and more encompassing. The bond becomes a safe refuge where much of the stringent rules for being a man are bypassed, allowing a more unguarded relational experience to occur. The connection between man and dog may also be a powerful means for personal and sociocultural transformation allowing men to rethink dysfunctional ways of being masculine.

Readers will find chapters that include data driven projects, theoretical models, and applied programs that interface masculinity and HAI. The assumption in each case is that man's best friend adds something unique to the lives of males across the life span. Many of these same works also offers a special glimpse into other contextual areas, factors that add additional psychological strain. This includes but is not limited to the difficulty of being a homeless youth, males that have been part of the judicial system, ones in the military, others facing age-related transitions such as boys becoming men, middle-aged men facing declining social support, and the elderly struggling to juggle health-related issues and still maintaining good care for their animal companions. Pulling back the layers of contextual meaning(s) offer a unique glimpse into the lives of males. Sometimes the most revealing investigations occur when a person is in transition, or under duress. These contexts become a gateway for understanding more about the relationship between man and dog.

Explaining the psychological significance of the human–animal bond in males' lives is a complex endeavor. Part of the bond's importance is derived from the various psychological roles animal companions play in our lives (Brown, 2004, 2007), and yet, one cannot accurately presuppose that each and every individual experiences human–animal connectedness in the exact way (Blazina et al., 2011). Some may struggle with loneliness, or at the extreme, be unable to connect with other people, yet able to sustain a meaningful tie with an animal companion. Others perceive the HAI as a generative if not healing presence (Brown, 2004, 2007). Still others experience the bond as a key part of a community that includes both human and animal companions. These familiar types of profiles reflect only a portion of those encountered; there are many largely unexplored contextual variables found at the cultural, familial, and personal levels that shape one's own phenomenological experience (Blazina et al., 2011). Only by developing a deeper more integrative perception of the potential factors involved in the HA bond will clinicians and researchers be able to better understand the complexity and depth of these themes. Just as in relationships with other people, each human animal bond/ relationship will have a unique meaning developed from one's own personal history. One key contextual variable includes the influence of masculinity, creating the need to explore this aspect in more detail. Therefore, the present project begins the contextual dialogue of how masculinity influences the meaning and impact of the HA bond in males' lives across the life span.

References

Addis, M. E., & Cohane, G. H. (2005). Social scientific paradigms of masculinity and their implications for research and practice in men's mental health. *Journal of Clinical Psychology, 61*, 633–647.

Barbee, A. P., Cunningham, M. R., Winstead, B. A., Derlega, V. J., Gulley, M. R., Yankeelov, P. A., et al. (1993). Effects of gender role expectations on the social support process. *Journal of Social Issues, 49*(3), 175–190.

Beck, A. M., & Katcher, A. H. (1996). *Between pets and people: The importance of animal companionship*. Purdue University Press.

Blazina, C. (2001). Analytic psychology and gender role conflict: The development of the fragile masculine self. *Psychotherapy, 38*, 50–59.

Blazina, C. (2011). Life After Loss: Psychodynamic Perspectives on a Continuing Bonds Approach with Pet Companions. In C. Blazina, C.,D. Shen-Miller, & G. Boyraz, G. (Eds.)., *The Psychology of the Human-Animal Bond: A Guide for Clinicians' and Researchers*. New York: Springer.

Blazina, C., Boyraz, G., & Shen-Miller, D. S. (2011). *The psychology of the human–animal bond*. New York, NY: Springer.

Blazina, C., & Miller, D.S. (Eds.). (2010). *An international psychology of men: Theoretical advances, clinical conceptualizations, adn cases studies*. New York: Routledge.

Bowlby, J. (1969/1982). *Attachment: Attachment and loss* (Vol. 1). New York: Basic Books.

Brown, K. (2006). Pastoral concern in relation to the psychological stress caused by the death of an animal companion. *Mental Health, Religion & Culture, 9*(5), 411–422.

Brown, S. E. (2004). The human-animal bond and self-psychology: Toward a new understanding. *Society & Animals, 12*(1), 67–86.

Brown, S. E. (2007). Companion animals as self-objects. *Anthrozoos, 20*(4), 329–343.

Cain, A. O. (1983). A study of pets in the family system. In H. Katcher & A. M. Beck (Eds.), *New perspectives on our lives with companion animals* (pp. 72–81). Philadelphia, PA: University of Pennsylvania Press.

Doka, K., & Martin, T. (2010). *Grieving beyond gender: Understanding the ways men and women mourn*. New York: Routledge. Revised.

Enns, C. Z. (2008). Toward a complexity paradigm for understanding gender role conflict. *The Counseling Psychologist, 36*, 446–454.

Falmagne, R. J. (2000). Positionality and thought: On the gendered foundations of thought, culture and development. In P. H. Miller & E. Scholnick (Eds.), *Developmental psychology through the lenses of feminist theories* (pp. 191–213). New York: Routledge.

Folse, E. B., Minder, C. C., Aycock, M. J., & Santana, R. T. (1994). Animal-assisted therapy and depression in adult college students. *Anthrozoös, 7*(3), 188–194.

Garrity, T. F., Stallones, L. F., Marx, M. B., & Johnson, T. P. (1989). Pet ownership and attachment as supportive factors in the health of the elderly.*Anthrozoös, 3*(1), 35–44.

Good, G. E., & Wood, P. K. (1995). Male gender role conflict, depression, and help-seeking: Do college men face double jeopardy? *Journal of Counseling and Development, 74*, 70–75.

Herzog, H. A. (2007). Gender differences in human-animal interactions: A review. *Anthrozoös, 20*(1), 7–21.

Klass, D., Silverman, P. R., & Nickman, S. (1996). *Continuing bonds: New understandings of grief*. New York: Taylor & Francis.

Kidd, A. H., & Kidd, R. M. (1985). Children's attitudes toward their pets. *Psychological Reports, 57*, 17–31.

Klass, D., & Silverman, P. R. (1996). Introduction: What is the problem? In D. Klass, P. R. Silverman, & S. L. Nickman (Eds.), *Continuing bonds: New understandings of grief*. New York: Taylor & Francis.

Kurdek, L. A. (2008). Pet dogs as attachment figures. *Journal of Social and Personal Relationships, 25*(2), 247–266.

Kurdek, L. A. (2009). Pet dogs as attachment figures for adult owners. *Journal of Family Psychology, 23*(4), 439–446.

Liu, W. M. (2005). The study of men and masculinity as an important multicultural competency consideration. *Journal of Clinical Psychology, 61*(6), 685–697.

Levant, R. F. (1995). Toward the reconstruction of masculinity. In R.F. Levant, F. Ronald, & W.S. Pollack (Eds.), *A new psychology of men* (pp. 229–251). New York, NY: Basic Books.

Levinson, B. M. (1972). *Pets and human development*. Charles C Thomas, Springfield, IL.

Muschel, I.J. (1984). Pet therapy with terminal cancer patients. Social Casework: *The Journal of Contemporary Social Work, 65*(8), 451–458.

O'Neil, J. M., Helm, B., Gable, R., David, L., & Wrightsman, L. (1986). Gender role conflict scale (GRCS): College men's fears of femininity. *Sex Roles, 14*, 335–350.

O'Neil, J. M. (2008). Summarizing 25 years of research on men's gender role conflict using the gender role conflict scale: New research paradigms and clinical implications. *The Counseling Psychologist, 36*, 358–445.
O'Neil, J. M. (2013). Gender-role conflict research thirty years later: An evidenced based diagnostic schema. *Journal of Counseling and Development, 91*, 498–499.
O'Neil, J. M. (2015). *Men's gender role conflict: Psychological costs, consequences, and an agenda for change*. Washington, DC: APA Books.
Pleck, J. (1981). *The myth of masculinity*. Cambridge, MA: MIT Press.
Pollack, W. (1995). No man is an island: Toward a new psychoanalytic psychology of men. In R. Levant & W. Pollack (Eds.), *A new psychology of men* (pp. 33–67). New York: Basic Books.
Prato-Previde, E., Fallani, G., & Valsecenchi, P. (2006). Gender differences in owners interacting with pet dogs: An observational study. *Ethology, 112* (1), 64–73.
Ramirez, M. (2006). "My dog's just like me": Dog ownership as a gender display. *Symbolic Interaction, 29*(3), 373–391.
Robin, M., & Bensel, R. T. (1985). Pets and the socialization of children. *Marriage & Family Review, 8*(3–4), 63–78.
Roth, B. (2005). Pets and psychoanalysis: A clinical contribution. *Psychoanalytic Review, 92*, 453–457.
Sharkin, B. S., & Knox, D. (2003). Pet loss: Issues and implications for the psychologist. *Professional Psychology: Research and Practice, 34*(4), 414.
Stewart, A. J., & McDermott, C. (2004). Gender psychology. *Annual Review of Psychology, 55*, 519–544.
Triebenbacher, S. L. (1998). Pets as transitional objects: Their role in children's emotional development. *Psychological Reports, 82*(1), 191–200.
Vacha-Haase, T., Wester, S. R., & Christianson, H. (2010). *Psychotherapy with older men*. New York: Routledge.
Voith, V. L. (1985). Attachment of people to companion animals. *Veterinary Clinics of North America: Small Animal Practice, 15*, 289–295.
Wester, S. R. (2008). Male gender role conflict and multiculturalism: Implications for counseling psychology. *The Counseling Psychologist, 36*, 294–324.
Zarski, J. J. (1984). Hassles and health: a replication. *Health Psychology, 3*(3), 243.

Chapter 2
Gender Role Conflict Theory, Research, and Practice: Implications for Understanding the Human–Animal Bond

James M. O'Neil, Robyn Denke and Chris Blazina

In December 2014, the Jesuit pope, Francis made comments that suggested that animals have souls and would be welcomed in heaven. This single comment activated a 150-year-old debate in Vatican on whether animals have souls like humans and has significant implications for theology and anyone bonded to a pet. If animals have souls and human beings bond with them, then the animal bond has significant spiritual–religious dimensions. In this way, animals become not only agents of psychological growth and soothing for people (Blazina et al. 2013) but spiritual partners like human beings. In this context, the animal–human bond becomes more than fringe topic but a critical one that needs to be more vigorously studied.

Men's relationships with dogs deserve study because limited knowledge exists on how gender role socialization affects men's intimate relationships with animals. "Men's Best Friend," an endearing way to capture people's relationship to dogs suggests that there is something special about the human–dog connection. What this special connection means and how dog bonds mediate men's intrapersonal and

J.M. O'Neil (✉)
Department of Educational Psychology, Neag School of Education,
University of Connecticut Storrs, 249 Glenbrook Road Box U-3064,
Mansfield, CT, 06268, USA
e-mail: JIMONEIL1@aol.com

R. Denke
University of Connecticut Storrs, 45 Cavalry Hill Road, Wilton, CT 06897, USA
e-mail: robyndenke@gmail.com

C. Blazina
Department of Counseling and Educational Psychology MSC 3CEP,
New Mexico State University, College of Education, PO Box 30001,
Las Cruces, NM 88003, USA
e-mail: cblazina@nmsu.edu

C. Blazina and L.R. Kogan (eds.), *Men and Their Dogs*,
DOI 10.1007/978-3-319-30097-9_2

interpersonal processes deserve analysis and theorizing. In this chapter, we explore how men's gender role socialization and gender role conflict (GRC) may interact with men bonding with dogs.

First, GRC theory and definitions are presented to provide a theoretical perspective on how men's attachment to animals can be understood. Only a brief summary of GRC is given here to contextualize the animal–human bond. In-depth description of the GRC concepts is found in previous publications (O'Neil 1981a, b, 1990, 2008a, b, 2015; O'Neil et al. 1995). After the theory is presented, a new GRC conceptual model is described that depicts how GRC relates to men's psychological problems with both human and animal bonding. The model depicts 15 contextual concepts that explicate how human and animal attachment relates to men's GRC and to a gender role transformational process. Next, how GRC is measured using the Gender Role Conflict Scale (GRCS, O'Neil et al. 1986) is discussed and a summary of the GRC research is presented in 16 areas where GRC has been correlated with men's intrapersonal and interpersonal problems.

In subsequent sections of the chapter, criticism of the GRC construct is summarized and new theoretical conceptualizations are presented elucidating how GRC may relate to the man–dog bonding process. How GRC is operationalized as real experiences in men's lives are presented next by defining the gender role journey phases, gender role transitions and schemas, and the gender role transformation process. Next, the chapter integrates human attachment, GRC, and psychosocial development in the context of mastering developmental tasks and resolving psychosocial crises. In order to fill a conceptual gap between men's GRC and animal bonding, two questions are posed at the end of the chapter related to how human and animal bonding are different and how the patterns of GRC may stimulate bonds with animals. The chapter concludes with research areas that need exploration and an initial dog assistance curriculum that can be used to help men transform themselves.

Gender Role Conflict Theory and Definitions

GRC is defined as a psychological state in which socialized gender roles have negative consequences for the person or others. It occurs when rigid, sexist, or restrictive gender roles result in personal restriction, devaluation, or violation of others or oneself (O'Neil 2008a, b). The ultimate outcome of this kind of conflict is the restriction of the human potential of the person experiencing it or a restriction of another person's potential. GRC has been operationally defined by four psychological domains, three situational contexts, and three personal and interpersonal experiences. How this definition, the domains, contexts, and experiences of men's GRC relate to the animal–human bond is the primary focus of the chapter.

The psychological domains of GRC imply problems that occur at four overlapping and complex levels—cognitive, emotional (affective), behavioral, and unconscious—and are caused by restrictive gender roles learned in sexist and patriarchal societies. These same domains are part of the animal–human bond dynamics because thoughts, feelings, behaviors, and unconsciousness dynamics operate when humans enter the animal world. Furthermore, GRC is conceptualized as occurring in four general contexts (or categories) that give the construct a simple explanation and form. These contexts are defined as GRC within the man (intrapersonal), GRC expressed toward others (interpersonal), GRC experienced from others (also interpersonal), and GRC during gender role transitions. All of the contexts have relevance to understanding how GRC is a relevant construct to understand how men bond with animals.

The intrapersonal and interpersonal processes that contribute to men's GRC are explained in three contexts that affect men's relationship with themselves and others. The first of the three personal contexts is gender role devaluation. Such devaluations are negative critiques of oneself or others when conforming to, deviating from, or violating stereotypical gender role norms of masculinity ideology. The second of the three personal and interpersonal experiences is gender role restriction, which implies that sex-typed gender roles and GRC confine the man or others to stereotypical norms of masculinity ideology. Gender role restrictions also result in attempts to control people's behavior, limit their potential, and decrease human freedom. Gender role violations represent the most severe kind of GRC. They occur when men harm themselves, harm others, or are harmed by others because of destructive gender role norms of masculinity ideology. To be violated means to be victimized and abused, resulting in emotional and physical pain and, sometimes, gender role trauma strain, which can result in severe, negative outcomes for psychological functioning.

Gender role devaluations, restrictions, and violations are the personal and interpersonal experiences of GRC and are critical to understand how men become conflicted with their gender roles and may find comfort bonding with animals. In sum, men who have experienced gender role devaluations, restrictions, and violations may find bonding with animals safer than bonding with humans.

Restrictive Masculinity Ideology

Restrictive masculinity ideologies predict GRC and cause it. Masculinity ideology is a cofactor of GRC that describes how men are socialized to masculine stereotypes and has been operationalized by the concepts of masculine norms and roles (Levant et al. 1992; Thompson and Pleck 1986) and masculine conformity and nonconformity (Mahalik et al. 2003). Masculinity ideology represents the primary values and standards that define, restrict, and negatively affect boys' and men's lives (Levant et al. 1992; Mahalik et al. 2003; Pleck 1995; Pleck et al. 1993). Masculinity ideology also refers "to beliefs about the importance of men adhering to culturally defined standards for male behavior" (Pleck 1995, p. 19) and involves "the individual's endorsement and internalization of cultural belief systems about masculinity and male gender, rooted in the structural relationships between the sexes" (Pleck 1995, p. 19). Masculinity ideologies are primary ways that boys and men live out patriarchal and sexist values and have negative consequences in interpersonal relationships (Levant and Richmond 2007; O'Neil 2010, 2012, 2015; O'Neil and Crapser 2011). The negative outcomes of adhering to or deviating from culturally defined and restrictive masculinity ideologies can produce distorted gender role schemas and patterns of GRC that are potentially damaging to men and others (Mahalik 1999a, b; O'Neil and Nadeau 1999; O'Neil 2008b; Pleck 1995). How men's masculinity ideologies impact bonding with animals or cruelty toward them has not been explored in the social science literature. This chapter contributes initial ideas about how masculinity ideologies relate to the animal–human bond.

Fear of Femininity (FOF)

The fear of femininity (FOF), is a strong, negative emotion associated with feminine values, attitudes, and behaviors and regarded as inferior, inappropriate, and immature—in short, a devaluation of all that is feminine (O'Neil 1981a, 1982). Jung (1953) believed that men's difficulties with femininity were archetypal, passed down over the centuries, and outside the consciousness of the man. Despite the prominence of the subject in the psychoanalytical circles in the early 1900s (Connell 2005), the centrality of femininity in men's lives has been limited in psychology and only recently it has been conceptualized and discussed (Blazina 1997a, b; Kierski and Blazina 2009).

The FOF is endorsed by patriarchal societies that profit from it (Kierski and Blazina 2009; Norton 1997; O'Neil 2015) and is learned during early childhood socialization, when gender identity is being formed and in later years by physical maturation, developmental changes, and life events. FOF develops in men before, during, and after experiencing GRC and can be conscious or unconscious affecting gender role identity and a man's masculinity ideology. Boys learn to avoid most stereotypical feminine qualities in response to both peers and parents' displeasure at their deviation from masculine norms. The rejection and repression of the feminine parts of their personalities from an early age can produce a lifelong aversion to any quality perceived as feminine; a constant striving for the ways to be masculine; a male image that prohibits open expression of feelings and feminine characteristics; and an emotional and physical distance among men because of feared homosexuality. The unconscious aspect of FOF and its relationship to GRC are critical issues in understanding men's gender role socialization, GRC, and the animal–human bond.

Patterns of Gender Role Conflict

Four patterns of GRC have been empirically derived and the *Gender Role Conflict Scale* (*GRCS*) has documented that these patterns relate to men's psychological problems in many studies (O'Neil 2008a, b, 2015). The pattern of Success/Power/Competition (SPC) describes personal attitudes about success pursued through competition and power. Restrictive emotionality (RE) is defined as having restrictions and fears about expressing one's feelings, as well as difficulty in finding words to express basic emotions. Restrictive affectionate behavior between men (RABBM) represents restrictions in expressing one's feelings and thoughts with other men and difficulty in touching them, and conflict between work and family relations (CBWFR) reflects the experience of restrictions in balancing work, school, and family relations, resulting in health problems, overwork, stress, and a lack of leisure and relaxation. The four patterns of GRC predict men's psychological and interpersonal problems as well as attachment problems that may explain men's closer relationships to dogs rather than humans.

Measuring GRC: The *Gender Role Conflict Scale* (*GRCS*)

The *GRCS* has been developed to assess four patterns of GRC through item generation and reduction, content analysis of items, factor analysis, and tests of reliability (O'Neil et al. 1986; O'Neil 2008a, b, 2015). Four empirically derived factors of GRC have been determined with higher scores on the *GRCS* indicating greater degree of conflict regarding the GRC factors. The four factors are: Success, Power, Competition, (SPC), 13 items, e.g., "I worry about failing and how it affects my doing well as a man"; Restrictive Emotionality (RE), 10 items, e.g., "I have difficulty expressing my tender feelings"; Restrictive Affectionate Behavior Between Men (RABBM), 8 items, e.g., "Affection with other men makes me tense"; and Conflict Between and Family Relations (CBWFR), 6 items, e.g., "My work or school often disrupts other parts of my life: home, health, or leisure."

The GRCS uses a six-point Likert scale of highly agree to highly disagree with higher scores on the *GRCS* indicating greater degree of conflict regarding the GRC factors. Research results indicate that the *GRCS* has good construct, divergent, and convergent validities. Twenty-four factor analyses have been completed on the *GRCS* to document its factorial validity (O'Neil 2015) and overall, the factor analyses with American college students and diverse samples of men living in the United States and all over the world have supported the early GRC model (O'Neil 1981a, b, 1982; O'Neil et al. 1986).

There have been three adaptations of the *GRCS* that have increased its validity or made it more useful to younger boys or women. The Gender Role Conflict Scales for Adolescents was developed (GRCS-A, Blazina et al. 2005) and a short form of the scale was developed in 2012 (GRCS-SF, Wester et al. 2012). A slightly altered version of the GRCS has been developed for women (O'Neil 2015). These adaptations of the GRCS allow the measure to be used with a variety of samples of humans who might bond with animals.

Conceptual Model Linking Human and Animal Attachment to Gender Role Conflict and Men's Psychological and Interpersonal Problems

The primary theoretical model used to summarize the premises of GRC dates back to the early 1980s (O'Neil 1981a, 1990, 2008b; O'Neil et al. 1995). Figure 2.1 depicts a newer model that shows gender-related contexts and men's psychological problems related to human attachment and the human–animal attachment. This new model also shows the process-oriented factors of men's attachment as well as how transformation can occur. A brief description of the new model provides a summary of ideas about GRC in the context of the animal–human bond.

The human and animal attachment processes are shown in the circle in Fig. 2.1. Fifteen contexts are depicted on the outside of the circle. At the top of Fig. 2.1 are shown three precursor processes that affect gender role development over the life span including being in a certain phase of the gender role journey, experiencing gender role transitions, and having distorted gender role schemas. As shown with the bold arrows at the top, these processes affect the human and animal bonding and interact with a man's gender role socialization. At the bottom of Fig. 2.1 is shown the gender role transformation process. These processes are changes in

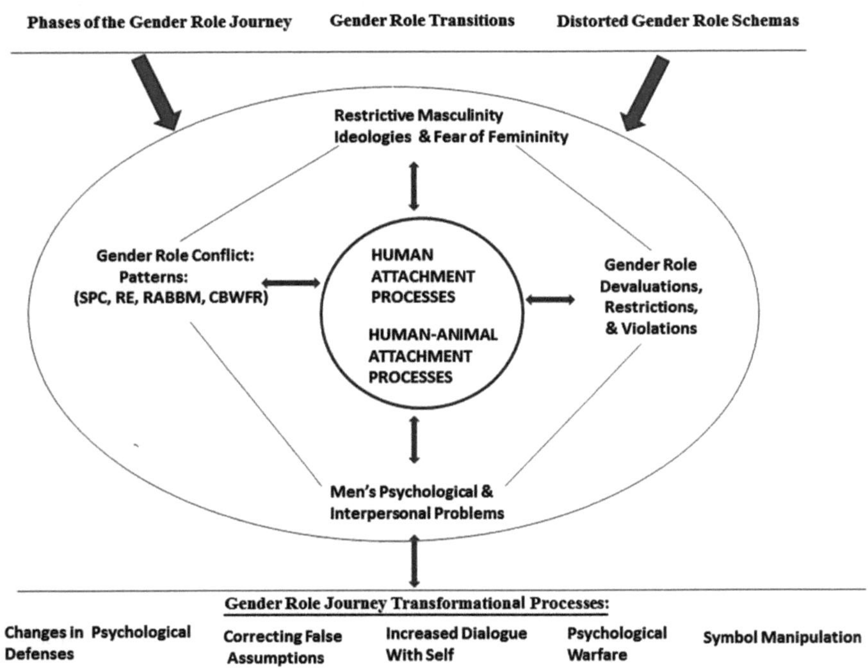

Fig. 2.1 A model to understand men's human and animal attachment in the context of gender role conflict

psychological defenses, correcting false assumptions, increased dialogue with self, psychological warfare, and symbol manipulation. These processes represent how the transformation and growth can occur for men whether the bond is with human or animals.

On different sides of the circle are shown gender-related contexts including the patterns of GRC, restrictive masculinity ideologies, the fear of femininity, and gender role devaluations, restrictions, and violations. Also shown are men's psychological and interpersonal problems. These contexts are connected by straight lines implying that they theoretically relate to each other. Each of these contexts are also shown with bidirectional arrows implying that the gender-related contexts and men's problems have a reciprocal relationship with both animal and human attachment processes. What is unknown is how both human and animal attachments relate to men's psychological and interpersonal problems in the context of GRC and restricted masculinity ideologies. The concepts in Fig. 2.1 represent an advance organizer for the rest of the chapter as well as a depiction of the theoretical, research, and practical issues related to men and their animal bonds.

Review of GRC Research: What Has GRC Been Correlated with?

Thirty years ago the first authors' assertion was that: "….men are also oppressed and restricted by rigid gender role socialization that limits their potential to be fully functioning and whole human beings" (O'Neil 1981a, b, p. 205). What empirical evidence exists that men's human potential has been negatively affected by restricted gender roles? Over the last three decades, the GRC research program has provided evidence (over 350 studies) that men's psychological problems do relate to restrictive gender roles. A man's restricted thoughts, feelings, and behaviors about masculine gender roles predict significant psychological and interpersonal problems.

Table 2.1 lists 16 areas where GRC has been correlated with men's psychological or interpersonal problems. The intrapersonal categories are: (a) depression, anxiety and stress, low self-esteem, shame, and guilt, (b) alcohol and substance abuse, self-destructiveness, hopelessness, and suicide, (c) help seeking and stigma. GRC in an interpersonal context (expressed toward others) is shown in the following areas: (a) attachment, family individuation, intimacy, self-disclosure, relationships, and fathers, (b) marital satisfaction, family dynamics, and couple relationships, (c) stereotyping, attitudes toward women, equalitarianism, homophobia, and racial bias, (d) negative attitudes, interpersonal and sexual violence toward women and others. For GRC from others the categories are: (a) perceived racism, internalized homophobia, internalized heterosexism, perceived discrimination, internalized oppression, (b) attachment, bonding, and family individuation. Only brief summaries of the 16 research areas are summarized and more extensive

Table 2.1 GRC studies correlated with psychological and interpersonal problems by problem category

Dependent variables significantly correlated with GRC	Number of studies
Depression	34
Anxiety and stress	9
Help seeking attitudes	35
Low self-esteem	35
Alcohol and substance abuse	15
Shame and guilt	7
Stigma	6
Intimacy, self-disclosure, and relationship with father	15
Marital dissatisfaction, family dynamics, and couples' GRC	12
Discrimination and internalized oppression	6
Negative attitudes, abuse, and violence toward women	23
Attachment, bonding, family individuation	15
Hopelessness, self-destructiveness, and suicide	6
Traditional attitudes toward women	5
Stereotyping and sex role egalitarianism	10
Bias against sexual and racial minorities	6

discussion of the studies is found in previous publications (O'Neil 2008a, b, 2015; O'Neil and Denke 2015). Specific references for each category that documents the psychological problems in Table 2.1 can be found on the Gender Role Conflict Research Web Page (jimoneil. uconn.edu) in the file "O'Neil and Denke references Table 3 citations and references."

GRC's relationship to depression has been assessed in 34 studies. All of the patterns of GRC have significantly correlated with depression and RE has been the most consistent predictor suggesting that restricted emotions may be a marker for a depressed man. These results have been found for diverse groups of men including men of color, gay men, and men from different cultures. Stress and anxiety have been significantly correlated with all the patterns of GRC in 32 studies. Even with these studies, the specific situations and interactions that link GRC to stress and anxiety remain unknown. Twenty-one studies have assessed self-esteem and GRC and 90 % of them have shown low self-esteem significantly correlated with all of the GRC patterns. Furthermore self-esteem has been negatively correlated with GRC across seven diversity groups including: White, college American students; Japanese, Korean, African American, Mexican American, Asian American men, and gay men. Seven studies have assessed GRC's relationship to shame or guilt. In these studies, all the patterns of GRC significantly correlated with shame with RE and CBWFR being the most strongly correlated. Fifteen studies have assessed the relationship between men's GRC and substance use and abuse and eleven of theses studies showed significant relationships. The overall results of these studies indicate that problems with increased alcohol use or substance abuse are significantly related to SPC, RE, RABBM, and other variables. Thirty-five studies have found that men's negative help-seeking attitudes significantly relate to GRC with adult men. Like with depression, these results have indicated that men of different races, nationalities, and sexual orientations report GRC to be significantly correlated with negative attitudes toward help seeking. Negative attitudes toward help seeking may explain why men seek solace with dogs that cannot talk back but provide unconditional regard without the control and power dynamics inherent in most human relationships. All of these studies have relevance to the animal–human bond because depression, anxiety, shame/guilt, substance abuse, and negative attitudes toward help seeking may contribute to men's decision to distance themselves for human relations and seek comfort with animals.

Attachment to parents and GRC has been investigated in fifteen studies. All the patterns of men's GRC have significantly correlated with attachment problems to both mothers and fathers. The initial studies on attachment suggest that GRC is complexly related to bonding and separation from parents. Eleven studies have found both college age and adult men's GRC to be negatively related to intimacy. Becoming close to others is difficult if the man has restricted emotions or problems with power, control, and vulnerability. Twenty-three studies have assessed whether GRC relates to men's negative or violent attitudes toward women. Collectively, these studies indicate that GRC has been significantly correlated with sexually aggressive behaviors, likelihood of forcing sex, abusive behaviors, coercion, threats and intimidation, dating violence, hostile sexism, hostility toward women, rape myth acceptance, positive attitudes toward and tolerance for sexual harassment, and self-reported violence and aggression. What is unknown is whether higher levels of GRC predict men's animal abuse and can be an area to be explored in the future. Finally, six studies have found that GRC correlates with internalized homonegativity, internalized homophobia, heterosexist discrimination, and negative feelings about being gay. All of these empirical relationships between GRC and interpersonal variables could be related to men's decisions to bond with animals and avoid the complexity of human contact.

Gender Role Devaluations, Restrictions, and Violations

Psychological problems that have significant relationship to *GRCS* subscales (SPC, RE, RABBM, and CBWFR) defined as gender role devaluations, restrictions, and violations have been assessed. Sixty-six specific psychological problems have been empirically correlated with SPC, RE, RABBM, and CBWFR (O'Neil 2013, 2015). Forty-seven of the psychological problems relate to men's possible self-devaluations, restrictions, and violations. Another 19 problem areas relate to men's devaluation and violation of others. With violations of others, as reported earlier, GRC has been correlated to 13 ways to hurt other human beings including violence against women, sexual harassment, sexually aggressive behavior, likelihood of forced sex, hostility toward women, dating violence, hostile sexism, rape myths, abusive behavior, and coercion.

A review of the studies also found that self-devaluations, self-restrictions, and self-violations were significantly related to negative psychological outcomes for racially and ethnically mixed groups of males, men from five countries, and also gay men. In 26 studies, 19 psychological symptoms were correlated with gender role devaluations, restrictions, and violations. Five symptoms that defined self-devaluations were correlated with GRC including: internalized homonegativity and heterosexism, negative feelings about being gay, racism-self-hate, depression, low self-esteem, and shame. Self-restrictions correlated with GRC and psychological problems were coping, anxiety, stress, alexithymia, hopelessness, limited intimacy, and negative attitudes toward help seeking. There were fewer studies that related GRC to self-violations for diverse men but correlations were found with eating disorder symptomology, substance abuse, chronic self-destructiveness, suicidal attempts or risk behavior, and coercion.

Summary of Empirical Evidence Related to GRC

The research indicates that GRC significantly relates to men's psychological problems, is experienced in both the intrapersonal and interpersonal contexts, and has relevance for men's home and family life. The psychological domains of GRC (cognitive, affective, behavioral, and unconscious) have empirical support. Substantial support exists relating GRC to men's cognitive and affective processes. The affective aspects of GRC are evident from significant correlations with men's reports of anxiety, depression, homonegativity, negative identity, anger, and low self-esteem. The cognitive aspects of GRC are evident by significant correlations with traditional attitudes toward women, stereotyping, antigay attitudes, homophobia, and low sex role egalitarianism. In the behavioral domain significant correlations exist between GRC and hostile behavior, spousal criticism, sexually aggressive behaviors, and health risk behaviors. The unconscious domain of GRC has gone unexplored. All of the GRC results may influence men to avoid human connections and seek comfort with animals.

Additionally, the situational contexts of GRC have been supported by research indicating that GRC is related to intrapersonal processes (within the man) and in an interpersonal context in families and couple relationships (Alexander 1999; Breiding 2004; Breiding et al. 2008; Rochlen and Mahalik 2004). There is also evidence for men's personal experiences of GRC (gender role devaluations, restrictions, and violations) (O'Neil 2013). The research also indicates that GRC relates to men's potential to restrict, devalue, or violate themselves and others.

Overall, the empirical research provides support for the GRC constructs developed over 30 years ago. There is now considerable empirical research indicating that men's psychological problems relate to conflict with restricted gender roles. The research findings support new directions for future study and more elaborate

GRC theory and research paradigms in new contextual domains including the human–animal bond. New directions for GRC have been recommended by past critics of the research program as described below.

Past Criticism of the GRC Paradigm and the Gender Role Conflict Scale (GRCS)

Over the years much critique has shaped the GRC paradigm (O'Neil 2008a, b) and produced revisions and adaptations of the *GRCS* (Blazina et al. 2005; Wester et al. 2012). Extensive criticism of the GRC construct is found elsewhere (O'Neil 2008a, b, 2015) and only critiques relevant to this chapter's topic of situational GRC are presented here. The fundamental question is whether any of the past criticism supports studying how GRC relates to men's bonds with animals. First, the research program has failed to assess GRC longitudinally by identifying development tasks and contextual demands that interface with men's socialization and psychosocial development (Enns 2000; Heppner 1995; Smiler 2004). Without developmental perspectives, how GRC occurs and can be changed remain unknown. Furthermore, the research program has not assessed how GRC impact others and how it is experienced from others (Rochlen and Mahalik 2004). For example, does men's GRC result in animal bonds and how do animals mediate men's GRC? Additionally, there has been criticism that the *GRCS* measures a limited number of behavioral domains and does not assess important areas like men's sexuality, performance, homophobia, and health issues (Thompson and Pleck 1995). The critics are correct about the limited number of behavioral domains and therefore further scale development is needed as well as exploring the situational dynamics of GRC both theoretically and empirically. Furthermore, the GRCS has been described as a trait base construct and measure that is limited in implementing situational and contextual research (Addis et al. 2010; Jones and Heesacker 2012). The definitions of GRC do not imply innate traits and whether the GRCS is trait-based measure is controversial and complicated (O'Neil 2014).

Two major critiques of the GRC research have occurred (Addis et al. 2010; Jones and Heesacker 2012) and both are important in expanding the options for researchers to study the contextual and situational GRC. Addis et al. (2010) describes the previous GRC research as limited and recommends a gendered social learning approach and Jones and Heesacker (2012) make a case for micro-contextual research with GRC (see Chap. 3). Both Addis et al. (2010) and Jones and Heesacker (2012) are suggesting similar directions for masculinity research in the future. Using different terminology, they are arguing for research that is contextual, micro-contextual, situational, and studying environmental cues and factors that affect GRC or men's behavior. We agree with this analysis and encourage research where GRC is the dependent variable. All the criticism suggests expanding the GRC theory to include a macrosocietal, developmental, and situational perspectives.

New Theoretical Assumptions About Men's GRC

Bases on these critiques, the new GRC theory was summarized in a single text (O'Neil 2015) with fourteen new GRC assumptions that explain how restricted gender role may affect men's lives. The new GRC assumptions are summarized here to provide a theoretical basis for the understanding of men's animal bond in a situational context. First, descriptive and situational contexts can explain men's GRC and possibilities for healthy positive masculinity. This assumption implies that there are situational precursors and contingencies that can activate men's GRC or help resolve it. Second, healthy development and GRC are hypothesized to occur over the life span during gender role transitions and when mastering developmental tasks and psychosocial crises. From this perspective, psychosocial theory needs to be integrated with GRC theory and research. Furthermore, the theory states that journeying with gender roles is part of resolving GRC and seeking positive and healthy masculinity. These first three assumptions convey that contexts for GRC can be negative, situational, developmental, and positive but how restricted gender roles are part of these processes has not been conceptualized.

The new theory also assumes that society (the macrosocietal context) is based on patriarchal values that foster stereotypes and sexist ways of thinking that cause GRC and psychological problems for men, women, and children (Enns 2000, 2008). Furthermore, restricted gender roles and GRC are theoretically connected to patriarchy, sexism, restrictive stereotypes, oppression, social injustices, and the differential socialization of boys and girls to sexist masculinity and femininity ideologies. Acknowledging the relationships between these social/political realities can put men's problems in a new and provocative light. Moreover, gender role identity can be negatively affected by the macrosocietal contexts and many other situational contingencies creating contextual complexity in understanding men. The perils of sexist and patriarchal societies are assumed to interact with a multitude of indices that produce dysfunctional psychological health for men. Whether men's bonds with animals can mediate these macrosocietal influences is an important empirical question.

Furthermore, the new theory enumerates gender-related contexts that negatively affect men's gender role identity including restrictive and sexist masculinity and femininity ideologies, fears of femininity, distorted gender role schemas, patterns of GRC, defensiveness, and vulnerability to gender role devaluations, restrictions and violations. All of these contexts emanate from macrosocietal level and men's restrictive gender role socialization in families and can cause internalized oppression, psychological and interpersonal problems, social injustice, and violence, and therefore are critical mental health issues for both sexes. The gender-related contexts represent important dimensions of the animal–human bond focused on in this chapter.

Another theoretical assumption is that micro-contextual and situational contexts of men's lives need to be studied to document more specifically the outcomes and consequences of GRC. For example in this chapter, the situational context is men's bonds with animals and discussed later in the chapter. Finally, therapeutic and psychoeducational interventions need to be developed for boys and men experiencing GRC. The use of dogs to help men cope with their interpersonal problems and trauma is commonplace but has not been fully researched.

A more extensive explanation of these assumptions is found elsewhere (O'Neil 2015) and for this chapter these premises provide a theoretical foundation for studying the animal–human bond in the context of men's GRC. For this study to be advanced, more information is needed about how men experience GRC as psychological processes and these issues are discussed below.

Explaining GRC Processes: The Gender Role Journey, Gender Role Transitions, Gender Role Schemas, and the Gender Role Transformational Process

Gender Role Journey Transformation Processes

How men experience GRC in situational contexts is a current topic in the psychology of men (Addis et al. 2010; Jones and Heesacker 2012). Very little is known about how men are gender role conflicted during their psychosocial development. In order to understand the animal–human bond, concepts are needed to explicate how men respond to sexism, GRC, and restricted gender roles. In this section, we provide conceptual information that gives insight into how GRC is experienced and worked through.

The Gender Role Journey

The gender role journey is metaphor that helps people understand how restricted gender roles, sexism, and adherence to gender role stereotypes may negatively affect their lives personally, professionally, and politically (O'Neil and Egan 1992a; O'Neil et al. 1993a, b). The gender role journey provides a framework for evaluating thoughts, feelings, and behaviors about gender roles, sexism, and GRC by promoting a retrospective analysis of early family experiences with gender roles, assessment of how sexism is currently experienced, and decision-making about how gender roles will shape one's behavior in the future.

Three empirically derived phases of the gender role journey are: (a) acceptance of traditional gender roles; (b) gender role ambivalence, confusion, anger, and fear, and (c) personal and professional activism (O'Neil et al. 1993a, b). Part of the journey is gaining an understanding of which phase you are in and how GRC and distorted gender role schemas develop in the family as well as identifying gender role transitions that occur across the life span (O'Neil and Egan 1992b, c; O'Neil and Fishman 1992; O'Neil et al. 1987). Journeying with gender roles and bonding with people and animals are usually complexly related and deserve analysis and explanation.

For example, men who have attachment problems may endorse Phase 1 (acceptance of traditional gender roles) because it is the expected, easily explained, and psychologically familiar even though it is restrictive and limits options. The gender role journey in Phase 1 may be attractive to men who need the sexist structure to survive and avoid emasculation. Men who learn distorted gender role schemas (i.e., power, control, emotionality, winning), their interpersonal relationships maybe more likely to bond with animals and endorse Phase 1.

Furthermore, unattached men may also vacillate between Phase 1 and 2 of the gender role journey. Phase 2 of the journey is experiencing ambivalence, confusion, anger, and fear related to gender role issues. For men who insecure attachments or unresolved GRC, gender role ambivalence, confusion, anger, and fear may contribute bonding with animals to avoid the complexity of human interaction.

Phase 3, personal and professional activism means changing oneself by resolving the conflict and making commitments to reduce sexism in one' own life as well as doing something to reduce sexism in other people's lives. Personal and professional activism occurs when there is the positive attachment to oneself and others and attachment to dogs can promote both types of activism. Using dogs to improve or soothe yourself is now well established in therapeutic circles (Blazina et al. 2013; Blazina 2011a, b). Becoming an animal rights activist, by protecting animals from harm is an example of the last phase of the gender role journey (references here). The overall theoretical premise is that men consciously and unconsciously journey with their gender roles when bonding with animals.

Gender Role Transitions

Gender role transitions stimulate GRC and can facilitate resolving issues during the gender role journey. Gender role transitions are events in a person's gender role development that produce changes in his or her gender role identity and self-assumptions. Understanding gender role transitions across the life span by journeying with them is one way to understand GRC and develop the healthy positive masculinity. In the midst of them, men and women demonstrate, resolve, reevaluate, or integrate new or old conceptions of masculinity and femininity—as West and Zimmerman (1998) put it, they are "doing gender" or "redoing gender." Our position that is explored later in the chapter is that bonding with animals is a gender role transition that affects gender role ideologies and schemas played out during psychosocial development.

Gender role transitions are also hypothesized to relate to mastering developmental tasks and resolving psychosocial crises. The most salient gender role transitions relevant to this chapter are human attachment or the human–animal attachment.

Bonding can produce positive growth or confusion, anxiety, and despair but failure to resolve gender role transitions may stimulate GRC and other emotional problems.

A major inhibitor of gender role transitions is the fear of femininity (FOF), a strong, negative emotion associated with feminine values, attitudes, and behaviors, which are regarded as inferior, inappropriate, and immature—in short, a devaluation of all that is feminine (Blazina 1997a, b; Kierski and Blazina 2009; O'Neil 1981a, 1982). FOF is primarily learned during early childhood socialization, when gender identity is being formed by input from parents, peers, and societal institutions and also occurs in later years through physical maturation, developmental changes, and life events. How the FOF relates to men's bonding with animals has not been discussed in the previous literature and therefore we discuss it in later sections of the chapter.

A second inhibitor to men's gender role transitions is homophobia and the presumed relationship between feminine values and homosexuality. Homophobia is the fear of homosexuals or worries about appearing to be homosexual. In our dualistic culture, femininity and homosexuality and masculinity and heterosexuality have been erroneously linked. If you are male and act feminine, the assumption is you are not a real man. If you are not a man, you are like a woman, and this means you are a homosexual because stereotypically gay men are viewed as feminine.

This illogical reasoning is the source of destructive heterosexism, homophobia, and homonegativity. Homophobia is a form of sexism that inhibits men from exploring their femininity and masculinity and completing gender role transitions over the life span. Homophobia contributes significantly to distorted gender role schemas and hypermasculine attitudes and behavior. How the FOF relates to men's bonding with animals has not been discussed in the previous literature and we hypothesize that bonds with animals can be gender role transitions or they can facilitate them as men evaluate and redefine masculinity ideology.

Gender Role Schemas and Distorted Gender Role Schemas

Other theoretical constructs that promote our understanding of GRC and animal–human bond are gender role schemas and distorted gender role schemas. Personal changes and modifications in gender role values are not completed in a vacuum and thoughts and feelings that get demonstrated, resolved, reevaluated, or integrated is the critical question. In order for boys and men to complete gender role transitions, there are usually cognitive and affective processes operating that facilitate for the completion of the transition. With human–animal bonding the cognitive and affective processes at both the conscious and unconscious levels are just beginning to be explored by scholars. One hypothesis is that these gender role transitions are experienced in the context of certain gender role schemas.

Gender role schemas are cultural definitions of maleness and femaleness that organize and guide an individual's perception of masculinity and femininity based on sex and gender roles. Examples of salient gender role schemas are control, achievement, personal worth, communication, sexuality, intimacy, performance, dependence, and power to just name a few. Gender role schemas relate to the person's self-concept and are used to evaluate his or her personal adequacy as male or female. The issue of personal adequacy to meet the demands of restrictive gender roles schemas is part of the gender role strain and conflict that both men and women experience. Gender role schemas are considered when boys or men demonstrate, resolve, reevaluate, or integrate masculinity and femininity during gender role transitions. On a cognitive and affective level, gender role schemas are what men struggle with during gender role transitions. The gender role schemas with animals are hypothesized to be the same schemas that men experience with humans, but very little information exists on this topic.

Many men have learned gender role schemas that are distorted and based on sexist stereotypes. Distorted gender role schemas are exaggerated thoughts and feelings about masculinity and femininity as applied to major life issues. The distortion occurs because of perceived or actual pressure to meet stereotypical notions of masculinity, resulting in fears and anxieties about not measuring up to traditional gender role expectations. These distorted gender role schema are part of the man's restricted masculinity ideology that produce GRC and may contribute to precarious manhood (Vandello and Bossom 2013; Vandello et al. 2008). Example of distorted gender role schema for competition is "I have to always win to feel good." For power the distortion is "Without my power, I am less of man." How distorted gender schemas affect men's relational capacities and bonding with animals has previously gone unexplored and therefore we hypothesize that gender role schemas and distorted schemas as well are "in play" when men bond with animals. For example, a distorted schema might be: "I have to be a provider because others depend on me and dogs help me fulfill this role by giving me comfort and a sense of control."

Gender Role Journey Transformational Processes

The critical question is how to journey with gender roles, resolve GRC and gender role transitions, and effectively redefine distorted gender role schemas to enrich one's life. This process is challenging and relates to transformations that include men's attachment to humans and animals. Gould (1978, 1980) defined transformation as expanding one's self-definition to produce inner freedom without conflict or anxiety, thereby internalizing a maximum sense of personal security. Likewise, gender role transformation can produce a redefinition of masculinity and femininity, decreased gender role conflict, greater freedom with gender roles, and increased self-confidence. Gould posited four processes of the transformation process that have relevance to explaining the internal dynamics of the gender role journey including (a) changes in psychological defenses, (b) facing and dealing with false assumptions, (c) increases in internal dialogue with self, (d) internal psychological warfare. Journeying with one's gender roles and managing gender roles and transitions follow these same processes in both intrapersonal and interpersonal realms.

Gender Role Journey Transfomational Processes

A bond with an animal can be part of man's transformational process with their masculinity. The critical question is how to journey with gender roles, resolve gender role transitions, and effectively redefine distorted gender role schemas to enrich one's life. This process is challenging and relates to transformations (See the bottom of Figure). Gould (1978, 1980) defined transformation as expanding one's self-definition to produce inner freedom without conflict or anxiety, thereby internalizing a maximum sense of personal security. Likewise, gender role transitions can produce a redefinition of masculinity and femininity, decreased gender role conflict, greater freedom with gender roles, and increased self-confidence. Gould posited numerous properties of the transformation process that have relevance to explaining the internal dynamics of gender role transitions and the gender role journey including (a) changes in psychological defenses, (b) facing and dealing with false assumptions, (c) increases in internal dialogue with self, (d) internal psychological warfare. We add to this list manipulation of symbols as central to transforming ourselves. Each of these is elaborated in the context of men's gender role transitions and the animal–human bond.

When people struggle to change their fundamental conception of gender roles, the defensive structure of their personality may need alteration to foster more functional and expansive ways to live. Many men have a defensive posture in relationships because they fear losing control and power and therefore appear invulnerability and tough. At various points in a man's life the established defenses may no longer function fully and new psychological mechanisms are needed to enhance coping and promote the transformation. Defensive structures vary greatly, but repression, projection, regression, and reaction formation are quite common. The essence of most defense mechanisms is the inability to face emotions and feelings and therefore an emotional leveling or shutdown. Emotions relevant to one's gender role identity can be intellectualized, denied, represses, and projected in anger and hostility toward others. Therefore, gender role transitions may require a fundamental change in men's psychological defense system and new ways of experiencing deep emotions as part of the gender role journey. When men cannot change their defenses in human relationships, they may turn to animals where fewer, if any, are needed. Having no defenses in animal relationships, the man can discharge emotions, be himself, and be human in ways that may ultimately transfer to human relationships without their defensiveness.

Furthermore, false assumptions or illusions about gender roles may help maintain a defensive posture. Before the transformation occurs, false ideas about gender role stereotypes from childhood consciousness usually establish the functional boundaries of a sexist self-definition. These stereotypes are usually internalized at an early age to establish men's and women's gender role identities. These functional boundaries are maintained until the false ideas are disconfirmed and the stereotypes are disconfirmed. For example, beliefs that real men always have to be strong, successful, powerful, unemotional, and in control of all relationships are gender role illusions that reflect societal stereotypes. The insecurely attached man may extend these stereotypes by concluding that no one can be trusted and getting close in relationship is risky. Animals may be a safe alternative to having one's intimacy needs met. Willingness to challenge these false ideas may depend on obtaining new information, deep emotional awakenings, and political awareness that sexism violates women and men in a capitalist society. Animal relationships may be a stimulus to revaluate long held stereotypes that keep men distant and unfulfilled in human relationships.

More important, gender role transitions stimulate an internal dialogue in the context of the new, emerging gender role identity. This internal dialogue may inhibit transformation, since the false ideas may produce anxiety and feelings of psychological regression. Usually, the false self-assumptions prohibit the gender role transition process and maintain personal anxiety and gender role conflict. If men and women can face these false assumptions and feel support, they can begin the internal dialogue necessary to deconstruct gender roles and prompt gender role change. Communing with animals can be a safe place to have this internal dialogue that promotes psychological and interpersonal growth.

This internal dialogue may bring about psychological warfare between the person and their external world or between the old self and the new, emerging human identity. During gender role transitions, "enemies of the self" are sometimes identified from the intense emotions, especially anger and fear. Yet, who these enemies are may be unclear. Women, other men, parents, children, and institutional structures may be targeted as the enemy to be attacked or avoided. Men may identify a weakened sense of themselves as the enemy, in terms of their self-imposed restrictions, devaluations, and personal limitations. Identifying the "enemy within" usually produces low self-esteem, anxiety, anger, and defensiveness that destabilize the person. Again, animals may be positive mediators of this war with man by providing nurturance and hope for better human relationships.

Adding to Gould's definition of transformation, gender role transitions may require a manipulation of symbols and the use of metaphors for change and healing. Cherished masculine stereotyped success, status, control, and power can be replaced with transformative myths, metaphors, symbols, and images. Past interest in mythology (Campbell 1988; Johnson 1986) represents an evolving person's desire to use symbolic representation to find greater meaning in life. Johnson (1986) indicated that the "most rewarding mythological experience you can have is to see how it lives in your own psychological structure" (p.x). Myths offer us the truth about ourselves and dispel the hardened illusions that we have based our lives on.

The use of metaphors, images, and symbols gives men an opportunity to redefine their gender perspectives. In gender role journey workshops (O'Neil 1996, 2015; O'Neil and Roberts Carroll 1988), I have seen the power of symbols and metaphors in promoting transformation. For example, if the symbols (i.e., stereotypes) of power and control have been rigidly internalized as money, status, authority, and power over others, then a new conceptualization of power and control can be developed. Power could be redefined as the symbolic and real activity of empowering others. The symbol of "power over others" becomes transformed to "conscious empowerment of others" through service, leadership, and nurturing support.

Helping men manipulate symbols related to masculinity and femininity requires facing the illusions of gender role stereotypes. For gender role transitions to occur, the artificiality and illusions of gender role stereotypes need to be assessed through the deconstruction process. For example, one illusion is the value of highly sex-typed behavior and masculine and feminine stereotypes as a basis for healthy self-definition. For an evolving person who is seeking transformation, stereotypes no longer have the same power or utility in coping with life events. Men can recognize that stereotypic masculinity and femininity are not synonymous with health. This recognition represents a significant breakthrough toward a more substantial understanding of gender and human identity. The past gender role stereotypes are exposed as shallow and as not sustaining the person on a deeper, internal level. The illusions of the stereotypes need exploration if real growth is to occur over the life span. This process involves capturing deep emotions about masculinity and femininity and finding new meaning in them. Whether animals can be helpful to men in creating metaphors or manipulating symbols can be operationalized through future research.

A person who has an insecure or disorganized attachment will have difficulty trusting their transformative process and altering their defense mechanisms and rethinking their false assumptions about gender roles. Furthermore, self-processing and having useful positive dialogues with oneself and resolving psychological warfare may be more difficult if human bonding has not occurred. Whether, movement between the gender role journey phases and the four transformation processes can be altered by the man's attachment to animals is a critical and empirical question.

The GRC concepts discussed above provide a theoretical foundation to raise questions about men's relationships with animals in the context of gender roles. Speculation is needed on how animals and men have relationships and in the next section more theoretical and empirical background is provided that connects GRC with men's bonds with animals.

Filling the Conceptual Gap Between the Psychology of Men and the Human–Animal Bond

Theorizing that men's restricted gender roles affect their human relationships has been widely discussed for decades. Overall, the consensus is that restricted gender roles (i.e., GRC) limit men's behavioral repertoires in friendships, close relationships, and parenting roles. As reported earlier, the research also indicates that GRC is related to significant problems in men's lives. What has gone unexplored is how men's problems might relate to men's bonds with animals. Theoretical concepts are needed to help both practitioners and researchers theorize about how the human–animal bond might relate to men's gender role socialization. In the next sections, psychosocial concepts are presented to help connect GRC with how men bond with animals.

Psychosocial Theory and Attachment: Male Developmental Tasks and Psychosocial Crises

A new GRC assumption states that men's GRC needs to be studied in the context of psychosocial theory, specifically developmental tasks and psychosocial crises (O'Neil 2015). Developmental tasks elucidates the animal–human bond in extensive ways and are defined as "a set of skills and competencies that contribute to increased mastery over one's environment and what is healthy, normal development is at each age in a particular society" (Newman and Newman 2012, p. 11). The developmental tasks occur during sensitive periods when an individual is ready to acquire a new set of abilities that promote gains in physical, cognitive, emotional, social, and/or emotional skills that all affect a man's self-concept. The person needs to master specific developmental tasks to move on to the next stage of development and psychosocial growth. Many of the developmental tasks have implications for our relationships with animals, but in this chapter, we focus on one: human attachment. In infancy, attachment is the major developmental task and relevant to a child's and adult's intrapersonal and interpersonal functioning. Without human attachment, trusting others and oneself are compromised and many times resulting in withdrawal and delayed development. A brief review of attachment theory is provided here to explain how GRC is related to men's bonding with animals.

Attachment spans the life span just like gender role issues do. At each stage of development, attachment plays a different role because different psychosocial tasks and responsibilities are encountered. Bowlby's theory of attachment stresses children's expectations about their caregivers and also that the parental bonding can contribute to children's interpersonal security during the early years and later in life (Kobak and Madsen 2008). Attachment styles are developed in infancy when a child is reliant on a caregiver for nurturance and security. Based on experiences with their caregivers, a child may develop a secure or insecure attachment style. Securely attached children have positive expectations about the availability of their caregiver and are hopeful about finding satisfaction in human contact (Kobak and Madsen 2008). Insecure attachment styles are expressed either as avoidant or ambivalent style. Children with avoidant styles expect rejection from their parents, while children with ambivalent styles are uncertain about what to expect from their caregivers (Kobak and Madesen 2008). A third pathological style is disorganized style of attachment where the child may learn to perceive their caregiver as frightened or frightening (Kobak and Madesen 2008). If the child's fear in an attachment relationship can be worked through, an increased sense of security can occur, particularly if basic needs are met. However, if the fear is left unresolved or left for the child to resolve it on their own, a child's functioning in emotional or interpersonal domains may be negatively impacted. Children and adults with attachment problems may seek bonds with animals to find their meaning, identity, and personal security.

Attempts to master developmental tasks produce a "psychosocial crisis" at each stage of development (Newman and Newman 2012) and these challenges are need to be resolved for growth and development to continue. Psychosocial crisis refers to a normal set of stressors and coping strategies associated with exerting psychological effort to adjust to the conditions of a new level of maturity and growth. The individual makes the adjustment by integrating personal needs, skills, and social demands that vary from stage to stage. At the end of each stage, the person resolves the crisis by translating the societal demands into personal change, producing a state of tension that is experienced in terms of polarities or opposites—for example, trust versus mistrust or autonomy versus shame. Both polar ends foster development, but the tension between them must be reduced for the person to proceed to the next stage and meet new challenges.

Problems with attachment may inhibit the resolution of psychosocial crises needed for ongoing growth and development. When secure attachment is not accomplished, the psychosocial crises of trust versus mistrust in infancy may not be resolved with parents, resulting in infant withdrawal, lost mutuality with a caregiver, and limited hope for psychosocial growth and intimacy with others (Newman and Newman 2012). Furthermore, early attachment problems may contribute to not resolving the psychosocial crises, autonomy versus shame/guilt in toddlerhood, inferiority versus industry in middle childhood and identity issues that can cause alienation in early and late adolescence (12–22 years). These early problems may affect interpersonal communication, sensorimotor intelligence, emotional development, and the subsequent mastery of developmental tasks of toddlerhood, early school age, middle childhood periods. Furthermore, psychosocial delays with attachment during these formative years may affect capacities for intimacy and positive relationships in adulthood.

Men who have attachment or relational deficits with humans may bond with animals to help master developmental tasks and resolve psychosocial crisis. Furthermore, efforts to master the developmental tasks and resolve psychosocial crises can activate GRC consciously or unconsciously. Animal bonds can help men master developmental tasks and resolve psychosocial crises, specifically when human bonds are difficult or threatening. Attempts to resolve tasks and crises can promote psychosocial growth but failed attempts to connect with animals can also result in animal abuse, loneliness, and greater isolation.

Finally, boys and men who bond with dogs can experience positive psychosocial growth that facilitates mastering the developmental tasks. How attachment problems and psychosocial development contribute to boys and men's problems in interpersonal and intimate relationships is a critical topic to be explored in the future. For example, knowledge and research about men's attachment and GRC can help provide information on men's bonding with animals.

Summary

Psychosocial theory postulates that human attachment is a developmental task of infancy and for this bonding to occur there must be mutuality between the parent and child. The result of this bonding is hope for the child and being able to trust others. Without attachment, trust, and hope the child is vulnerable to withdrawal and social detachment. If attachment and trust of other human beings are difficult or impossible, bonding with objects and animals may be the only way to define oneself and have positive self-esteem.

Psychosocial development can be enhanced by the animal–human bond because the canine relationship can be a laboratory for positive attachment, mastering developmental tasks, and resolving psychosocial crises. Mastering developmental tasks with animals can provide confidence and beliefs that learned skills can be used in human relationship and developmental delays can be reversed and changed. The psychosocial development of humans through animal bonds represents an exciting new area for theory development and empirical research.

Attachment and Gender Role Conflict Theory and Research: What Is Known?

Little evidence exists to support gender-specific theories in attachment, but Grossmann et al. (2008) report that child–mother attachment plays a role in young children's behavior. They found that securely attached children were found to behave in less gender-stereotypic ways than insecurely attached children (Grossmann et al. 2008). This result could suggest that parents who conform to rigid notions of masculinity and femininity, engage in sexist parenting. Restrictive views of masculinity and femininity by parents can influence boys and girls to endorse in restrictive gender roles themselves promoting insecure attachment to their caregiver(s).

Attachment, bonding, and family individuation problems have conceptualized in the psychology of men using concepts like disidentification with the mother, the fragile masculine self, and a traumatic abrogation of the early holding pattern (Blazina 2001; Blazina and Watkins 2000; Pollack 1995a, b). Researchers have argued that early parent–son dynamics impact male bonding that contribute to problems with attachment, separation, individualization, disidentification, and conflictual independence (Blazina and Watkins 2000; DeFranc and Mahalik 2002; Fischer and Good 1998; Schwartz et al. 2004).

Very few studies have assessed the relationship between attachment and men bonding with animals but attachment to parents and GRC has been investigated in 15 studies (Blazina et al. 2008; Blazina and Watkins 2000; Cachia 2001; Covell 1998; DeFranc and Mahalik 2002; Fischer 2007; Fischer and Good 1998; Griffin 2011; James 2006; Land et al. 2011; Napolitano et al. 1999; Schwartz et al. 2004; Selby 1999; Siffert 2012). All the patterns of men's GRC have significantly correlated with attachment to both mothers and fathers. Siffert (2012) found autonomy from parents and affective attachment to be correlated negatively with RE, RABBM, and CBWFR. Six studies used either canonical correlations or structural equation modeling to assess GRC's relationship to attachment (Blazina and Watkins 2000; DeFranc and Mahalik 2002; Fischer 2007; Fischer and Good 1998; Napolitano et al. 1999; Selby 1999). Complex and significant findings were found between GRC and measures of attachment, separation, individuation problems (Blazina and Watkins 2000), affective attachment (Siffert 2012), attachment quality (Fischer 2007), attachment styles (Blazina et al. 2008; Cachia 2001; Schwartz et al. 2004; Selby 1999), perceptions of father's GRC (DeFranc and Mahalik 2002), conflicts with mothers (Fischer and Good 1998), and identity development (Napolitano et al. 1999). For example with a sample of college men, Blazina and Watkins (2000) found that as GRC increases, so do problems of attachment, separation, and individuation with parents. In another study, higher levels of SPC, RE, and RABBM were significantly related to fearful and avoidant attachment styles (Cachia 2001) and increases in GRC predicted higher attachment avoidance scores. Siffert (2012) found autonomy from parent and affective attachment to be correlated negatively with RE, RABBM, CBWFR. He also studied self-object dimensions and found that maladaptive self-object orientation was associated with the gender role conflict patterns. Land et al. (2011) found the GRC total score GRC negatively predicted maternal bonding care and parental bonding and that GRC did not mediate the relationship between maternal bonding care and adult attachment avoidance. Finally, with African American men's all GRC patterns were related to unhealthy attachment styles (Blazina et al. 2008). Finally, a nonsignificant mediational effect of GRC on the relationship between attachment insecurity and sexual compulsivity was found by Griffin (2011).

The initial studies on attachment suggest that GRC is complexly related to attachment and separation from parents. The overall results of these studies do support greater attention to the developmental aspects of gender roles being studied in the context of GRC. More study is needed to explore how early parent–child bonding affects gender role development and GRC. Theory on how psychosocial issues affect developmental tasks and psychosocial crises could be useful to future researchers and practitioners helping men.

Moreover, there is very limited information about how human attachment to animals develops and the reasons why. A more comprehensive view of how attachment, GRC, and the animal–human bond are needed and in this chapter a new conceptualization is presented. Furthermore, we argue that men who have few attachment problems can increase their relational competency by their bonds with animals. How attachment problems and psychosocial development contribute to boys and men's GRC in interpersonal and intimate relationships is a critical topic to be explored in the future.

Exactly what happens in the animal–human attachment has not been extensively studied and even less is known on what role gender roles play in the bonding. Our overall premise is that animal–person bond is a significant focal point for men to journey with their gender role. As discussed earlier the transformation process of journeying with gender roles includes changing psychological defenses, facing false assumptions, increasing internal dialogue. Boys and men who have insecure or disorganized attachment may have difficulty working with this transformation process and forming effective interpersonal relationships. Resisting or avoiding transformation can produce maladaptive coping and psychological problems (such as GRC) that can restrict behavior and stunt psychosocial and interpersonal growth.

Specifically, when important attachment and gender roles issues go unresolved, distorted gender roles schema can be played out causing GRC and significant psychological costs to the man and others. Skewed schemas related to personal worth, control, power, communication, safety, and interpersonal competence may affect relational capacities of men to manage the complexity of interpersonal relationships. Distorted gender role schemas may need to be corrected and if they are not, men are likely to bond with animals. We hypothesize that corrective animal–human bonding may increase a man's capacity to communicate with humans.

Closing the Conceptual Gap: Between Animal–Human Bond and GRC

We theorize that the animal–human bond, psychosocial development, and the journey with gender role conflict are intimately connected. Two critical questions help focus the connection of these concepts (a) how does men's bonding with people differ than their bonding with animal? and (b) how do men's patterns of gender role conflict (SPC, RE, RABBM, and CBWFR) cause interpersonal problems and stimulate intimate bonds with animals? The other way also.

Regarding the first question, relationships with animals may not be perceived by men "as gendered" or if they are, it is usually not in a negative or threatening way. Second, homophobia or threats to gender role identity usually do not operate with the animal bond; sex and sexual orientation are not driving dynamic in the human–animal bond as they might be in human relationships. Third, with dogs, men do not have to prove their masculinity and their authentic sleeves, transcending the norms of the restrictive patriarchal structure. Furthermore, as noted earlier, masculinity ideologies and norms may be suspended or altered with animal interactions, since the threat to one's gender role identity is nonexistent or significantly lessened. Fears of femininity (FOF) and worries about emasculation may be inoperative in the human–animal bond and the degree of GRC may be less or nonexistent with animals compared to humans. Moreover, the powerful gender role schemas operative in most human relationships (power, control, safety, esteem, and intimacy) may have different meaning with animal interactions. Distorted schemas can be altered, corrected, and redefined in positive and functional ways with animals. Finally, animals can be safe objects/subjects to project on, without any negative consequences.

In summary, the differences in human versus animal bonds provide a theoretical foundation for asking more focused questions related to men's relationships with dogs. Examples of these questions are addressed later in the chapter and more elaborate conceptualizations are found in this chapter of this volume.

The second question is how do the patterns of gender role conflict (SPC, RE, RABBM, and CBWFR) cause interpersonal problems for men that may promote intimate bonds with animals? As presented earlier in the chapter, much empirical research shows that GRC is correlated with men's depression, low self-esteem, shame and guilt, attachment problems, marital dissatisfaction, intimacy problems, and negative and abusive attitudes toward women. What is missing is research that links GRC to men's intimate connection with animals. To begin to answer the question of why and how men bond with animals, we speculate on how SPC, RE, RABBMN, and CBWFR may theoretically relate, moderate, or mediate both the human and animal bonds.

For SPC the issue is how men seek success, power, control, and competition to stabilize their human masculine identities rather than human qualities like mutuality, cooperativeness, emotionality, compassion, honesty, admitting error, sharing power, and vulnerability. Overall, men who are obsessed with SPC objectify others and subordinate them in interpersonal relationships to prove their masculinity. Without human qualities, the man has a restrictive behavioral repertoire that restricts interpersonal communication and can cause stress and conflict. Many men who have unresolved interpersonal conflicts either withdraw to avoid the conflict or lash out with abuse or sometimes even violence. Either way their relational needs go unmet and isolation and loneliness are many times the outcome. Bonds with animals can fill this relational void in men's lives since the power, control, and competition issues with animals are different and unlikely to stimulate the same degree of GRC as in human relationships (more elaboration).

When men have high restrictive emotionality (RE) interpersonal relations can also be problematic. Specifically, when men view emotions as feminine rather than human qualities, feelings can become a source of conflict and pain. Rational problem solving and intellectualization have their limitations in solving life's problems and many times emotional expression is needed for resolutions and breakthroughs to occur. If the man has no outlet for his emotions, then feelings are repressed, many times causing depression, stress, and substance abuse. Dogs can be "the go to" relationship where emotions can be expressed without the fear of being emasculated or appearing feminine. Animals do respond to human affect (need some sources here) and are primary sources of emotional support for many people. In this way, animals can be corrective experiences for men who have repressed their emotions their whole lives because of fears of femininity and potential emasculations from others.

RABBM is another pattern of GRC that constrains men's interpersonal and human capacities. Affection is a positive and intimate way to communicate one's care and affirmation of others. Unfortunately, expressing affection can be experienced as letting down one's competitive guard with other men. The risk is that your affection might not be accepted, reciprocated, or stimulated a change of power in the relationship. For some men, affection and intimacy may become confused with sexuality and therefore touching other men may activate a distorted schema around touch that implies sexual attraction or desire. In these situations unresolved homophobia is activated; better not to touch or show affection, fearing that it will be construed as making a sexual advance. Even though this makes no logical sense, these processes exist probably at an unconscious and intrapsychic level.

Restricted affectionate behavior with women may operate because touching will be construed as making a sexual advance or come on. These days touching anybody is risky business because of the widespread realities of sexual harassment and sexual abuse. In this way, GRC dehumanized both men and women and represents how affection as a human quality has been ruined by patriarchal values and misinformation. This unfortunate development requires constant education about the differences between sexuality, human intimacy, and affection. With both sexes, many men decide to inhibit their positive affection both verbally and physically because it is too risky which only contributes to increasing dehumanization that plagues our violence-ridden world.

Men's affection with animals is a completely different dynamic. Men pet and hug animals in highly emotional ways and get their relational needs met through the animal bond. There is a striking difference between how men show affection to animals versus humans and some of the difference has to do with GRC and masculine gender role socialization. Recently, the first author was discussing the human–dog bond with a colleague and she described how her husband is highly emotional, affectionate, vulnerable, and intimate with their dog. She said: "I wished I could get more of that from him in our relationship; I need that too!"

Many men have CBWFR as they balance competitive work situations, providing for their families, and managing family dynamics. Feeling stressed and sometimes out of control with many unresolved problems with both family and work is common for many men. Actually taking care of an animal can add to the CBWFR because pets do require care and attention. When there is conflict and particularly marital stress from the problems, animals can be the mediators of men's stress and a safe haven to sort out the issues with limited negative consequences or further loss of control. It is unknown how often men discuss their stressors, think about their problems with their animals, or project their problems onto their pets to find comfort and soothing. Our view is that these conversations are frequent but only research can verify our hypothesis.

Future Research Directions, Hypotheses, and Perspectives

Research questions need to be generated to promote a more empirically informed understanding of the animal–human bond and GRC. Both quantitative and qualitative research are needed to assess how bonding with dogs can enhance men's lives and relationships. One of the first research priorities can be qualitative interviews with men about the meaning of their relationships with dogs. These interviews could identify topics that can be operationalized through empirical research. For example, how does a man's GRC predict the probability of developing an animal bond and how do these relationships affect his capacity to have human bonds? How does the human–animal bond mediate or moderate GRC? Moreover, what actually happens in the animal–human bond that mediates GRC and other psychological problems? Does the animal–human bond reduce men's GRC and what mechanism operates to make this happen.

Are there precursor conditions that promote men's bonding with animals? For example, do insecure attachments to humans promote the animals bond? How does failure to master major developmental tasks like attachment predict closer bonds with animals compared to humans? Does unresolved loss promote men's bonding with animals or help them recover from the grief and enhance attachment to humans? Do animal bonds help men who have a fear of intimacy or help men who have been dehumanized by trauma, discrimination, and violence. How do the patterns of GRC and masculinity ideologies relate to men's bonding with animals? Additionally, are restrictive norms of masculinity ideology suspended or altered when men bond with animals?

What are men's emotional experiences with animals and how do these experiences differ than in human interaction? For example, do men have less RE in animal interactions and if so, does this help men experience, express, and discharge emotion in human relationships? Does affectionate and petting animals help men with their restricted affectionate toward humans? Can men learn to be more emotionally intelligent and empathic because of their relationships with animals and can this learning impact developing more functional human relationships? Can bonds with animals help men correct distorted gender role schemas and resolve patterns of gender role conflict (SPC, RE, RABBM, CBWFR)?

Implications of GRC Theory for Practice with Men and Dogs

Animal bonds and GRC are fertile ground for helping men understand how sexism has negatively affected their lives and attachment to dogs can be part of the healing process. In this section of the chapter some psychoeducational approaches are discussed to help men who have bonds with their dogs. The heuristic value of a theory is demonstrated by its application within an applied setting. GRC theory can be used by practitioners to deepen both their bonds with animals and human beings.

Animal assistance professionals can use the premises of gender role journey therapy (O'Neil 2015) when working with men and their animals. With gender role journey therapy, deepening (Rabinowitz and Cochran 2002) and transtheoretical perspectives (Brooks 2010) are integrated with the three phases of the gender role journey. With this kind of therapy, a man's readiness to change is one the most critical diagnostic categories as specific processes in each phase guide the man as he makes changes and solves his problems. Readiness for a man's change is complex and beyond the scope of this chapter, but critical transformational processes (See bottom of Fig. 2.1) are discussed. A complete summary of gender role journey therapy is discussed elsewhere (O'Neil 2015).

Rather than specifying how to implement a **complete animal assistance program**, a broader psychoeducational curriculum is presented using the contextual variables in Fig. 2.1. The practical question of any dog assistance curriculum is how do men change to achieve healthy masculinity and positive psychological growth? How men change has rarely been addressed in the psychology of men and few empirically validated interventions exist that help men transform themselves (Cochran 2005). Research has documented that men have gender role-related problems (O'Neil 2008a, b, 2015), but the contextual conditions that help men change are still mostly unknown. Animal bonds, as a contextual condition for changing men, deserve psychoeducation experimentation and research. Six curricular areas to help men deepen their dog bonds and understand their gender role conflict are discussed.

Psychoeducational Information and Setting Positive Expectancies

Many men need information on how to recover from their sexist gender role socialization and recognize that animal bonding can liberate them from restricted gender roles. Printed information, mini lectures, self-help books (Blazina 2008;), and DVD documentaries can provide the necessary background on the challenges growing up male in America. Moreover, many men are unaware of how dogs can facilitate their gender role transformation and improve their human relationships. Imbedded within the present volume are examples or case studies of how animals have helped males across the life span. Chapters also present new research demonstrating the value of animal-assisted interventions impacting males in positive psychological ways. However, these results are preliminary and it is prudent to be critical of any intervention that professes to gain men's confidence.

Positive expectancies can be established about how the animal bond can bring greater pleasure in life without the burdens of restricted gender roles. In very simple terms, men can be told "if you talk to your dog, you are likely talking about yourself in some way and therefore the animal relationship is an opportunity for your own growth and personal self-exploration." However, the further value of the human–animal bond for men's well-being may lie in the relational context of the man and dog interaction; the bond may promote men's health, or at least, be more free of gender role restraint.

Gender Role Vocabulary: Gender Role Journey and Patterns of GRC

A bond with an animal can be explained as a journey with one's gender roles where gender role transitions can occur that prompt significant questions about psychosocial growth and opportunities for improved intrapersonal and interpersonal relationships (unclear). Many men will need a gender role vocabulary to begin thinking about how gender role socialization has affected them. One way to introduce this vocabulary could be to administer the GRCS or the Gender Role Conflict Checklist or the Gender Role Journey Measure for a quick assessment of how restricted gender roles operate in the man's life. The results could be important but maybe what is most important is that the man begins to think about how gender roles affect his life. Knowledge about the phases of the gender role journey or the patterns of GRC (SPC, RE, RABBM, CBWFR) can expand how a man sees his masculinity identity and help him ask significant psychosocial questions.

Defensiveness

Another important psychological concept in the curriculum could be human defensiveness. Defenses could be explained as helping people feel safe or avoid uncomfortable emotions. Defense mechanisms could also be defined as both conscious and unconscious and examples could be given so that the man begins to understand his own defensive postures. How defenses are functional could be explained but also how defenses can inhibit growth and development would be emphasized.

One critical question is whether there are differences in men's defensiveness with humans versus animals? Do most men drop or suspend defenses when interacting with animals? This question can stimulate further exploration about how defenses operate in human relationships and whether it really promotes safety or inhibit his interpersonal growth and development? The goal of discussing defensiveness is to find a portal to men's deeper processing of their emotional life (Rabinowitz and Cochran 2002). Likewise, the human–animal bond may provide a means of accessing men's inner worlds.

Increased Self-Dialogue and False Assumptions

When a man understands that he is not defensive with his dog and has greater human vulnerability in its presence, then there can be increased possibilities for self-dialogue, self-processing, and overall communication. This change can be invigorating and exciting as new dimensions of the man's interior self become apparent.

With less defensiveness and increased self-dialogue, the stage is set for possible discussions about the false assumptions of masculine and feminine stereotypes and the lies about the benefits of high sex-typed behavior including control, power, competition, and restrictive emotionality. Sexist and distorted gender role schemas are analyzed and new definitions of what it means to be human can be explored. When this happens with animals, the parallel processes with humans can follow with significant implications for greater intimacy.

Consciousness About Differences in Human and Animal Relationships

An important part of the process is observing any differences in how the man communicates with animals compared to humans. For example, numerous questions occur when differences are observed. Does the man express more emotions with his dog or show greater affection and vulnerability than in human relationships? If there are differences, then the question might be "what do these communication differences mean?" For example, "Is it less risky to be your authentic self with animals than with humans and if so, why? Are there differences in masculine roles, control, and power in the two relational contexts?" Do gender role schemas or distortions operate differently in the two situations and if so, why? If the man is freer with animals, can he conceptualize his emotional and interpersonal problems as they relate to restrictive gender roles and GRC?

Psychological Warfare and Symbol Manipulation

All of this deconstruction of gender roles may create insecurity in the man as the old self is diminished to make room for the new self, free from the shackles of sexist masculinity. The man may experience psychological warfare from his new consciousness that collides with the sexist values of the patriarchal world. The man may experience psychological warfare as his masculine identity and sense of self-change. He may feel a weakened sense of self (the enemy within himself) that produces low self-esteem, defensiveness, anxiety, and anger and the ultimate goal is to turn these negatives into positives. The animal bond and safe places are where these issues can be sorted out and continuing the transformative process.

Sometimes symbols and metaphors emerge that help the man redefine his masculinity ideology and face his GRC that blocks his future growth. When the sexist vales of masculinity ideology are deconstructed and the illusion and artificiality of gender role stereotypes are known (and rejected), there is a "meaning gap" that can be filled with myths, metaphors, and symbols that bring powerful new way to find meaning in life. These metaphors and symbols help us tell the truth about ourselves and dispel the illusions that have been erroneously thrust into our lives. Animals can be part of the symbols and metaphor making because animals represent authentic relationships that men can trust.

A Final Word

The curricular issues described above represent just one way to explain how men may journey with their gender roles in the context of their bond with dogs. Other creative approaches could be developed and since every man is different much experimentation is recommended. This might include the human–animal bond as being rich in symbolism in traditional therapist settings, helping to address males' issues of attachment and loss. The bond may also be present in more structured animal-assisted interactions/interventions that men may not be fully aware that personal and greater gender role transformations are occurring amidst the development of the bond with an animal companion. Practitioners' tasks involve helping to become more aware of these processes and integrating them into the sense of self.

In conclusion, from the gender role journey workshops completed over three decades (O'Neil and Roberts Carroll 1988; O'Neil 1995, 2015), what is apparent to us is that change occurs most frequently when men see their self-interests are "at stake" in terms of living fuller life. Second, change occurs when the social injustices against women, men, and sexual minorities are understood as occurring from sexist and patriarchal values in society that are oppressive. A caring, social conscience develops and anger at how society oppresses people is expressed and many times results in personal and professional activism. When conscious raising from deconstructing distorted gender role stereotypes occurs, finding equity with women and closeness with men becomes an attractive option compared to restricted gender roles that deaden the human spirit. Bonds with animals can be a stimulus for this kind of gender role journey. Men come to realize that the bond is an asset within their lives.

Put another way, when consciousness is raised and men see that the sexist society sets them up to be oppressed, confused, and conflicted about gender roles, breakthroughs and transformations become a real possibilities. With this single insight, men can stop blaming themselves and others for their GRC, sexism, and other oppressions. Men can let themselves off the "sexist hook" and consider how to recover through personal growth and societal activism. Bonds with animals can be stimulators of personal transformation and that is why the chapters in this book are so important to men, women, and children.

References

Addis, M. E., Mansfield, A. K., & Sydek, M. R. (2010). Is "masculinity" a problem: Framing the effect of gendered social learning in men. *Psychology of men and Masculinity, 11*, 77–90.

Alexander, P. E. (1999). The relationship between masculinity ideology and gender role conflict to parenting and marital issues (Doctoral dissertation, University of Missouri-Columbia). *Dissertation Abstracts International, 59*, 3678.

Blazina, C. (1997a). The fear of the feminine in the western psyche and the masculine task of disidentification: Their effect on the development of masculine gender role conflict. *Journal of Men's Studies, 6*, 55–68.

Blazina, C. (1997b). The fear of the feminine in the western psyche and the masculine task of disidentification: Their effect on the development of masculine gender role conflict. *Journal of Men's Studies, 6*, 55–68.
Blazina, C. (2001). Analytic psychology and gender role conflict: The development of the fragile masculine self. *Psychotherapy, 38*, 50–59.
Blazina, C. (2008). *Secret lives of men*. Deerfield, FL: HCI.
Blazina, C., Guler Boyraz, G., Shen-Miller, D. (2011a). *The psychology of the human-animal bond: A resource for clinicians and researchers*. New York: Springer.
Blazina, C., Guler Boyraz, G., Shen-Miller, D. (2011b). Introduction: Using context to inform clinical practice. In C. Blazina, G. Guler Boyras, D. Shen-Miller (Eds.), *The psychology of the human-animal bond: A resource for clinicians and researchers* (pp 3–24). New York: Springer.
Blazina, C., & Watkins, C. E. (2000). Separation/individuation, parental attachment, and male gender conflict: Attitudes toward the feminine and the fragile masculine self. *Psychology of Men and Masculinity, 1*, 126–132.
Blazina, C., Pisecco, S., & O'Neil, J. M. (2005). An adaptation of the Gender Role Conflict Scale for adolescents: Psychometric issues and correlates with psychological distress. *Psychology of Men and Masculinity, 6*, 39–45.
Blazina, C., Novotny, M. L., Stevens, D. N., & Hunter, M. (2008, August). Man's best friend: Pet companions, gender role conflict, attachment, and loss. In J. M. O'Neil & G. E. Good (chairs), *Four studies assessing the contextual complexity of the gender role conflict construct*. Boston, MA: Symposium conducted at the American Psychological Association.
Blazina, C., Boyraz, G., & Shen-Miller, D. (Eds.). (2013). *The psychology of human-animal. A resource for clinicians and researchers*. New York: Springer.
Breiding, M. J. (2004). Observed hostility and observed dominance as mediators of the relationship between husbands' gender role conflict and wives' outcomes. *Journal of Counseling Psychology, 51*, 429–436.
Breiding, M. J., Windle, C. R., & Smith, D. A. (2008). Interspousal criticism: A behavioral mediator between husband's gender role conflict and wife's adjustment. *Sex Roles, 59*, 880–888.
Brooks, G. (2010). *Beyond the crises of masculinity: A transtheoretical model for male-friendly therapy*. Washington, D.C.: American Psychological Association.
Cachia, P. (2001). *The interplay of gender role conflict and adult attachment*. Unpublished Master thesis, University of Malta, Malta.
Campbell, J. (1988). *The power of myth*. New York: Doubleday.
Cochran, S. V. (2005). Evidence based assessment with men. *Journal of Clinical Psychology, 61*, 649–660.
Connell, R. (2005). *Masculinities* (2nd ed.). Berkeley: California Press.
Covell, A. (1998). Characteristics of college males who are likely to sexually harass women: A test of a mediated model (Doctoral dissertation, University of Southern California, 1998). *Dissertation Abstracts International, 60*, 2400.
DeFranc, W., & Mahalik, J. R. (2002). Masculine gender role conflict and stress in relation to parental attachment and separation. *Psychology of Men and Masculinity, 3*, 51–60.
Enn, C. (2000). Gender issues in counseling. In S. Brown & R. Lent (Eds.), *Handbook of counseling psychology* (3rd ed., pp. 601–638). New York: Wiley.
Enns, C. Z. (2008). Toward a complexity paradigm for understanding gender role conflict. *The Counseling Psychologist, 36*, 446–454.
Fischer, A. R. (2007). Parental relationship quality and masculine gender role strain in young men: Mediating effects of personality. *The Counseling Psychologist, 35*, 328–358.
Fischer, A. R., & Good, G. E. (1998). Perceptions of parent-child relationships and masculine role conflicts of college men. *Journal of Counseling Psychology, 45*, 346–352.
Gould, R. L. (1978). *Transformation and change in adult life*. New York: Simon & Schuster.
Gould, R. L. (1980). Transformation during early and middle adult years. In N. Smelser & E. Erikson (Eds.), *Themes of work and love in adulthood* (pp. 213–237). Cambridge, MA: Harvard University Press.

Griffin, J. A. (2011). *Sexual compulsivity among sexual minorities: Relations to attachment orientations and gender role conflict*. Master's Thesis, Loyola University Maryland, Baltimore, MD.
Grossman, K., Grossman, K. E., Kindler, H., Zimmerman, P. (2008). View of attachment and explanation: The influence of mothers and fathers on the development of psychological security from infancy to your adulthood. In J. Cassidy & P. Shaver (Eds.), *Handbook of attachment: Theory, research, and clinical applications* (pp. 595–63). New York: Guilford Press.
Heppner, P. P. (1995). On gender role conflict in men: Future directions and implications for counseling. *Journal of Counseling Psychology, 42*, 20–23.
James, S. D. (2006). Gender role conflict, attachment style, interpersonal problems, and help seeking in adult men (Doctoral dissertation, University of Alberta, Canada, 2006). *Dissertation Abstracts International, 44*, 2006.
Johnson, R. (1986). *He: Understanding masculine psychology*. New York: Harper & Row.
Jones, K., & Heesacker, M. (2012). Addressing the situation: Some evidence for the significance of microcontexts with the gender role conflict construct. *Psychology of Men and Masculinity, 13*, 294–307.
Jung, K. (1953). *Animus and anima*. Collected Works (Vol. 7). New York: Pantheon.
Kierski, W., & Blazina, C. (2009). The male fear of femininity and its effect on counseling and psychotherapy. *The Journal of Men's Studies, 17*, 155–172.
Kobak, R. & Madsen, S. (2008). Disruptions in attachment bonds: Implications for theory, research, and clinical interventions. In J. Cassidy & P. Shaver (Eds.), *Handbook of attachment: Theory, research, and clinical applications* (pp. 3–24). New York: Guilford Press.
Land, L. N., Rochlen, A. B., & Vaugh, B. K. (2011). Correlates of adult attachment avoidance: Men's avoidance of intimacy in romantic relationships. *Psychology of Men and Masculinity, 12*, 64–74.
Levant, R. F., & Richmond, K. (2007). A review of research on masculinity ideologies using the Male Norm Inventory. *The Journal of Men's Studies, 15*, 130–146.
Levant, R. F., Hirsch, L., Celentano, E., Cozza, T., Hill, S., MacRachorn, M., et al. (1992). The male role: An investigation of contemporary norms. *Journal of Mental Health Counseling, 14*, 325–337.
Mahalik, J. R. (1999a). Incorporating a gender role strain perspective in assessing and treating men's cognitive distortions. *Professional Psychology: Research and Practice, 30*, 333–340.
Mahalik, J. R. (1999b). Incorporating a gender role strain perspective in assessing and treating men's cognitive distortions. *Professional Psychology: Research and Practice, 30*, 333–340.
Mahalik, J. R., Locke, B. D., Ludlow, L. H., Diemer, M. A., Scott, R. P., Gottfried, M., et al. (2003). Development of the conformity to masculine norms inventory. *Psychology of Men and Masculinity, 4*, 3–25.
Napolitano, J. M., Mahalik, J. R., & Kenny, M. E. (1999, August). *Relation of gender role strain and attachment to men's psychosocial development*. Paper presented at the American Psychological Association, Boston, MA.
Newman, B., & Newman, P. (2012). *Development through life: A psychosocial approach*. Belmont, CA: Wadsworth Publishing.
Norton, J. (1997). Deconstructing the fear of femininity. *Feminism & Psychology, 7*, 441–447.
O'Neil, J. M. (1981a). Male sex-role conflict, sexism, and masculinity: Implications for men, women, and the counseling psychologist. *The Counseling Psychologist, 9*, 61–80.
O'Neil, J. M. (1981b). Patterns of gender role conflict and strain: Sexism and fear of femininity in men's lives. *Personnel and Guidance Journal, 60*, 203–210.
O'Neil, J. M. (1982). Gender role conflict and strain in men's lives: Implications for psychiatrists, psychologists, and other human service providers. In K. Solomon & N. B. Levy (Eds.), *Men in transition: Changing male roles, theory, and therapy* (pp. 5–44). New York: Plenum Publishing Co.
O'Neil, J. M. (1990). Assessing men's gender role conflict. In D. Moore & F. Leafgren (Eds.), *Men in conflict: Problem solving strategies and interventions* (pp. 23–38). Alexandria, VA: American Association for Counseling and Development.

O'Neil, J. M. (1995). The gender role journey workshop: Exploring sexism and gender role conflict in a coeducational setting. M. Andronico (Ed.), *Men in groups: Insights, interventions, psychoeducational work* (pp. 193–213). Washington, D.C.: APA Books.

O'Neil, J. M. (1996). The gender role journey workshop: Exploring sexism and gender role conflict in a coeducational setting. In M. A. Andronico (Ed.), *Men in groups: Insights, interventions, psychoeducational work* (pp. 193–213). Washington, DC: APA Books. *Bond: A resource for clinicians and researchers*. New York: Springer.

O'Neil, J. M. (2008a). Special issue. Men's gender conflict: 25 year research summary. *The Counseling Psychologist, 36*, 358–476.

O'Neil, J. M. (2008b). Special Issue: Summarizing twenty-five years of research on men's gender role conflict using the Gender Role Conflict Scale: New research paradigms and clinical implications. *The Counseling Psychologist, 36*, 358–445.

O'Neil, J. M. (2010). Is criticism of generic masculinity, essentialism, and positive-healthy-masculinity a problem for the psychology of men? *Psychology of Men and Masculinity, 11*, 98–106.

O'Neil, J. M. (2012). The psychology of men. In E. Altmaier & J. Hansen (Eds.), *Oxford handbook of counseling psychology*. New York: Oxford University Press.

O'Neil, J. M. (2013). Gender-role conflict research thirty years later: An evidenced based diagnostic schema. *Journal of Counseling and Development, 91*, 498–499.

O'Neil, J. M. (2014). *Trait issues assessment of GRC theory and the GRCS from national authorities*. Storrs, CT: Department of Educational Psychology, University of Connecticut.

O'Neil, J. M. (2015) *Men's gender role conflict: Psychological costs, consequences, and an agenda for change*. Washington, D.C.: American Psychological Association.

O'Neil, J. M., & Crapser, B. (2011). Using the psychology of men and gender role conflict theory to promote comprehensive service delivery for college men: A call to action. In J. Laker & T. Davis (Eds.), *Masculinities in higher education: Theoretical and practical considerations*. New York: Routledge Publishers.

O'Neil, J. M., & Egan, J. (1992a). Men and women's gender role journeys: A metaphor for healing, transition, and transformation. In B. Wainrib (Ed.), *Gender issues across the life cycle* (pp. 107–123). New York: Springer Publishing Co.

O'Neil, J. M., & Egan, J. (1992b). Men's gender role transitions over the life span: Transformations and fears of femininity. *Journal of Mental Health Counseling, 14*, 305–324.

O'Neil, J. M., & Egan, J. (1992c). Men's gender role transitions over the lifespan: Transformation and fears of femininity. *Journal of Mental Health Counseling, 14*, 306–324.

O'Neil, J. M., & Fishman, D. (1992). Adult men's career transitions and gender role themes. In H. D. Lee & Z. B. Leibowitz (Eds.), *Adult career development: Concepts, issues, and Practices* (2nd ed., pp. 132–162). Alexandria, VA: ACA Press.

O'Neil, J. M., & Nadeau, R. A. (1999). Men's gender-role conflict, defense mechanism, and self-protective defensive strategies: Explaining men's violence against women from a gender-role socialization perspective. In M. Harway & J. M. O'Neil (Eds.), *What causes men's violence against women?* (pp. 89–116). Thousand Oaks, CA: Sage Publications.

O'Neil, J. M., & Roberts Carroll, M. (1988). A gender role workshop focused on sexism, gender role conflict, and the gender role journey. *Journal of Counseling and Development, 67*, 193–197.

O'Neil, J. M., Helm, B., Gable, R., David, L., & Wrightsman, L. (1986). Gender role conflict scale (GRCS): College men's fears of femininity. *Sex Roles, 14*, 335–350.

O'Neil, J. M. & Denke, R. (2015). An Empirical review of the gender role conflict research: New conceptual models and research paradigms. In J. Wong and S. Wester (Eds.), *APA Handbook of the Psychology of Men and Masculinities* (pp 51–80). Washington, D.C.: APA Books.

O'Neil, J. M., Fishman, D. M., & Kinsella-Shaw, M. (1987). Dual-career couples' career transitions and normative dilemmas: A preliminary assessment model. *The Counseling Psychologist, 15*(1), 50–96.

O'Neil, J. M., Egan, J., Owen, S. V., & Murry, V. (1993a). The gender role journey measure (JRJM): Scale development and psychometric evaluations. *Sex Roles, 28*, 167–185.

O'Neil, J. M., Egan, J., Owen, S. V., & Murry, V. M. (1993b). The gender role journey measure (GRJM): Scale development and psychometric evaluations. *Sex Roles, 28*, 167–185.
O'Neil, J. M., Good, G. E., & Holmes, S. (1995). Fifteen years of theory and research on men's gender role conflict: New paradigms for empirical research. In R. Levant & W. Pollack (Eds.), *The new psychology of men* (pp. 164–206). New York: Basic Books.
Pleck, J. H. (1995). The gender role strain paradigm: An update. In R. F. Levant & W. S. Pollack (Eds.), *A new psychology of men* (pp. 11–32). New York: Basic Books.
Pleck, J. H., Sonenstein, F. L., & Ku, L. C. (1993). Masculinity ideology and its correlates. In S. Oskamp & M. Costanzo (Eds.), *Gender issues in social psychology* (pp. 85–110). Newbury Park, CA: Sage Publications.
Pollack, W. (1995a). No man is an island: Toward a new psychoanalytic psychology of men. In R. Levant & W. Pollack (Eds.), *A new psychology of men* (pp. 33–67). New York: Basic Books.
Pollack, W. (1995b). No man is an island: Toward a new psychoanalytic psychology of men. In R. Levant & W. Pollack (Eds.), *A new psychology of men* (pp. 33–67). New York: Basic Books.
Rabinowitz, F. E., & Cochran, S. V. (2002). *Deepening psychotherapy with men*. Washington, DC: American Psychological Association.
Rochlen, A., & Mahalik, J. R. (2004). Women's perceptions of male partner's gender role conflict as predictors of psychological well-being and relationship satisfaction. *Psychology of Men and Masculinity, 5*, 147–157.
Schwartz, J. P., Waldo, M., & Higgins, A. J. (2004). Attachment styles: Relationship to masculine gender role conflict in college men. *Psychology of Men and Masculinity, 5*, 143–146.
Selby, B. W. (1999). The relation of attachment, adjustment, and narcissism to masculine gender role conflict (Doctoral dissertation, University of North Texas, 1999). *Dissertation Abstracts International, 61*, 5005.
Siffert, K. J. (2012). *A structural equation model investigating parental relationships and gendered-functioning among men: Links to Kohut's self psychology (unpublished doctoral dissertation)*. Houston, TX: University of Houston.
Smiler, A. P. (2004). Thirty years after the discovery of gender: Psychological concept and measures of masculinity. *Sex Roles, 50*, 15–26.
Thompson, E. H., & Pleck, J. H. (1986). The structure of the male norms. *American Behavioral Scientist, 29*, 531–543.
Vandello, J. A., & Bossom, J. K. (2013). Hard won easily lost: A review and synthesis of theory and research on precarious manhood. *Psychology of Men and Masculinity, 14*, 101–113.
Vandello, J. A., Bossom, J. K., Cohen, D., Burnaford, R. M., & Weaver, J. R. (2008). Precarious manhood. *Journal of Personality and Social Psychology, 95*, 1325–1339.
West, C., & Zimmerman, D. H. (1998). Doing gender. In B. M. Clinchy & J. K. Norem (Eds.), *The gender and psychology reader* (pp. 104–124). New York: New York University Press.
Wester, S. R., Vogel, D. L., O'Neil, J. M., & Danforth, L. (2012). Development and evaluation of the Gender Role Conflict Scale Short Form (GRCS-SF). *Psychology of Men and Masculinity, 13*, 199.

Chapter 3
A New Understanding of Man's Best Friend: A Proposed Contextual Model for the Exploration of Human–Animal Interaction Among Insecurely Attached Males

Chris Blazina, James M. O'Neil and Robyn Denke

My own (Chris Blazina) interest in the bond between man and dog is longstanding, tracing its origins to my youth. When my family's little house was filled with ten or more people, and felt particularly cramped, I would take a seat on the back steps and talk things over with our gentle German shepherd. I remember him sitting very still, alert, and attentive, almost like he was on point, but with a much calmer demeanor. As I recounted sometimes the frustrating events occurring on the other side of the brick wall, he would occasionally glance in my direction. As I talked and eventually felt some release, I would pet him as a token of thanks. We would then go to play. These exchanges influenced my aspirations for how I thought a good listener and then a psychologist should be. A calming, steady presence can be impactful. I have even unwittingly adopted a similar demeanor in my work counseling, a catch-and-release style of looking and then glancing away. However, I did not realize until recently that these exchanges also held significance for what I thought a man could be. Even with the influences of traditional male socialization's being prevalent across much of my formative years, being in the presence of dogs offered by contrast a different and unique encounter.

C. Blazina (✉)
Department of Counseling and Educational Psychology,
New Mexico State University, College of Education,
MSC 3CEP, PO Box 30001, Las Cruces, NM 88003, USA
e-mail: cblazina@nmsu.edu

J.M. O'Neil
University of Connecticut, Mansfield, USA
e-mail: JIMONEIL1@aol.com

R. Denke
University of Connecticut, 45 Cavalry Hill Road, Wilton, CT 06897, USA
e-mail: robyndenke@gmail.com

C. Blazina and L.R. Kogan (eds.), *Men and Their Dogs*,
DOI 10.1007/978-3-319-30097-9_3

I was surprised to discover there had not been a systematic psychological study of the bond between males and their dogs. While some research does exist, it is often inconclusive in terms of why males of various ages and life experiences find a special tie with animal companions. Besides my personal anecdotes with dogs that extend to the current day, over the years in my clinical practice I have also witnessed male clients discussing their ties with dogs in a special way. The male–dog bond is complex and needs to be understood within its own unique context. Context adds to the explanatory power of both clinical and research understanding, and is utilized throughout this chapter.

The bond with animal companions, just as in the case of human relationships, can be influenced by numerous contextual factors including age, socioeconomic status, race, religion, etc. (Blazina et al. 2011). How these dynamics occur as a main effect or interact with other variables has begun to be explored especially in regard to health and well-being. Human–animal interaction (HAI) has been previously associated with facilitation of recovery after a heart attack (Friedmann et al. 1980), and increasing physical activity (Dembicki and Anderson 1996; Serpell 2010). The presence of animal companions have also been shown to reduce levels of stress, anxiety, depression, and loneliness (Brown 2004, 2007; Garrity et al. 1989; Zarski 1984) as well as ameliorate the effects of potentially stressful life events (Folse et al. 1994), and enhance feelings of autonomy, competence, and self-esteem (Beck and Katcher 1996; Kidd and Kidd 1985; Levinson 1972; Robin and Bensel 1985; Triebenbacher 1998).

There are other variables of interest in need of attention among the HAI literature. This chapter explores the influence of male gender roles socialization. Further, more work needs to be done in understanding the role the bond plays in males' lives, especially those that experience psychological distress as the result of limiting definitions of traditional forms of masculinity. For example, researchers and theorists have identified some of the limiting effects of restricted forms of male gender roles (O'Neil 1981a, b; O'Neil et al. 1986, 1995, 2015) leading to conflict and dysfunction in both areas of work and love. O'Neil created the concept of *gender role conflict* to represent when restrictive socially constructed gender role do harm to the individual and those in their immediate circle, the ultimate result is a restriction of human potential causing psychological harm. Understanding more about the presence of animal companions in gender role conflicted males' lives across the life span is a needed contextual inquiry. The bond therefore deserves scholarly exploration, especially as a potential health-promoting agent. In order to understand more about gender and HAI, a contextual approach can be further expanded to include how the psychology involved in socializing males is interfaced with other key variables such as attachment related issues.

Attachment theory (see Bowlby 1969, 1982; Ainsworth 1978) has provided a heuristic model to not only understand various human dyads such as parent–child and romantic relationships (see Hazan and Shaver 1987) but also has become the leading research paradigm among HAI (Pachana et al. 2005; Sharkin and Bahrick 1990). This includes a focus upon those that claim a special relationship with animal companions. In several research studies, between 87 and 99 % of pet owners defined their pets as being "like a friend or family member" (Cain 1983; Voith 1985). However, there is no universal agreement regarding male's relationships with pets. Inquiries examining to what degree males attach to animal companions is a work in progress, and much remains unclear. Some research suggests that taken as a whole, males show lower levels of attachment (Kidd and Kidd 1985), while others find no gender differences (Prato-Previde et al. 2006; Ramirez 2006). Part of the problem with this line of inquiry is it does not always adequately account for male socialization as a contextual variable. Likewise, Herzog (2007) suggested it is the within-group differences among men (and women) that also accounts for some of the potential gender confusion regarding attitudes toward the bond. That is, simply comparing the average female to male on attitudes about animal companions does not consider a wide range of contexts and depositions toward HAI, which include both health and unhealthy influences. Even in North America, we assume that males are not a single homogenous sample but instead there will be expected individual differences in their experiences and expression of traditional male roles and also that of HAI (Blazina and Kogan in press).

There is also an expected variability regarding willingness to freely report experiences concerning an animal companion because they involve reactions that are both personal and private (Blazina and Kogan in press). Some males may deem this information as off-limits to discuss. To do otherwise may lead to the violation of stringent male norms regarding restricted emotionality, and self-sufficiency. We see these same potential influences beginning to shape male behavior toward the bond at a young age. In one study examining boys and girls levels of attachment to their animal companions, as measured through the likelihood of expressing love to them, saying they were loved by them, and reporting missing them when apart, boys reported significantly lower levels (Kidd and Kidd 1985). The researchers concluded that male socialization may have influenced boy's willingness to report their actual feelings, because when examining the actual behaviors shown toward their animal companions, there were no gender differences.

Therefore, to begin understanding gender role-related factors within the context of HAI means accounting for a number of potentially divergent variables. One way to form a more integrated picture is by taking established gender role paradigms and applying each variable of interest in a systematic fashion. More specifically, in keeping with the psychology of men and masculinity, we wish to explore how males that experience gender role conflict (GRC) and the challenges of an insecure attachment history, respond in positive ways to their bond with canine companions—man's best friend. If we begin mapping these various factors and their potential interfaces in a nuanced way, we are better able to make both descriptive and prescriptive statements regarding how males across the life span experience their attachment bonds with animal companions.

This chapter is a theoretical exploration of how the GRC paradigm and attachment history is related to the human–animal bond. More precisely, can males that have experienced insecure types of attachment with human companions, family, friends, and significant others have those experiences ameliorated by a positive secure bond with an animal companion? Further, can males' *relational capacity*, the ability to make and sustain meaningful bonds with both human and animal companions, also be subsequently affected?

While attachment theory is one of the more contemporary psychoanalytic approaches emphasizing an innate and hardwired need to bond with others, it is our perspective that sexist gender roles restrict men's relational capacity and dehumanize both men and women. That is, male gender roles can thwart the innate attaching tendency, making a male feel as if forming emotional bonds is a violation of what it means to be a man. Many times, men's problems are not just personal failures but result from constricting values in the larger society (the macrosocietal context) that degrade men and discourage close intimate relationships. These macrosocietal contexts include patriarchal structures, restrictive stereotypes, oppression, social injustices, and the sexist socialization of both sexes (see O'Neil 2008a, b, 2015). From a GRC perspective, restricted gender roles potentially limit meaningful attachment with both humans and animals and help explain why some men have limited relational encounters, even violent ones, with animals and humans. When men have deficits in relational skills, there are fewer options for dealing with frustration, primitive emotions, less behavioral opportunities, and greater tendencies for skewed versions of power and control, and unhealthy aggression as tools.

Our general position is that many males can experience the human–animal bond as exception to the rule regarding getting close, being attached or vulnerable with another. Males not only developing deep and lasting attachment ties but also carrying the possibility of increasing the relational capacity with a range of others, both human and nonhumans. What makes this possible is in part that animal companions can be a "safe haven" and "safe base." Bowlby (1982) identified these as key dimensions of an attachment figure that facilitates a sense of safety when under duress and allows for continued personal growth. It is suggested this process occurs because a different set of gender role and attachment norms operate within the human–dog dyad, allowing for at least a temporary relaxing of stringent male norms. Moreover, bonds with animals may help men validate or repudiate dysfunctional aspects of their masculinity ideologies and identities. There is also something exceptional found within the relational context of the man–dog bond that promotes men to grow in numerous other ways, once that initial prerequisite bond has been established. Themes of males' personal growth are explored in this chapter and include but are not limited to: searching for existential meaning, turning one's attention to matters of transcendence, and advocacy for others.

How male's bonds with animals can foster psychological development and interpersonal competence is a critical question that has far reaching implications across numerous disciplines. In this regard, the chapter supports the notion that the human–animal bond can directly impact the fostering of a positive, healthy sense of masculinity for males (see Kiselica and Englar-Carlson 2010) with insecure attachment styles. That is, the bond can act as a compensatory way of dealing with attachment needs that are the result of human bonding gone awry both in the formative years and then later as an adult. The human–animal bond leads to at least one safe and secure type of attachment scenario for males. These contextual concepts are developed throughout the chapter within the framework of a proposed model with implications for research and clinical practice. Next, we turn to the summary of our model.

Proposed Model

How masculinity ideology and GRC affects men's relationships with animals raises a number of provocative questions. How do masculine norms and stereotypes play out in men's relationship with animals and are the expected gender role stereotypes, typical in human interactions, suspended and altered when men interact with animals and if so, why does this happen? Is animal bonding easier than human bonding for some men because worries about power, control, competition, and potential for devaluations and violations are not operating in animal relationships? Furthermore, a bond with an animal may be involved in a gender role transition, where a man changes his self-assumptions and world views about gender roles, thereby changing his behaviors. In this case, distorted gender role schemas may be mediated and changed with animal interaction, promoting healthy human development. Whether the animal–human bond facilitates men's journey with their gender roles and helps them deconstruct stereotypic views of masculinity and femininity is an empirical question. How the processes occur and how men change their relational capacities through animal interaction deserves study.

Our proposed model (see Fig. 3.1) suggests there will be an intersection of multiple contextual factors directly influencing males' experience of both human–human interaction (HHI) and human–animal interaction (HAI). Figure 3.1 depicts a model that expands our understanding of the animal–human bond by focusing numerous contexts, processes, and outcomes. At the bottom of the figure are four contextual parameters that include the actual attachment experiences, moderators, and mediators of the human/animal processes that include restricted masculinity ideology and GRC, and psychological outcomes that include concepts like generalization, compensation, and positive and negative psychological outcomes.

Located above the parameters is one way to map the contextual factors that influence the animal–human bond in both positive and negative ways. On the left in the rectangle is shown a men's insecure human attachment history that produce a variety of different bonding experiences. The most common attachment experiences have been described using the following terminology: secure/insecure, avoidant/ambivalent, anxious-ambivalent, and disorganized. The degree of insecurity in the human bonding processes predicts a man's relational capacity with both humans and animals.

Moving to the right, in the first circle, the HAI processes are hypothesized to be moderated and mediated by restricted masculinity ideology and GRC. The bidirectional arrow implies that a man's insecure attachment history, masculinity ideologies, and GRC have a reciprocal relationships, each potentially influencing each other.

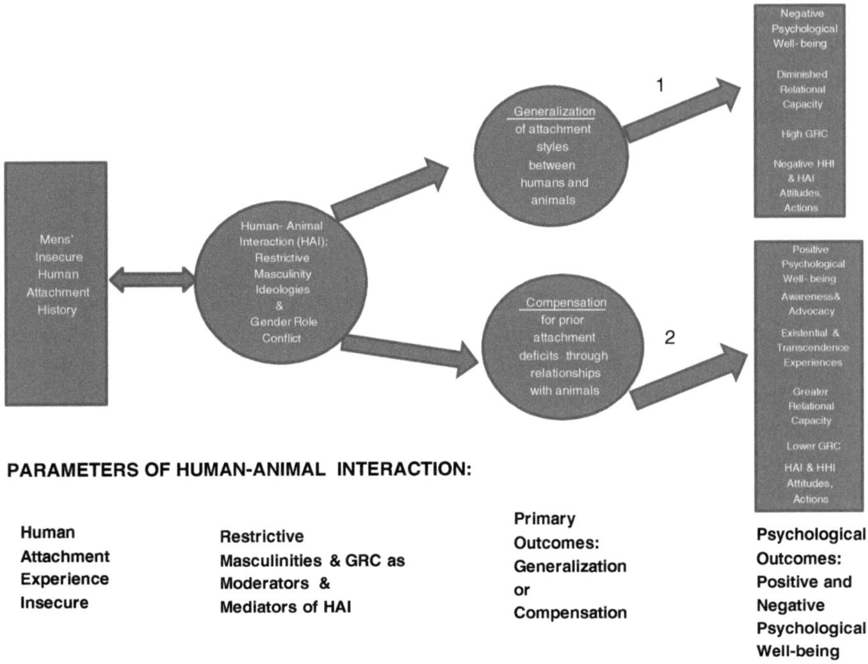

Fig. 3.1 Relationship between human and animal

The two circles in the middle of the diagram are defined as the primary attachment outcomes between animals and humans including generalization and compensation. These outcomes are defined as two bonding patterns based on prior attachment experiences and suggest variability in how attachment to humans and animals are played out in real life. In keeping with ideas discussed earlier, there is a range of variability and individual differences among men with insecure attachment histories, leading to at least two possible outcomes regarding the human–animal bond (especially with dogs). One possibility is that insecure attachment experience is generalized to most if not all attachment experiences (i.e., generalization). The other outcome involves how an animal companion can offset those with attachment challenges leading to improved quality of life through deeper more meaningful attachment bonds (i.e., compensation). Generalization implies that one's prior insecure attachment process with humans can be negatively replicated with animals mirroring one another. For example, insecure bonding with humans will be repeated with animals and yield negative psychological outcomes, low relational capacity, higher GRC, and strained relationships with both human and animals (see the long arrow labeled number 1 in Fig. 3.1).

The second outcome involves compensation. Compensation means that what attachment problems that men have with other humans can be ameliorated and changed through bonding with animals and produce positive psychological outcomes, greater relational capacity, lower GRC, awareness and advocacy for both humans and animals, greater potential for existential and transcendent experiences, and greater affirmation of both humans and animals (see arrow 2 Fig. 3.1). Each aspect of the model above is discussed in more detail with special attention paid to the theoretical rational and supporting research.

Generalization of Insecure Attachment Styles

The first trajectory involves the application of insecure attachment styles, attitudes, and behaviors from one type of attachment scenario to others, where patterns of interaction for humans and animals resemble one another. For example, if one has an insecure attachment disposition in one relational domain it will be generalized to humans or nonhumans. This makes for negative relational capacity affecting a wide range of other type of attachment scenarios. There is some research support for this generalized application, and it is consistent with the prevailing prescriptive and descriptive stereotype of men in North America, that investing in relationships is not considered masculine (Blazina 2001; David and Brannon 1976; Pollack 1995). One might argue that achieving core elements of traditional male socialization is tantamount to an avoidant or dismissive attachment style.

In terms of the HAI and HHI literature, Beck and Madresh (2008) found similarities when comparing subjects' insecure attachment scores for their pets versus romantic partners but ratings carried little or no statistical significance. Furthermore, relationships with pets were always rated as more secure. Zilcha-Mano et al. (2011) found a relationship between people's attachment orientations in human–pet relationships and their attachment orientations in human–human relationships. This included higher scores on attachment anxiety and/or avoidance in human–human relationships related to higher scores on the human–animal bond insecurity. Additionally, prevalent attachment insecurities seemed to counteract the beneficial regulatory effects of the presence of a pet. That is, attachment insecurities prevented the occurrence of the safe haven effect associated with being in the presence of an attachment figure. The disruptive occurrence was especially true for those with higher avoidant attachment styles toward pets. Persons who scored high on avoidant attachment viewed their pet in more negative terms such as perceiving them as unreliable, unsupportive, and expecting the pet not to be available and responsive to their needs.

In terms of these findings, a few considerations of Zilcha-Mano et al.'s (2011) work as it applies to this current chapter is in order. Their sample included mostly women and a mix of dog and cat owners. More research needs to be conducted given the contextual issues that have been highlighted regarding gender and those that have been previously found in terms of type of animal companion and attachment bond (e.g., cat attachment scores being lower than dogs) (see Zasloff 1996; Winefield et al. 2008). However, what seems most relevant are certain contextual factors that make an avoidant attachment style especially troubling for men with animals. With more severe forms of avoidant attachment elements, it may not only impact attachment expectations but also the ways gender roles are enacted. The end result is males' relational capacity may be severely limited, impacting self-monitoring, levels of empathy, perspective-taking beyond one's own experience, and may also include the use of violence, neglect and harm being perpetuated against others both human and animal.

DeGue (2011) discusses the potential *triad of family violence* in which adult males target romantic partners, children, and pets for domestic abuse. In this scenario, the perpetrator who has traditionally (but not exclusively) been an adult male may use violence as a mean of threatening or controlling others. However, gender in itself does not adequately explain the contextual nature of what can be viewed as a type of generalizing of attachment expectations and behaviors from people to animals. Ducan et al. (2005) found conduct disordered boys that abused animals differed significantly from those that did not, by their history of being the victim of physical or sexual abuse and/or being exposed to domestic violence. Gupta (2008) found that callousness was a significant predictor of college men's violence against women and pets in a nonclinical sample. McPhedran (2009) suggests there are several complex risk factors involved in adult intimate partner violence (IPV) such as low levels of empathy, lack of prosocial parenting experiences from the formative years, childhood exposure to violence, and perhaps other dynamics, all of which potentially interact leading to violence toward intimate partners and pets. Obviously this is an area in need of further examination with other contextual research. However, it does not suggest that all men who have an insecure attachment experience with human attachment figures will lead to these violent outcomes. To the contrary and discussed next, are the various emotionally corrective experiences with human and animal companions that can offset these early attachment hurdles.

Compensation for Males' Insecure Attachment Experiences

The second trajectory in our proposed model involves males with insecure attachment histories regarding human attachment figures that have corrective bonding occurrences with animal companions. It is our argument that some males that may have had less than satisfactory attachment experiences with human attachment figures may find compensation for prior attachment deficits in the company of animal companions.

There is the notion of an *earned secure attachment* among human attachment figures, where early difficult attachment experiences can be compensated by others that provide a different type of bonding experience (see Wallin 2007). An earned type of security emphasizes the level of accompanying work involved in transforming an insecure attachment schema into a secure one. This occurrence is a fundamental change in one's general attachment orientation where attachment figures are seen in more benign if not benevolent perspectives. We argue that one's animal companion may be among those attachment figures that supply rudimentary bonding that helps reorient males toward more generally secure types of general attachment perspectives. However, even this secure attachment bond is also earned through hard work; the context of the human–animal bond may allow males more flexibility and freedom to be relational.

We also recognize that not all males with insecure attachment orientations who have corrective human–animal bond experience will have an overall general schema change with attachment. Rather, some males may only see animal companions as a viable attachment figure and other possible human attachments as less favorably. This scenario leads to simultaneous competing perspectives of attachment within a male's mind, and with it, very different outlooks for animals versus humans.

The notion that we may have somewhat different or competing attachment models within our attachment repertoire is in keeping with recent evidence for human dyads (Klohnen et al. 2005) and has been referred to as *layering* of attachment expectations (see Wallin 2007) or hierarchical structuring of attachment figures (see Mikulincer and Shaver 2001, 2003). We also argue that different attachment scenarios for those that experience insecure human relations versus more secure animal companions can lead to very divergent perspectives. For some, the result is the development of a competing perspective of who is safe and trustworthy (i.e., humans are not to be trusted but animal companions are). For others, these attachment perspectives become more aligned and generalized from one scenario to another. While one might mark the ends of an attachment continuum with certain males that only feel safe bonding with animal companions versus those who are able to reconsider human companions in the same positive light. No doubt there will be many others who find their place in between.

So, not every insecurely styled male that has a positive bonding experience with an animal companion will develop a positive point of view with human companions. However, we argue the one good attachment figure be it in the context of animal and human companions carries with it the possibility of promoting psychological wellness in a number of ways that are outlined next in the chapter.

The Basis for Psychological Wellness

Figure 3.1 also shows how psychological wellness can be the product of a compensatory attachment HAI history. In the human–animal attachment dyad, it is possible for males to have a unique experience affecting attachment expectations but also further affecting other domains of one's life.

The premise that dogs are agents of emotional support and even healing is based upon recent research that suggests canines are unique in the animal kingdom (along with chimpanzees) to show a mutual gaze with humans (Horowitz 2009, 2011). Horowitz (2011) suggests that dogs possess a "rudimentary theory of mind." Furthermore, dogs even outshine man's closest genetic cousin, on the "left gaze bias," an essential step in reading emotions (Guo et al. 2009). The left side (from the observers' perspective) gives much more unfiltered information about how people feel (see Ekman 2007). When a dog looks at a human face this includes scanning the right side of the face, (which is actually the left side from the dog's perspective) for tell-tale signs of emotional cues. Until recently, it was thought that only humans showed this type of gaze bias given that the human face is lopsided in displaying microexpressions related to displaying emotions. In the same vein, dogs have shown evidence for social referencing of their owner's facial expressions when encountering novel stimuli, utilizing the gaze as a means to process information and subsequently direct behavior (Merola et al. 2011, 2012). Likewise, there is indication for dogs displaying migraine-alerting behaviors on behalf of human companions (Marcus and Bhowmick 2013); a dog's ability to discriminate the emotional expressions of human faces (Müller et al. 2015), and a dogs' gaze being tuned to human communication (Téglás et al. 2012). There is also recent support for the hypothesis that dogs are capable of showing empathy (Silva and de Sousa 2011), and empathic responses to strangers in distress (Custance and Mayer 2012), and even more intense reactions to their own human companion in the same condition.

Research also indicates human physiological changes due to HAI. The tactile experience of canine companions can be experienced as emotionally soothing. Research supports blood pressure and heartbeat decrease when petting and stroking an animal's fur (Charnetski et al. 2004; DeMello 1999; Nagengast et al. 1997). Research on oxytocin, sometimes referred to as the "bonding hormone," has been shown to increase in a number of scenarios that involve the presence of dogs (Handlin et al. 2011; Miller et al. 2009; Odendaal and Lehmann 2000; Odendaal and Meintjes 2003) and when owners' mutual gaze with dogs (Nagaswa et al. 2009, 2015). Increase in oxytocin level is important in human health, as oxytocin may be a mechanism for the stress-buffering effects of social support (Heinrichs et al. 2003). There is also evidence for HAI decreasing the stress hormone cortisol even in short-term exposure to a dog (Polheber and Matchock 2014).

Furthermore, some scholars have argued that the power and value of the human–animal relationship is based on the psychological experience of nonjudgmental emotional support (Allen et al. 2002; Corson and Corson 1980). Nieburg and Fischer (1982) referred to this concept as one of "unqualified love and acceptance." Both Freud and his daughter Anna wrote of their personal experiences with dogs and how this affiliation taught them about "pure love" relationships (Roth 2005). Likewise, Brown (2004, 2007) suggests animal companions play psychological roles on our behalf such as the perceived sense we are worthy of care.

It is argued in contemporary psychodynamic theories (see attachment theory, object relations, etc.) that human beings are predisposed to make and sustain attachments throughout the life span. In fact, not having these connections leads to disruption in initial psychological development, and later continued growth and wellness. We suggest human beings respond to those companions (human and animal) that perform (or approximate) basic attachment-like cues. The attachment cues indicate that the human or animal companion is a viable attachment figure. The cues may involve our physiological changes (e.g., increase of oxytocin, decrease of cortisol levels with HAI interaction), and sensations (when petting fur the tactile sense of connecting). Cues may also include interactions with those that accompany us on day-to-day exploits (psychological accompaniment) and those we perceive as being in sync with our mood states and physical changes (psychological attunement) derived from mutual gaze, left gaze bias experiences, alerting responses, and the perceived psychological roles animal companions play in our lives. Each of these approximates our bonding cues with human companions prompting us to attach with animal companions. While HAI science has not progressed to the point of definitively offering dictums like dogs are "good listeners," we can suggest that many of their behaviors are what humans recognize as attachment cues, ones that prompt building a potentially strong attachment bond. In essence, we suggest that animal companions become agents of helping and healing through relational encounters, an especially important point for those that had unmet needs or experienced trauma, abuse, or neglect. It seems important to continue studying these underlying dynamics of HAIs in future research. Next, we turn to other possible outcomes as the result of the human–animal bond interaction.

Awareness and Advocacy

We suggest that a possible outcome of the compensatory nature of the HAI is the development of awareness and advocacy for human and nonhuman beings. That is, males call upon more positive masculine gender roles that can manifest in a number of ways: feeling protective of those they care about, standing firm in the face of opposition, and working toward long-term solutions leading to others' betterment. There can be a number of factors that make these changes possible, including a psychological shift from viewing animals as a less than pertinent topic. Instead, animals take on a new relevance regarding one's own life experience or identity; some even perceive key-shared commonalities or/and develop a sense of kinship. One in turn is more likely to advocate for another that shares similarities and certain fundamental characteristics, emotions, and experiences. Frequent examples include awareness raising concerning animals as sentient beings capable of pain, or discovering that nonhumans display emotions. The position of awareness and advocacy is not entirely altruistic in a nature though, because the stance betters the individual through helping another. Sometimes it is the satisfaction of helping, gaining new levels of awareness, and personal growth; other times, the reward is symbolically in nature, one is helping a cause that has a special meaning to the individual.

There are various examples of how males have gained awareness and then taken on an advocacy position in terms of nature, animals, and animal companions. Some of these are captured by fiction writers such as in the case of William Falkner's short story, *The Bear*. A boy discovers a new respect and kinship with the legendary bear that roamed the nearby woods. Other stories come from historical accounts. Aldo Leopold is the father of modern day ecology. In the 1870s he was involved in the wilderness land management principles of the day that included hunting wolves. In one of these instances, he shot a mother wolf and her cubs, and personally witnessed a "... fierce green fire dying in her eyes ... I realized then, and have known ever since, that there was something new to me in those eyes—something known only to her and the mountains" (p. 130). After that encounter, Leopold went on to champion "The Land Ethic" emphasizing the interdependence of humans and the natural world and a call to respond in ethical ways.

Consistent with our proposed model is the notion one can demonstrate psychological well-being through social advocacy as a reflection of Alfred Adler's concept of *social interest*. Adler (1938) suggested that social interest is an attitude or outlook toward furthering the welfare of others. He also theorized that social interest as "a feeling of community, an orientation to live cooperatively with others, and a lifestyle that values the common good above one's own interests and desires" (Guzick et al. 2004; p. 362). Adler assumed that social interest promotes better coping and a healthier attitude toward stressful situations (Crandall and Putman 1980).

Social interest is compared to another of Adler's concepts, *Masculine protest*—"The desire to be above, like a real man." While social interest allows a male to expand his focus beyond his own interest, by comparison masculine protest limits involvement in the betterment of others. Adler believed that in a patriarchal, masculine-dominated culture what we would refer to know as the stereotypical notion of the feminine was evaluated negatively. Therefore, many men feel they must hide those aspects of self by exaggerated stereotypical masculine attitudes and behaviors through overcompensation. This can lead to egotistical drives, including greed and overambition that not only cause continuous psychological conflicts but work against social interest. In more contemporary times *relational* could be appropriately substituted for Adler's notion of feminine. Males can assume a broader view of events and issues beyond their own self-interest. In our model, we extend the notion of social interest to include an awareness and potential advocacy of nonhuman animals. In essence, a position of awareness and advocacy ultimately leads to an understanding of the interconnectivity of living beings. This includes the knowledge of how the health of one entity within a system is impacted and in turn, influences others.

Wilson (1986) discussed the *biophilia hypothesis* arguing humans have an instinctive bond with other living systems. Theodore Roszak (1992) coined the term *ecopsychology* arguing that we find more than physical sustenance in the natural world. Ecopsychology attempts to scientifically understand nature's positive psychological impact on human beings. Ecopsychology researchers (see Roszak et al. 1995) suggest that an individual's connection to nature can improve physical health and mental functioning. It is part of the reason researchers argue humans are innately drawn to architecture and settings that reflect elements of nature, feeling enlivened by settings that let in natural light, include plants, and have wood and stone as part of the decor. Psychologists like Roger Ulrich have shown the effects of bringing nature indoors through studies that examine how we are soothed by looking at pictures of landscapes or watching a fish tank. A part of biophilia and ecopsychology is investigating the place of HAI.

While Western culture has traditionally struggled with the place of nonhuman animals and in some cases taking the benign stewardship position of overseeing the beasts of the field, in another cases nonhuman animals have fared far worse. Especially since the seventeenth century Cartesian mechanistic perspective built upon "I think therefore I am," placed nonhumans that were consider nonthinking animals at risk. In the Western viewpoint animals are reduced to little more than chattel, in some cases justifying abuse and neglect. Animals became soulless automatons that existed solely for man's use or misuse. Descartes explained away the pained sounds of animals during their live dissections as little more than a spring within a clock that was overwound. Various humane movements in the United States and England in the nineteenth and twentieth century lead to personal and societal changes (Wilson 2011).

Likewise, in the case of more contemporary research with dogs and their impact on human well-being, with each new study there is the possibility of not only gaining more scientific knowledge but also acquiring a reframing of societal viewpoints that have been detrimental, limiting, and violent toward animals. For example, in this text alone, there are several studies emphasizing how research subjects or clients training dogs to become more adoptable is a form of advocacy and awareness. It highlights the notion of perceived commonalities between man and dog bringing about changes in perspective. In addition, being in service to others occurs when one moves beyond the sole preoccupation of one's own needs and works toward a more generative position impacting others. However, it is not surprising these types of programs also seem to have mutually beneficial effects for dogs and the males helping them.

Transcendence

We suggest that HAI can also prompt growth in other ways and for some, this can lead to a focus upon *transcendence*—an awareness of mystery and the sacred. In short, transcendence involves the expanding of one's phenomenological experience or perception leading to the psychological occurrence of wholeness, calm, and wonderment. Searching for the transcendence prompts a higher level of awareness and attention to life; it may occur through a ritual, a personal awakening, or a deep meaningful interaction or encounter. It should be stated this type of encounter also can lead to an expansive feeling; one is connected to others, natural elements, animals, and even people in new ways. While there are numerous ways to achieve this state, being in the presence of nature and animal companions can increase our awareness of the ways living beings interact adding a unique appreciation of life and our place in it. Again, there are numerous examples of how one may achieve this state of transcendence influencing wellness.

Levinson (1969) was among the first to argue that it was animal companions, especially dogs, helped humans return to a more meaningful interface with nature as a means of restoring psychological balance. However, there are other traditions outside of psychology that also emphasis the transcendent promoting qualities of animals, some of which go back to medicinal practices in ancient Greece, or are part of totemic ceremonies, or even as spiritual guides within Native American rituals (Serpell 1996). Caedmon was a seventh century monk that had a spiritual awakening in the presence of animals who subsequently went onto to become England's first poet. Likewise, Francis of Assisi was inspired by animals and is noted for his compassion and gentleness toward them. He believed nature itself was the mirror of God, calling nonhuman creatures his "brothers" and "sisters." The emphasis in each of these examples is one where human beings are enhanced significantly by the presence of nonhuman animals. Beyond the monotheistic religions are various polytheistic traditions that emphasis a sacred connectedness among beings. Shinto religion argues that rocks, trees, animals, humans, and even geographical regions all have *kami*—sacred or divine spiritual essences. The Hindu tradition venerates animals, a core belief that the divine exists in all living beings, both human and nonhuman. Buddhists try to show loving-kindness to all beings. They also believe animals possess a *Buddha nature* and therefore have the potential for enlightenment. Outside formalized religions and approaches are those that experience the sacred in nature in other ways. Henry David Thoreau was among the American transcendentalists of the nineteenth century that found nature and his frequent walks in it, a source of wonder and awakening. John Muir, the cofounder of the Sierra Club, talked about the trees of the forest delivering sermons to those who were ready to hear their message.

Above are all examples of a type of search for transcendence leading to the further actualization of the individual. In our model, transcendence allows us to see human and nonhumans as part and parcel of a larger framework. In this context, the human–animal bond becomes more than fringe topic within psychology but instead one of critical importance that needs more vigorous study. Some men that perceive their dogs as animal companions will be prompted to consider how the bond plays a vital role in a unique appreciation of life.

Existential Meaning

Another potential outcome of our model suggests that males' bond with animal companions can draw attention to existential concerns, and the search for deeper meanings. While existential issues are encountered in a number of places within the life cycle, facing the loss of a beloved attachment figure is certainly one of the more difficult challenges. For men who perceive their pets as animal companions it is understandable they may experience an inward turning, reflection, and life assessment. The research examining males' attachment to animal companions and the intensity of grief when lost is a work in progress. The research from the past has left some with the impression that men do not grieve the loss of an animal companion as much, or on average perhaps do not feel all that attached in the first place. However, these results need to be viewed in context and alongside the pressures of male gender role socialization to not grieve openly in the ways mental health professions usually deems as optimal. The reluctance to disclose vulnerable material research studies makes it difficult to measure HAI accurately.

Doka and Martin (2010) argue many men feel socialized to adopt an instrumental approach to grief. The instrumental approach emphasizes "mastery" over "oneself," the "environment," and "one's feelings." Here the accent is on dealing with loss in a more private, introspective fashion, channeling reactions into mental or physical activity. For instance, the griever may retreat to the wood shop, work out at the gym, or even take action in support of some type of related cause after loss has occurred. But it is not just the way men may be socialized to grieve that is an issue, it is also the meaning found in the loss.

Blazina (2011) has discussed previously the importance of placing both secure and insecure attachment histories in the context of losing a beloved animal companion. Melanie Klein (1940/2002) and Bowlby (1960) discussed how losses in adulthood are particularly challenging when the current lost object took over an essential psychological role from another in an earlier timeframe, such as a caregiver. However, one can expand the significance of the lost love object to include adult friends, family, romantic partners, and animal companions in the role of a significant object, as well.

For the male experiencing an animal companion as such an attachment figure, the psychological importance may seem similar to the contributions and connections of other generative persons (or animal companions) from the past. In this case, one attachment figure may have taken on some of the duties of the other(s) that followed suit. However, even with the perceived similarity with former relations, it is important to recognize that an animal companion is experienced as a unique relationship in its own right. This kind of attachment figure is not only a generative presence like others but also has his or her own distinctive contribution in one's inner world. If there is a history of secure, satisfying relations, one might expect a male to approach loss with more potential resources in hand, although he may still need assistance working toward forming a *continued bond* after loss (see Packman et al. in press). That is, a way to sustain a permanent connection even in the face of loss.

For others with differing developmental histories, an animal companion can offset certain needs that were never fulfilled in childhood or the ensuing years. In this case, the HAI serves in part as a compensatory function, making up for prior attachment deficits. In the best situation, the animal companion altered one's internal world, relationships, and self for the better. When the transformation of the inner world occurs in the context of the animal companion, the existential issue of continuing bonds and existence of hope are particularly important. Fairbairn (1952) discussed how children go to great lengths to preserve a perception of some goodness in the world when growing up in dire familial circumstances. To not preserve hope means developing skewed relational perceptions, rigid defenses, and even extinguishing the expectancy of having any satisfying relations. For those who view the connection with an animal companion as such a tether to hope, they may be in danger of feeling the world has become bereft of any goodness. If the bond is not preserved in a meaningful way, males that possess extremely divergent attachment expectations regarding HAI and HHI, may feel at the mercy of previous damaging experiences. That is, one is left to contend with the residual from previously unsatisfying connection(s), but now, without the access to the special attachment figure. Pondering these types of dynamics can lead to a reexamination of our personal narrative and with it our affixed meaning.

Neimeyer (2001) comments on a relational constructivist view, where we are shaped by both attachments and subsequent losses sustained. The loss prompts the revision of our life story along many potential lines of meaning. Neimeyer suggests that when loss or death occurs, especially in an unexpected or violent way and seemingly for no good purpose, it can cause uncertainty about previously held assumptions that the world is predictable. Instead, it seems random, dangerous, or unjust. However, even when deaths are nonviolent, they can challenge a person's core beliefs. A protracted and painful illness that claims the life of a loved one may also cause the bereaved to question if the world is indeed safe or fair. The survivor may begin a chain reaction of reexamining once deeply held assumptions: "I will have to face my own mortality one day"; "How much control is there really in life?"; "Do people really get what they deserve?"; "Is there an afterlife?" The griever may in turn set out on a quest for new meaning(s). The most fundamental questions are asked, "Who am I really?" and "What does all this mean?" Neimeyer says that regardless of whether a minor update or a major overhaul to one's personal sense of meaning and beliefs is needed; there is an attempt to resolve the inconsistencies that do not make sense anymore after the experience of significant loss. While not every loss will spur the need for a drastic reexamination, not embarking on re-sorting one's personal perspective when needed is associated with complicated grief reactions and an identity that no longer makes sense.

Understanding the existential meaning of the bond in men's lives is no small undertaking. If the connection held a place of significance, or the bond was lost through difficult means, then it can cause one to reexamine long-held perspectives and one's sense of personal meaning. In some cases, it leads to the revision of the deepest beliefs, a journey that is embarked upon that can include gender role transitions, a move toward more relational focus, and a reexamination of previously held rigid beliefs that were connected to being a man. The existential issues connected to the human–animal bond and human attachment figures challenges males to rethink, reprioritize, and rewrite personal narratives as men.

Future Research Directions, Hypothesizes, and Perspectives

The proposed model is one where HAI and HHI are interfaced, having implications for the psychology of men and masculinity. However, the bond with animal companions does not guarantee a panacea for males with difficult attachment histories and so certain caveats need to be considered. One involves males that feel a strong sense of kinship with nature and animal companions but still have difficulty transitioning from the rigidity of traditional male roles and ideology. Will males of various ages be able to enact masculine role norms in a new ways within the context of HAI, and possibly generalize these ways of being a man when interacting with human companions, peers, family, and friends? The temptation may be to reuse old prescriptive dictums now applied in new contexts.

A parallel example may involve *ecowarriors*, or those that have utilized many of the male roles of traditional Western mythos, just generalizing them to the defense of nature (Gibson 2009). Ecowarriors have been known to engage in a range of activities from peaceful environmental protest to wanton destruction of property sometimes on the large scale such as fire bombs, destruction of ski resorts, car dealerships that sale SUV's, etc. Within these examples are aspects of some of the traditional male ideology that are valued by men and society that include a desire to protect and a willingness to stand firm in the face of opposition. However, we are also suggesting that those experiencing a positive generalization of attitudes and behaviors regarding HAI and HHI may need to seek new solutions through a change in dysfunctional male gender role schemata. Could it be the case that a subpopulation of men who value the bond with animal companions also becomes a type of ecowarrior on the behalf of pets and animal companions? This may manifest itself on one hand as rescuing stray dogs or standing up for their rights on various cultural levels. On the other, it may involve utilizing the 'leader of the wolf pack' mentality that has become erroneously associated with proper dog training. The metaphor has perspective traditional male gender roles embedded within as one assumes the role of an *alpha* in relating to one's animal companions, emphasizing a rigid hierarchy, dominance, or even violence.

The 'leader of the wolf pack' mentality may also extend challenges to relating with human beings that do not share the same HAI values and vehemently attaching them on social media, in print, and in person. These men may be viewed within our proposed model as wrestling with new solutions for both HAI and HHI. It should be noted the intersection of attachment and gender roles expectations make for a difficult personal and societal transformation. For men, rethinking core masculine beliefs is something profoundly personal and an impetus to do so involves events and encounters that are highly significant and life changing. We argue one starting place for insecurely attached males (though certainly not limited to this category of men) is found within the relational realm amide the bond with animal companions.

Placing prior research findings regarding gender and HAI in proper perspective also leads us to the following conclusion: seeking to compare the average male versus female on levels of attachment and/or loss regarding to animal companions is not the most beneficial way to interface masculine gender roles with HAI. In fact, we can lose contextual meaning by prioritizing those types of research studies. Instead, the context of how attachment and loss are both reported and underreported, as well as, their meaning in men's lives is more a viable avenue.

Another example of a future line of inquiry is based on findings that suggest men that enact traditional gender roles seem to have smaller social support networks (Barbee et al. 1993), and how middle-aged males turn to their animal companions as a significant source of emotional soothing when under duress (Kurdek 2009). In these types of scenarios, it is important to understand if there are real cohort differences in the ways males turn to animal companions for soothing. It may also be the case that there is a cumulative effect of negative life experiences due to failed attachments with human companions. It would seem reasonable that after so many failed attempts on the part of attachment challenged males, that an animal companion seems like a viable and secure form of emotional bonding. However, stating again that the power of the bond is not limited to males with difficult upbringings or have experienced some form of loss or trauma. Future research should also focus on how males that have found satisfaction in work and love may find very similar levels of meaning, purpose, and transcendence due in part to the animal bond.

Each potential trajectory of our proposed model, whether it involves transcendence, existential meaning, or various forms of advocacy, all derives meaning from a significant relationship with someone other than ourselves. As mentioned previously, traditional male ideology emphasizes a strictly go-it-alone mentality, and has been critiqued for a level of self-absorption (Pollack 1995). These dynamics make relational endeavors challenging if not at odds with men enacting traditional masculinity in Western culture especially in North America. Yet, if we consider that in the healthiest relational context there is enough psychologically space for a strong sense of self (not the same thing as a narcissistic self-absorption) and an equally well-equipped relational capacity, then it permits one to relate with another in a meaningful way. In these circumstances the two dynamics of self and being in relationship with another that are often so easily viewed as mutually exclusive facets in masculine world, instead become complementary parts. Perhaps this is one of the reasons man's best friend is valued so highly even if not all men can verbalize that sentiment. The bond allows males to experiment and experience the dynamic tension of self-other in a unique way. When males are truly connected to their animal companions a relational encounter emerges that is less buffered with psychological defenses. That is, males feel less threatened of losing their identities within this connection.

It is also paramount to understand more about how men response to grief when animal companions are lost; this includes the intensity, duration of symptoms, and how they are expressed. It involves helping males understand more about ongoing bonds with animal companions as a way of sustaining meaningful ties and a retaining a source of emotional support. Both self-report measures and qualitative research need to be pursued by interviewers that are culturally sensitive to male contextual dynamics. Acknowledging publically there is an emotional reliance upon a companion cuts against much of traditional male socialization, and so does expressing substantial feelings of grief when an animal companion is lost. Men's felt but often unspoken meaning(s) regarding the bond with animal companions needs to be uncovered in forthcoming studies.

Another aspect of the needed work involves ways to measure the various variables in the proposed model. This may include an instrument that assesses both HAI and HHI simultaneously. While there have been various attempts to restructure measures from one content area to another (e.g., attachment strength and style for people and then applied to pets), to date there has few efforts to develop an instrument solely for these purposes (see Zilcha-Mano et al. 2011). New measures may include elements of attachment strength to human and animal companions, as well as, purported behaviors.

Our model attempts to offer an initial way to contextually conceptualize and operationalize elements of male gender roles, attachment history, and HAI. Moving the field in this direction expands the various related variables of interest and provides a heuristic for both researchers and clinicians. However, attempting to do so will not be done without resistance or criticism that may involve anthropomorphizing or that an already fringe area of inquiry has now taken a few further steps in that direction. This new line of investigation must be accountable and held to stringent standards. Many of us have experienced the power of the bond. We honor those connections by exploring them with scientific rigor, all the while not losing sight of their emotional significance.

References

Adler, A. (1938). *Social interest: A challenge to mankind.* (J. Linton and R. Vaughan Trans.). London: Faber and Faber Ltd.

Ainsworth, M. D. S., Blehar, M. C., Waters, E., & Wall, S. (1978). Patterns of attachment: A psychological study of the strange situation. Hillsdale, NJ: Erlbaum.

Allen, K., Blascovich, J., & Mendes, W. B. (2002). Cardiovascular reactivity and the presence of pets, friends, and spouses: The truth about cats and dogs. *Psychosomatic Medicine, 64*(5), 727–739.

Barbee, A. P., Cunningham, M. R., Winstead, B. A., Derlega, V. J., Gulley, M. R., Yankeelov, P. A., & Druen, P. B. (1993). Effects of gender role expectations on the social support process. *Journal of Social Issues, 49*(3), 175–190.

Beck, A. M., & Katcher, A. H. (1996). *Between pets and people: The importance of animal companionship.* West Lafayette: Purdue University Press.

Beck, L., & Madresh, E. A. (2008). Romantic partners and four-legged friends: An extension of attachment theory to relationships with pets. *Anthrozoos, 21*, 43–56.

Blazina, C. (2011). Life After Loss: Psychodynamic Perspectives on a Continuing Bonds Approach with Pet Companions. In C. Blazina, D. Shen-Miller & G. Boyraz (Eds.), *The Psychology of the Human-Animal Bond: A Guide for Clinicians' and Researchers.* New York: Springer.

Blazina (2001). Analytic psychology and gender role conflict: The fragile masculine self. *Psychotherapy: Theory, Research, Practice, Training, 38*, 50–59.

Blazina, C., Boyraz, G., & Shen-Miller, D. S. (2011). *The psychology of the human-animal bond.* New York, NY: Springer Publishing.

Blazina, C., Novotny, M. L., Stevens, D. N., Hunter, M. (August, 2008). Man's best friend: Pet companions, gender role conflict, attachment, and loss. In J. M. O'Neil, & G. E. Good (chairs) (Eds.), *Four Studies Assessing the Contextual Complexity of the Gender Role Conflict Construct.* Boston, MA: American Psychological Association.

Blazina, C., & Watkins, C. E. (2000). Separation/individuation, parental attachment, and male gender conflict: Attitudes toward the feminine and the fragile masculine self. *Psychology of Men and Masculinity, 1*, 126–132.
Bowlby, J. (1960). Separation anxiety. *International Journal of Psychoanalysis, 41*, 89–113.
Bowlby, J. (1969/1982). Attachment and Loss: Volume 1: Attachment. 2nd edition. New York: Basic Books.
Breiding, M. J. (2004). Observed hostility and observed dominance as mediators of the relationship between husbands' gender role conflict and wives' outcomes. *Journal of Counseling Psychology, 51*, 429–436.
Breiding, M. J., Windle, C. R., & Smith, D. A. (2008). Interspousal criticism: A behavioral mediator between husband's gender role conflict and wife's adjustment. *Sex Roles, 59*, 880–888.
Brown, S. (2004). The human-animal bond and self-psychology: Toward a new understanding. *Society and Animals, 12*(1), 67–86.
Brown, S. E. (2007). Companion animals as self-objects. *Anthrozoos, 20*(4), 329–343.
Cachia, P. (2001). *The interplay of gender role conflict and adult attachment.* Unpublished Master thesis, University of Malta, Malta.
Cain, A. O. (1983). A study of pets in the family system. In H. Katcher & A. M. Beck (Eds.), *New perspectives on our lives with companion animals* (pp. 72–81). Philadelphia, PA: University of Pennsylvania Press.
Charnetski, C. J., Riggers, S., Brennan, F. X. (2004). Effect of petting a dog on immune system function. *Psychological Reports, 95*(3), 1087–1091.
Corson, S. A., & Corson, E. O. (1980). Pet animals as nonverbal communication mediators in psychotherapy in institutional settings. In S. A. Corson & E. O. Corlson (Eds.), *Ethology and nonverbal communication in mental health* (pp. 83–110). Oxford: Pergamon Press.
Covell, A. (1998). Characteristics of college males who are likely to sexually harass women: A test of a mediated model. (Doctoral dissertation, University of Southern California, 1998). *Dissertation Abstracts International,* 60, 2400.
Crandall, J. E., & Putman, E. L. (1980). Relations between measures of social interest and psychological well-being. *Source Journal of Individual Psychology, 1980*(20), 156–168.
Custance, D., & Mayer, J. (2012). Empathic-like responding by domestic dogs (Canis familiaris) to distress in humans: an exploratory study. *Animal Cognition, 15*(5), 851–9
David, D., & Brannon, R. (Eds.) (1976). The forty-nine percent majority. Reading, MA: Addison-Wesley.
Defranc, W., & Mahalik, J. R. (2002). Masculine gender role conflict and stress in relation to parental attachment and separation. *Psychology of Men and Masculinity, 3*, 51–60.
DeGue, S. (2011). A Triad of Family Violence: Examining Overlap in the Abuse of Children, Partners, and Pets. In C. Blazina, D. Shen-Miller & G. Boyraz (Eds.), *The Psychology of the Human-Animal Bond: A Guide for Clinicians' and Researchers.* New York: Springer.
Del Giudice, M. (2011). Sex differences in romantic attachment: A meta-analysis. *Personality and Social Psychology Bulletin, 37*(2), 193–214.
Dembicki, D., & Anderson, J. (1996). Pet ownership may be a factor in improved health of the elderly. *Journal of Nutrition for the Elderly, 15*(3), 15–31.
DeMello, L. R. (1999). The effect of the presence of a companion-animal on physiological changes following the termination of cognitive stressors. *Psychology & Health, 14*(5), 859–868.
Doka, K., & Martin, T. (2010). Grieving Beyond Gender: Understanding the Ways Men and Women Mourn, Revised Edition. New York: Routledge.
Ducan, A., Thomas, J. C., & Miller, C. (2005). Significance of Family Risk Factors in Development of Childhood Animal Cruelty in Adolescent Boys with Conduct Problems. *Journal of Family Violence, 20*(4), 235–239.
Ekman, P. (2007). Recognizing faces and feelings to improve communication and emotional life. In *Emotions revealed* (2nd edn.). New York: Holt Paperbacks.
Fairbairn, D. (1952). An object relations theory of personality. New York: Basic Books.

Fischer, A. R. (2007). Parental relationship quality and masculine gender role strain in young men: Mediating effects of personality. *The Counseling Psychologist, 35*, 328–358.

Fischer, A. R., & Good, G. E. (1998). Perceptions of parent-child relationships and masculine role conflicts of college men. *Journal of Counseling Psychology, 45*, 346–352.

Folse, E. B., Minder, C. C., Aycock, M. J., & Santana, R. T. (1994). Animal-assisted therapy and depression in adult college students. *Anthrozoös, 7*(3), 188–194.

Friedmann, E., Katcher, A. H., Lynch, J. J., & Thomas, S. A. (1980). Animal companions and one-year survival of patients after discharge from a coronary care unit. *Public Health Reports, 95*(4), 307–312.

Garrity, T. F., Stallones, L. F., Marx, M. B., & Johnson, T. P. (1989). Pet ownership and attachment as supportive factors in the health of the elderly. *Anthrozoös, 3*(1), 35–44.

Gentzler, A., & Kerns, K. (2006). Adult attachment and memory of emotional reactions to negative and positive events. *Cognition and Emotion, 20*(1), 20–42. doi:10.1080/02699930500200407.

Gibson, J. W. (2009). A Reenchanted World: The Quest for a New Kinship with Nature. NewYork: Metropolitan Books.

Gould, R. L. (1978). *Transformation and change in adult life*. New York: Simon & Schuster.

Gould, R. L. (1980). Transformation during early and middle adult years. In N. Smelser & E. Erikson (Eds.). *Themes of work and love in adulthood* (pp. 213–237). Cambridge, MA: Harvard University Press.

Griffin, J. A. (2011). *Sexual compulsivity among sexual minorities: Relations to attachment orientations and gender role conflict*. Master's Thesis, Loyola University Maryland, Baltimore, MD.

Gupta, M. (2008). Functional links between intimate partner violence and animal abuse: Personality features and representations of aggression. *Society and Animals, 16*, 223–242.

Guo, K., Meints, K., Hall, C., Hall, S., & Mills, D. (2009). Left gaze bias in humans, rhesus monkeys and domestic dogs. *Animal Cognition, 12*(3), 409–18.

Guzick, D. T., Dorman, W. J., Groff, T. S., Altermatt, E. R., & Forsyth, G. A. (2004). Fostering social interest in schools for long-term and short-term outcomes. *Journal of Individual Psychology, 60*(4), 361–378.

Handlin, L., Hydbring-Sandberg, E., Nilsson, A., Ejdebäck, M., Jansson, A., & Uvnäs-Moberg, K. (2011). Short-term interaction between dogs and their owners: Effects on oxytocin, cortisol, insulin and heart rate—an exploratory study. *Anthrozoos: A Multidisciplinary Journal of the Interactions of People and Animals*, *24*(3), 301–315.

Hazan, C., & Shaver, P. R. (1987). Romantic love conceptualized as an attachment process. *Journal of Personality and Social Psychology, 52*(3), 511–524.

Heinrichs, M., Baumgartner, T., Kirschbaum, C., & Ehlert, U. (2003). Social support and oxytocin interact to suppress cortisol and subjective responses to psychosocial stress. *Biological Psychiatry, 54*(12), 1389–1398.

Herzog, H. A. (2007). Gender differences in human-animal interactions: A review. *Anthrozoös, 20*(1), 7–21.

Horowitz, A. (2009). Inside of a Dog: What Dogs See, Smell, and Know. New York: Scribner.

Horowitz, A. (2011). Theory of mind in dogs? Examining method and concept. *Learning & Behavior, 39*(4) 314–317.

Kidd, A. H., & Kidd, R. M. (1985). Children's attitudes toward their pets. *Psychological Reports, 57*(1), 15–31.

Kierski, W., & Blazina, C. (2009). The male fear of femininity and its effect on counseling and psychotherapy. *The Journal of Men's Studies, 17*, 155–172.

Kiselica, M. S., & Englar-Carlson, M. (2010). Identifying, affirming, and building upon male strengths: The positive psychology/positive masculinity model of psychotherapy with boys and men. *Psychotherapy Theory, Research, Practice, and Training, 47*(3), 276–287.

Klein, M. (1940/2002). Mourning and its relationship to manic-depressive states. In Love, Guilt, and Reparation and Other Works. 1921–1945 (pp.344–369). New York: Free Press.

Klohnen, E. C, Weiler, J. A., Luo, L., & Choe, M. (2005). Organization and predictive power of general and relationship-specific attachment models: One for all, and all for one? *Personality and Social Psychological Bulletin, 31*, 1665–1682.

Kurdek, L. A. (2009). Pet dogs as attachment figures for adult owners. *Journal of Family Psychology, 23*(4), 439–446.
Land, L. N., Rochlen, A. B., & Vaugh, B. K. (2011). Correlates of adult attachment avoidance: Men's avoidance of intimacy in romantic relationships. *Psychology of Men and Masculinity, 12*, 64–74.
Leopold, A. (1949). *A sand county almanac, and sketches here and there*. Oxford: Oxford University Press.
Levant, R. F., Hirsch, L., Celentano, E., Cozza, T., Hill, S., MacRachorn, M., et al. (1992). The male role: An investigation of contemporary norms. *Journal of Mental Health Counseling, 14*, 325–337.
Levant, R. F., & Richmond, K. (2007). A review of research on masculinity ideologies using the male norm inventory. *The Journal of Men's Studies, 15*, 130–146.
Levinson, B. M. (1969). Pet-oriented child psychotherapy. Springfield, Illinois: Charles C Thomas.
Levinson, B. M. (1972). *Pets and human development*. Springfield, IL: Charles C Thomas.
Liu, W. M. (2005). The study of men and masculinity as an important multicultural competency consideration. *Journal of Clinical Psychology, 61*(6), 685–697.
Mahalik, J. R. (1999). Incorporating a gender role strain perspective in assessing and treating men's cognitive distortions. *Professional Psychology: Research and Practice, 30*, 333–340.
Marcus, D. A., & Bhowmick, A. (2013). Survey of migraine sufferers with dogs to evaluate for canine migraine-alerting behaviors. *The Journal of Alternative and Complementary Medicine, 19*(6), 501–508.
McPhedran, S. (2009) A review of the evidence for associations between empathy, violence, and animal cruelty. *Aggression and Violent Behavior, 14*, 1–4.
Merola, I., Prato-Previde, E., & Marshall-Pescini, S. (2011). Social referencing in dog-owner dyads? *Animal Cognition, 15*(2):175–85.
Merola, I., Prato-Previde, E., & Marshall-Pescini, S. (2012). Dogs' Social Referencing towards Owners and Strangers. *PLoS One, 7*(10), e47653. doi: 10.1371/journal.pone.0047653.
Mikulincer, M., & Shaver, P. R. (2001). Attachment theory and intergroup bias: Evidence that priming the secure base schema attenuates negative reactions to out-groups. *Journal of Personality and Social Psychology, 81*, 97–115.
Mikulincer, M., & Shaver, P. R. (2003). The attachment behavioral system in adulthood: Activation, psychodynamics, and interpersonal processes. *Advances in Experimental Social Psychology,* (35), 53–152.
Miller, S. C., Kennedy, C., DeVoe, D., Hickey, M., Nelson, T., & Kogan, L. (2009). An Examination of Changes in Oxytocin Levels in Men and Women Before and After Interaction with a Bonded Dog. *Anthrozoos, 22*(1), 31–42.
Müller, C. A., Schmitt, K., Barber, A. L. A., & Huber, L. (2015). Dogs can discriminate emotional expressions of human faces. *Current Biology, 25*(5), 601–605.
Nagasawa, M., Mitsui, S., En, S., Ohtani, N., Ohta, M., Sakuma, Y., et al. (2015). Oxytocin-gaze positive loop and the coevolution of human-dog bonds. *Science, 348*(6232), 333–336.
Nagasawa, M., Mogi, K., & Kikusui, T. (2009). Attachment between humans and dogs. *Japanese Psychological Research, 51*, 209–221.
Nagengast, S. L., Baun, M. M., Megel, M., & Leibowitz, M. J. (1997). The effects of the presence of a companion animal on physiological arousal and behavioral distress in children during a physical examination. *Journal of Pediatric Nursing, 12*(6), 323–330.
Napolitano, J. M., Mahalik, J. R., & Kenny, M. E. (1999, August). In *Relation of Gender Role Strain and Attachment to Men's Psychosocial Development.* Boston, MA: American Psychological Association.
Nieburg, H. A., & Fischer, A. (1982). Pet loss. New York: Harper & Row.
Niemeyer, R. A. (2001). The language of loss: Greif therapy as a process of meaning reconstruction. In R. A. Niemeyer (Ed.), *Meaning reconstruction & experience of loss* (pp. 261–292). Washington, DC: American Psychological Association.

Odendaal, J. S. J., & Lehmann, S. M. C. (2000). The role of phenylethylamine during positive human-dog interaction. *Acta Veterinaria Brno, 69*(3), 183–188.

Odendaal, J. S., & Meintjes, R. A. (2003). Neurophysiological correlates of affiliative behaviour between humans and dogs. *The Veterinary Journal, 165*(3), 296–301.

O'Neil, J. M. (1981a). Male sex-role conflict, sexism, and masculinity: Implications for men, women, and the counseling psychologist. *The Counseling Psychologist, 9*, 61–80.

O'Neil, J. M. (1981b). Patterns of gender role conflict and strain: Sexism and fear of femininity in men's lives. *Personnel and Guidance Journal, 60*, 203–210.

O'Neil, J. M. (1982). Gender role conflict and strain in men's lives: Implications for psychiatrists, psychologists, and other human service providers. In K. Solomon & N. B. Levy (Eds.), *Men in transition: Changing male roles, theory, and therapy* (pp. 5–44). New York: Plenum Publishing Co.

O'Neil, J. M. (1990). Assessing men's gender role conflict. In D. Moore & F. Leafgren (Eds.), *Men in conflict: Problem solving strategies and interventions* (pp. 23–38). Alexandria, VA: American Association for Counseling and Development.

O'Neil, J. M. (1995). The gender role journey workshop: Exploring sexism and gender role conflict in a coeducational setting. In M. Andronico (Ed.). *Men in groups: Insights, interventions, psychoeducational work* (pp. 193–213). Washington, DC: APA Books.

O'Neil, J. M. (2008a). Special issue. Men's gender conflict: 25 year research summary. *The Counseling Psychologist, 36*, 358–476.

O'Neil, J. M. (2008b). Special issue: Summarizing twenty-five years of research on men's gender role conflict using the gender role conflict scale: New research paradigms and clinical implications. *The Counseling Psychologist, 36*, 358–445.

O'Neil, J. M. (2010). Is criticism of generic masculinity, essentialism, and positive-healthy-masculinity a problem for the psychology of men? *Psychology of Men and Masculinity, 11*, 98–106.

O'Neil, J. M. (2012). The psychology of men. In E. Altmaier & J. Hansen (Eds.). *Oxford Handbook of Counseling Psychology.* New York: Oxford University Press.

O'Neil, J. M. (2013). Gender-role conflict research thirty years later: An evidenced based diagnostic schema. *Journal of Counseling and Development, 91*, 490–498.

O'Neil, J. M. (2015). Men's Gender Role Conflict: Psychological Costs, Consequences, and an Agenda for Change. Washington, D.C.: APA Books.

O'Neil, J. M., & Crapser, B. (2011). Using the psychology of men and gender role conflict theory to promote comprehensive service delivery for college men: A call to action. In J. Laker & T. Davis (Eds.), *Masculinities in higher education: Theoretical and practical considerations*. New York: Routeledge Publishers.

O'Neil, J. M., & Egan, J. (1992a). Men's gender role transitions over the life span: Transformations and fears of femininity. *Journal of Mental Health Counseling, 14*, 305–324.

O'Neil, J. M., & Egan, J. (1992b). Men and women's gender role journeys: A metaphor for healing, transition, and transformation. In B. Wainrib (Ed.), *Gender issues across the life cycle* (pp. 107–123). New York: Springer Publishing Co.

O'Neil, J. M., & Egan, J. (1992c). Men's gender role transitions over the lifespan: Transformation and fears of femininity. *Journal of Mental Health Counseling, 14*, 306–324.

O'Neil, J. M., Helm, B., Gable, R., David, L., & Wrightsman, L. (1986). Gender role conflict scale (GRCS): College men's fears of femininity. *Sex Roles, 14*, 335–350.

O'Neil, J. M., Egan, J., Owen, S. V., & Murry, V. (1993). The gender role journey measure (JRJM): Scale development and psychometric evaluations. *Sex Roles, 28*, 167–185.

O'Neil, J. M., & Fishman, D. (1992). Adult men's career transitions and gender role themes. In H. D. Lee & Z. B. Leibowitz (Eds.), *Adult career development: Concepts, issues, and practices* (2nd ed., pp. 132–162). Alexandria, VA: ACA Press.

O'Neil, J. M., Fishman, D. M., & Kinsella-Shaw, M. (1987). Dual-career couples' career transitions and normative dilemmas: A preliminary assessment model. *The Counseling Psychologist, 15*(1), 50–96.

O'Neil, J. M., Good, G. E., & Holmes, S. (1995). Fifteen years of theory and research on men's gender role conflict: New paradigms for empirical research. In R. Levant & W. Pollack (Eds.), *The new psychology of men* (pp. 164–206). New York: Basic Books.

O'Neil, J. M., & Nadeau, R. A. (1999). Men's gender-role conflict, defense mechanism, and self-protective defensive strategies: Explaining men's violence against women from a gender-role socialization perspective. In M. Harway & J. M. O'Neil (Eds.), *What causes men's violence against women?* (pp. 89–116). Thousand Oaks, CA: Sage Publications.

O'Neil, J. M., & Roberts Carroll, M. (1988). A gender role workshop focused on sexism, gender role conflict, and the gender role journey. *Journal of Counseling and Development, 67*, 193–197.

Pachana, N. A., Ford, J. H., Andrew, B., & Dobson, A. J. (2005). Relations between companion animals and self-reported health in older women: Cause, effect or artefact? *International Journal of Behavioral Medicine, 12*, 103–110.

Pleck, J. (1981). *The myth of masculinity*. Cambridge, MA: MIT Press.

Pleck, J. H. (1995). The gender role strain paradigm: An update. In R. F. Levant & W. S. Pollack (Eds.), *A new psychology of men* (pp. 11–32). NewYork: Basic Books.

Pleck, J. H., Sonenstein, F. L., & Ku, L. C. (1993). Masculinity ideology and its correlates. In S. Oskamp & M. Costanzo (Eds.), *Gender issues in social psychology* (pp. 85–110). Newbury Park, CA: Sage Publications.

Polheber, J. P., & Matchock, R. L. (2014). The presence of a dog attenuates cortisol and heart rate in the Trier Social Stress Test compared to human friends. *Journal of Behavioral Medicine, 37*, 860–867.

Pollack, W. (1995). No man is an island: Toward a new psychoanalytic psychology of men. In R. Levant & W. Pollack (Eds.), *A new psychology of men* (pp. 33–67). New York: Basic Books.

Prato-Previde, E., Fallani, G., & Valsecenchi, P. (2006). Gender Differences in Owners Interacting with Pet Dogs: An Observational Study. *Ethology, 112*(1), 64–73.

Ramirez, M. 2006. "My Dog's Just Like Me": Dog Ownership as a Gender Display. *Symbolic Interaction, 29*(3), 373–391.

Robin, M., & Bensel, R. T. (1985). Pets and the socialization of children. *Marriage and Family Review, 8*(3–4), 63–78.

Rochlen, A., & Mahalik, J. R. (2004). Women's perceptions of male partner's gender role conflict as predictors of psychological well-being and relationship satisfaction. *Psychology of Men and Masculinity, 5*, 147–157.

Roszak, T. (1992). The voice of the Earth: An exploration of ecopsychology. New York: Simon & Schuster.

Roszak, T., Gomes, M. E., & Kanner, A. D. (Eds.) (1995). Ecopsychology: Restoring the earth, healing the mind. San Francisco: Sierra Club Books.

Roth, B. (2005). Pets and psychoanalysis: A clinical contribution. *Psychoanalytic Review, 92*, 453–457.

Schwartz, J. P., Waldo, M., & Higgins, A. J. (2004). Attachment styles: Relationship to masculine gender role conflict in college men. *Psychology of Men and Masculinity, 5*, 143–146.

Selby, B. W. (1999). The relation of attachment, adjustment, and narcissism to masculine gender role conflict (Doctoral dissertation, University of North Texas, 1999). *Dissertation Abstracts International*, 61, 5005.

Serpell, J. (1996). *In the company of animals: A study of human-animal relationships*. Cambridge University Press.

Serpell, J. A. (2010). Animal-assisted interventions in historical perspective. In A. H. Fine (Ed.), *Handbook on Animal-Assisted Therapy: Theoretical foundations and guidelines for practice*. 3rd Ed. (pp. 17–32). San Diego, CA: Academic Press.

Sharkin, B. S., & Bahrick, A. S. (1990). Pet loss: Implications for counselors. *Journal of Counseling & Development, 68*(3), 306–308.

Silva, K., & de Sousa, L. (2011). 'Canis empathicus'? A proposal on dogs' capacity to empathize with humans. *Biology Letters, 7*, 489–92.

Téglás, E., Gergely, A., Kupán, K., Miklósi, A., & Topál, J. (2012). Dogs' gaze following is tuned to human communicative signals. *Current Biology*, (*22*)3, 209–212.
Triebenbacher, S. L. (1998). Pets as transitional objects: Their role in children's emotional development. *Psychological Reports, 82*(1), 191–200.
Vandello, J. A., & Bossom, J. K. (2013). Hard won easily lost: A review and synthesis of theory and research on precarious manhood. *Psychology of Men and Masculinity, 14*, 101–113.
Vandello, J. A., Bossom, J. K., Cohen, D., Burnaford, R. M., & Weaver, J. R. (2008). Precarious manhood. *Journal of Personality and Social Psychology, 95*, 1325–1339.
Voith, V. L. (1985). Attachment of people to companion animals. The Veterinary Clinics of North America. *Small Animal Practice, 15*(2), 289–295.
Wilson, E. O. (1986). The Biophilia Hypothesis. Cambridge: Harvard Press.
Wallin, D. J. (2007). Attachment in Psychotherapy: New York: Guilford press.
Wilson, D. A. H. (2011). British Animal Behaviour Studies in the Twentieth Century: Some Interdisciplinary Perspectives. In C. Blazina, D. Shen-Miller & G. Boyraz (Eds.), *The Psychology of the Human-Animal Bond: A Guide for Clinicians' and Researchers*. New York: Springer.
Winefield, H. R., Black, A., & Chur-Hansen, A. (2008). Health effects of ownership of and attachment to companion animals, in an older population. *International Journal of Behavioral Medicine, 15*(4), 303–310.
West, C., & Zimmerman, D. H. (1998). Doing gender. In B. M. Clinchy & J. K. Norem (Eds.), *The gender and psychology reader* (pp. 104–124). New York: New York University Press.
Wexler, D. B. (2009). Men in therapy: New approaches for effective treatment. New York, NY: WW Norton & Company.
Zarski, J. J. (1984). Hassles and health: A replication. *Health Psychology, 3*(3), 243.
Zasloff, L. R. (1996). Measuring attachment to companion animals: A dog is not a cat is not a bird. *Animal Behaviour Science, 47*, 43–48.
Zilcha-Mano, S., Mikulincer, M., & Shaver, P. R. (2011). Pet in the therapy room: An attachment perspective on Animal-Assisted Therapy. *Attachment & Human Development, 13*(6), 541–561.
Zilcha-Mano, S., Mikulincer, M., & Shaver, P. R. (2012). Pets as safe havens and secure bases: The moderating role of pet attachment orientations. *Journal of Research in Personality 46*(5).

Chapter 4
Street-Involved Youth and Their Animal Companions—Stigma and Survival

Michelle Lem

Should Homeless People Have Pets?

As a veterinarian who provides pro bono veterinary care for people who are homeless and vulnerably housed, the most common question asked by members of the public and media is "Should homeless people have pets?" Since my work is at the human–animal–environment interface—that is youth and their animal companions living within the street environment—it fits within the One Health model, which describes how the health of "humans, animals and the environment are inextricably linked" (van Helden et al. 2013).

One Health

The Centers for Disease Control and Prevention describes One Health as recognizing "that the health of humans is connected to the health of animals and the environment" (www.cdc.gov/onehealth/). One Health therefore also seeks to bridge historically independent disciplines and professions of human health, animal health, and environmental health. One Health's origins are in zoonoses (diseases transmitted between humans and animals), vector-borne diseases, and risks to human food supply and environmental or ecosystem health. The One Health model is slow to be adopted at the community health level and among the companion animal–human–environment relationship. Yet, the One Health model fits this context well, as the environment

M. Lem (✉)
PO Box 75, Carp, ON K0A 1L0, Canada
e-mail: michelle.lem@vetoutreach.org

C. Blazina and L.R. Kogan (eds.), *Men and Their Dogs*,
DOI 10.1007/978-3-319-30097-9_4

(e.g. urban vs. rural, housed vs. homeless) is inextricably connected to the health of both humans and animals in the relationship. Gaining an understanding of each of these three sectors and how they interact with each other allows us to fully understand the context in which these human–animal relationships exist. One Health has traditionally focused on disease and threats to the health of each sector; however, it can also be used to model the many beneficial effects of human–animal relationships. Among these are both the physical and psychosocial effects of companion animal ownership, which will be discussed in this chapter as we focus on the impact of the human–animal relationship among homeless youth within the street environment.

Throughout this chapter, we will seek to answer the question posed above. So to begin, let us first briefly review the general profile of homeless youth. In One Health terms, we will examine how youth homelessness is impacted by the interaction of individual factors (human sector) and the environment in which they come from (home, family) and leave to (the street).

Who Are Street-Involved Youth?

In the U.S. the Department of Housing and Urban Development's 2014 Annual Homeless Assessment Report stated that on a single night in 2014, over 194,000 youth and children were homeless, with children under 18 years of age representing 23 % of all homeless, and youth 18–24 years making up 10 % of the overall homeless population (Henry et al. 2014). In Canada, youth (16–24 years) represent 20 % of the over 35,000 homeless on any given night or 235,000 homeless in a year, with a 2:1 ratio of males to females (Gaetz et al. 2013, 2014; Government of Canada 2006). Young people between 18 and 24 years of age are almost twice as likely to report being homeless at some time compared to adults, are more likely to be "hidden homeless", and not engaged with emergency support systems (Gaetz et al. 2014). The number of homeless youth is typically underestimated in homeless and/or shelter counts, as many youth may utilize other forms of transient shelter, such as couch surfing and squatting, or engaging in prostitution for shelter (Evenson 2009; Government of Canada 2006; Kelly and Caputo 2007). The state of homelessness also encompasses those who are provisionally accommodated (e.g. incarcerated, hospitalized, in addictions treatment, or transitional housing), as well as those who are at risk of homelessness (Canadian Observatory on Homelessness 2012). Street-involved youth are described as youth who experience "precarious living conditions, which include poverty, residential instability and emotional and psychological vulnerability" (Government of Canada 2006). In this chapter, both terms "street-involved" and "homeless" are used to describe youth as homelessness is a state of transience, most if not all street-involved youth have experienced homelessness.

Contrary to popular belief, the vast majority of street-involved youth are not spoiled and lazy middle-class kids wanting a life of independence and who "choose" to live on the street. More accurately, street-involved youth represent a particularly vulnerable and growing subsection of the homeless population, typically between the ages of 16 and 24 years. While each person has their own individual experiences and path to homelessness, it is believed that it is the cumulative impact of structural factors (broad economic and social issues), institutional and systems failures (failures of systems of care and support), and individual and relational factors (circumstances affecting individuals at a personal level or within their family support system) that lead to homelessness (Gaetz et al. 2014).

Youths' path to homelessness is as varied as homelessness itself. Structural factors affecting youth homelessness include economic disparity, family poverty and deprivation (e.g. unemployment, housing affordability crises); institutional and systems failures include a failure to provide support and resources for youth discharged from jail or foster care; and individual and relational factors include youth who runaway, are parentally abandoned or kicked out (e.g. for substance abuse, disapproval of gender identification (LGBQT). Many homeless youth have histories of mental illness, domestic violence, sexual abuse, substance abuse, family and/or parental conflict, and/or parents involved in criminal activity (Kidd 2013; Rukmana 2010). Not surprisingly, predictors for adolescents who runaway include a history of substance abuse and depression (Tucker et al. 2011). In fact, adolescents with substance abuse have been found to have insecure attachments, weak family and social support, and low levels of parental acceptance and involvement (Aydogdu and Cam 2013). Tragically, the longer that youth remain on the street, the more likely they are to further suffer from both medical and mental health disorders, as well as criminalization and street victimization (Gaetz et al. 2010; Tyler and Beal 2010). Indeed, street life may be the cause of and/or exacerbate mental health issues, with many youth experiencing stress, trauma, and distress both prior to and while living on the street. For example, in a Canadian study of 102 homeless youth, the authors found that youth experienced a mean of seven traumatic or stressful events prior to becoming homeless and a mean of six events since becoming homeless, which included bullying (78 %), stressful isolation (63 %), assault (61 %), and fearing being injured or killed (61 %). Prior to becoming homeless, males experienced more physical types of violence (e.g. abuse, assault, muggings), and females experienced more sexual violence which continued after becoming homeless. Physical assault also continued after becoming homeless for both genders (62.7 %) (Coates and McKenzie-Mohr 2010). As the authors of this article state, "Youth left or were forced out of homes where most had experienced extensive trauma, only to find themselves experiencing severe and multiple forms of trauma 'on the street'".

The life of street-involved youth includes navigating street life in search of shelter, money, and safety while facing criminalization and victimization. In one study of 207 homeless or previously homeless youth in California, 75 % of youth reported regular and negative interactions with police (Bernstein and Foster 2008). Although street-involved youth are more likely to be involved in criminal activity than domiciled youth, O'Grady and Gaetz (2007) point out that while crimes are more likely to be committed by male youth, "theft and drug dealing are by no means dominant money-making activities". In the aforementioned California study, only 8 % of youth reported getting money from theft, 7 % from selling drugs, and 5 % from prostitution (Bernstein and Foster 2008). In the same study, 30 % of youth interviewed had slept outside, on the street, or in a car or vacant building the previous night, 28 % were couch surfing, 10 % were staying at a transitional shelter, and 8 % had spent the previous night in a shelter.

Street victimization includes being a victim of crime while on the street, but also the impact of public and social stigma and this has important implications as perceived social stigma by homeless youth has been found to be associated with low self-esteem, loneliness, and suicidal ideation (Kidd and Carroll 2007). Overwhelmingly, youth report that people's perception of them is negative with words often used to describe street youth that include "worthless", "junkie", "low-life", and "troublemaker", and yet over 90 % of these youth identified aspirations of specific career goals (Bernstein and Foster 2008). Public stigma of street-involved youth often serves to reinforce youth's sense of worthlessness further eroding their self-esteem and confirming their belief that they are "throwaways".

Companion Animals of Street-Involved Youth

Next, we will examine the "animal" component of the One Health model to further our understanding of companion animal ownership among the street-involved youth population. According to Rhoades et al. (2014), up to 25 % of America's homeless are pet owners, and of 398 homeless youth surveyed at two LA drop-in centres, 23 % were pet owners. Of these pet owners, just over 60 % were male, and 53 % of youth owned a dog (Rhoades et al. 2014). In a Canadian study of 89 street-involved youth who owned a total of 121 pets, 58 % were male, and 43 % of the total number of pets owned were dogs. Companion animals were obtained from numerous sources including street friends and street family (19.1 %), found as strays or rescued (14.9 %), adopted via newspaper and other ads (14.2 %), and left home with the pet (13.2 %); 26.4 % of the pets were obtained from other sources that included from a neighbour, a friend's pet who had a litter, a stranger, friends who were housed or other family members. One youth described obtaining his pet rat by saying "I paid $3 for him from a drug dealer" (Lem 2012). In a qualitative study of 25 youth who belonged to a group, of whom over a half of these youth belonged to a gang, Maher and Pierpoint (2011) found that over half of the dogs owned were bull breeds, including Staffordshire Bull Terriers, Bull Mastiffs, American Bulldogs, and crosses thereof.

Those who ask whether homeless people should have animals demonstrate concern for the welfare of the animal belonging to someone who does not likely have the means to care for an animal. Since this is not a chapter on animal welfare, I will not address this in detail. I will say, however, that based on over 12 years of experience in the field, and seeing thousands of animals belonging to those who are homeless and vulnerably housed in our veterinary outreach clinics, these pets are, for the most part, healthy and well-cared for. Anecdotally, I can say that in my

14 years of clinical practice and 12 years of outreach work, I have never seen an animal that has been brought to an outreach clinic that was in any worse condition than an animal owned by someone who is housed and employed and brought to a full service veterinary clinic. In other words, based on my experience the same health conditions and severity of disease (e.g. dental disease) exist in the housed pet population as in the homeless/vulnerably housed pet population.

In some aspects, the welfare of animals of those who are street-involved may actually be better than housed pets. For example, after systematically reviewing the medical records of over 300 of Community Veterinary Outreach patients (to veterinarians, animals are the "patients", and the pet owners are "clients"), we found that 73 % of our patients were in ideal body condition score, compared to the household pets in the U.S. where it is estimated that 52.6 % of dogs and 57.6 % of cats are clinically overweight (2013 National Pet Obesity Awareness Day Survey 2014). In fact, studies have shown that most homeless pet guardians do not have trouble feeding their animal companions (Irvine et al. 2012). In a survey of 332 homeless youth in Los Angeles, only 10.42 % of respondents indicated that it was hard to get pet food (Rhoades et al. 2014). Among the aforementioned Canadian study of 89 street-involved youth and 121 pets, we found that these pets were not left alone for extended periods of time; received a great deal of exercise and play (2–4 h/day for dogs; 1–2 h/day for cats); enjoyed constant companionship; were exposed to novel environments and stimuli; and received regular socialization with people and other animals. What we have observed is that these animals often have richer social and emotional lives, and increased physical activity and play than many housed pets.

Human–Animal Attachment—A Determinant of Health

Among homeless pet owners, a universally high level of attachment to their pets exists (Kidd and Kidd 1994; Singer et al. 1995; Taylor et al. 2004). A validated measure of human-companion animal attachment is the Lexington Attachment to Pets Scale (LAPS), which seeks to quantify attachment via Likert scale responses of agreement to a series of questions on pet owner's views of their relationship with their companion animal (Johnson et al. 1992). For example, LAPS was administered to 89 pet-owning street-involved youth in the Canadian study previously mentioned, and it demonstrated youth's strong attachment to their companion animals with a mean score of 58 (SD 9.5). Based on previous studies among the general population, a LAPS score of 54.9 or higher is considered "very attached" (Johnson et al. 1992). In this study, we found that male youth's LAPS scores were slightly lower than females with mean scores of 56.1 and 61.1, respectively (Lem 2012). Analysis of the LAPS administered to 389 Community Veterinary Outreach clients found a mean score of 61, with no significant difference between pet owner's gender (male/female) or between species owned (cat/dog).

It is important to consider the level of attachment between marginalized humans and animals, for not only the sake of animal health and welfare, as attachment is linked to willingness to care for and spend resources on an animal (Staats et al. 1996), but also for the impact that attachment can have on human health and welfare. A profound example of this is during natural disasters, where loss of human and animal life has been attributed to people failing to evacuate without their companion animals, or returning to retrieve their animal companion (Heath et al. 2000; Leonard and Scammon 2007). Therefore, human–animal attachment may drive decisions that impact the lives of both the human and the animal.

Companion animal ownership among those who are homeless and highly attached has benefits for both the human and animal. Yet it is important not to overlook the liabilities that can be associated with having a pet while being homeless. Among the liabilities, many homeless pet owners will refuse shelter or housing without their animals. Research has also shown that homeless people with pets have increased difficulty finding stable housing and are unable or unwilling to access shelter, healthcare, and other services where pets are not allowed (Lem 2012; Rhoades et al. 2014; Singer et al. 1995; Slatter et al. 2012; Taylor et al. 2004). For example, Rhoades et al. (2014) found that only 4 % of homeless youth with pets ($n = 76$) were staying in a shelter compared to 16.8 % of non-pet-owning youth ($n = 256$). This is consistent with the finding that non-pet owners were 2.5 times more likely to make use of shelter services than street-involved youth who had a pet (Lem 2012). In the same study, 89.9 % indicated that having a pet had made their life better and 87.6 % indicated that they would never give up their pet, despite the added difficulties of being a pet owner ($n = 89$). Youth forego opportunities to move off the streets because they are highly attached to their pet and unwilling relinquish their companion animal for opportunities of shelter and other supports.

Add to this that street-involved youth are typically difficult to engage in services (Carlson et al. 2006; Krüsi et al. 2010). For example in one study, only 50 % of the 229 street-involved youth interviewed had accessed medical care (Carlson et al. 2006), and in another study 57 % of 249 homeless youth interviewed had never received counselling services (Tyler et al. 2012). Through the lens of attachment theory this lack of engagement may be explained, in that "young people's attachment patterns may affect their reactions to offers of support or assistance"—youth who experience insecure attachment may consider service providers/social workers in a similar role as other adults and caregivers from their past experiences, and may not see those trying to help them as trustworthy and reliable (Vaughn Heineman 2010). For example, because many youth have developed attachment patterns stemming from trauma, whether physical and/or emotional, their response to adult figures may be reflected in their experience. For street-involved youth, insecure attachments and trauma often coexist, affecting mood, behaviour, attitudes as well as their capacity to self-regulate and self-sooth (Vaughn Heineman 2010). In a survey of 40 homeless and formerly homeless youth in California, 40 % said they felt safer since leaving home (Bernstein and Foster 2008). A sense of safety and security is paramount for youth who have experienced trauma, and dogs provide both the vehicle to self-sooth as well as a sense of security both physically and emotionally within the relationship (Kurdek 2009; Lange et al. 2006; Rew 2000; Rhoades et al. 2014; Thompson et al. 2006b). As Bowlby (1982) describes, a safe haven and opportunity for youth to experience consistent, unconditional and non-judgmental support are critical in engaging youth with insecure attachment patterns. The companionship of a dog provides this safe haven, especially for those who have been unable to attain this relationship with another person. Indeed, Zilcha-Mano et al. (2012) reported that pets can provide a safe haven by demonstrating lower participant blood pressure while performing a distress-eliciting activity when physically in the presence of their pet or cognitively thinking about their pet, compared to the control group (participants did not think about their pets and pets were not present). Similarly, in a web-based survey of 975 adult dog owners, males were more likely to turn to their dogs than to their mothers, sisters, best friends or children during times of emotional distress (Kurdek 2009). These human–animal relationships are trusting consistent relationships, without fear of punishment, retaliation or other negative consequences (e.g. abandonment). The following is a narrative from an interview with a Youth Drop-In Centre Manager (Lem 2012):

> There was one guy we were working with… he did a job training program with us … he got himself a dog … and the one thing that sticks out in my mind is he came in and he loves his dog and he was talking - that for the first time he understood what unconditional love was…because his dog loved him no matter who he was or what he was about and all that sort of stuff and so he tried to show that same kind of compassion back to his dog.

As previously discussed, for many youth with insecure attachment and given their past experiences, self-reliance may have been necessitated by the actions of adults in their lives. Resiliency among inner city adolescents and homeless youth has been negatively associated with social connectedness, suggesting that among marginalized youth resiliency may be attained from being independent and self-reliant (Kidd and Davidson 2007; Rew et al. 2001). The theme of self-reliance has also been shown to negatively impact service utilization (Garrett et al. 2008). In one study, 33 % of youth interviewed ($n = 40$) said that they would rely on themselves rather than parents, caregivers, service providers or other adults (Bernstein and Foster 2008). Among males, O'Neil (2008) describes how restrictive and oppressive North American gender role socialization further promotes this sense of self-reliance and self-sufficiency, and limits men "from being fully functioning human beings" (O'Neil 2008, 2015; O'Neil et al. 1995). Such gender role conflict and stress not only interferes with interpersonal attachments (e.g. parental) (Blazina 2001; Blazina and Watkins 2000) but also greater psychological distress including depression and anxiety, as well as less willingness to seek help, as this may be seen as weakness or vulnerability (Addis and Mahalik 2003; Leong and Zachar 1999; Mahalik et al. 2003).

A lack of resiliency has also been associated with loneliness, hopelessness, and life-threatening behaviours among homeless adolescents (Rew et al. 2001). Companion animal ownership among those who are homeless has been found to mitigate loneliness, provide a sense of responsibility and well-being, with animal companions serving as a source of emotional resilience (Rhoades et al. 2014;

Slatter et al. 2012; Wood et al. 2005). One case worker who refers clients to Community Veterinary Outreach describes the role of pets in the lives of her clients this way:

> All of my clients are living with compromised immune systems, less than 1/3rd of my clients have a pet. I've seen the quality of life change in every client who takes in a pet; I see increased energy, increased engagement in their community and increased quality of life - just by having the unconditional love of a pet. The clients I have who've had pets from before I began to work with them seem to have stronger support networks, greater confidence and more solid housing - having someone who 'needs' them as much as they need the pet seems to give greater meaning to living with a chronic condition.

This is consistent with findings among homeless youth whom describe the relationship with their pet as family, best friend or child-like (Lem 2013). One of Community Veterinary Outreach's youth clients described what his dog meant to him in this way: "I have Aspergers and have issues with relationships with people, and with Petey he is always there for me and I am there for him". Rew (2000) found that while friends/peers helped pass time and assisted in street survival, dogs helped homeless youth cope with loneliness, provided safety, unconditional love, and a reason to live in order to care for the dog. Dog-owning youth also reported feeling healthier because they got more exercise and their dogs kept them warm, and a desire to act more responsibly and make better choices for themselves and their dog (Rew 2000).

With high rates of emotional distress and mental illness, including major depressive disorder, post-traumatic stress disorder, multiple diagnoses, and comorbidity with substance abuse (Thompson et al. 2006), not surprisingly, street-involved youth are also at high risk for suicide. For example, Kidd and Carroll (2007) found that of 208 street-involved youth interviewed, 46 % reported making at least one suicide attempt, 40 % of whom were males; with 78 % of all attempters reporting more than one attempt (Kidd and Carroll 2007). In addition to a history of sexual and/or physical abuse, substance abuse, length of time on the street and victimization, low self-esteem has been found to be a predictor of suicide or suicidal ideation among homeless youth (Kidd and Kral 2002; Saade and Winkelman 2002). Self-worth, self-respect, and self-esteem have been found to be associated with positive outcomes of transitioning off the street, helping youth overcome adversity, and having a protective effect against the impact of fearful attachment on loneliness (Bender et al. 2007; Kidd and Shahar 2008; Thompson et al. 2013).

Despite the many barriers to establishing and/or maintaining self-esteem for street-involved youth, Irvine et al. (2012) have shown that pet ownership by homeless pet guardians helps to create a positive sense of self. Homeless pet owners described challenging public stigma of what good pet ownership looks like by demonstrating their ability to feed, care, and provide for their pets constant companionship and a freedom that housed pets are limited to. Through these confrontations with members of the public, marginalized pet owners established a "moral personal identity" that mitigates the stigma of pet ownership among those who are homeless (Irvine et al. 2012). In the aforementioned Canadian study of street-involved youth, the vast majority of pet-owning street-involved youth we interviewed (97.8 %) indicated that they were proud of being a good pet owner. Pet ownership may therefore buffer the negative effects of social stigma on mental health by empowering street-involved youth to self-identify as caring and responsible pet owners.

Pet ownership among homeless youth has also been associated with fewer symptoms of depression compared to non-pet-owning youth (Rhoades et al. 2014). Similarly, among the sample of 89 Canadian street-involved youth who owned pets (previously mentioned) and 100 youth who did not own a pet, this cross-sectional study revealed that the street-involved youth who did not own pets were three times more likely to be depressed than pet-owning youth, based on the Center for Epidemiologic Studies Depression Scale (Lem 2016). Among clients of our outreach programme, we ask "What does your pet mean to you?" and responses have included pets described to be therapeutic for depression and anxiety ("He helps keep me calm"), motivators to get outside and exercise ("I suffer from depression and he has changed my life—he has made me go out more and have more energy"), and to help with pain management ("Good company, sharing our lives together, and now that I have him I wouldn't be able to do without him...he knows when I am in physical pain and he comes to give me a kiss"). For some youth, their pets help them to self-monitor, as one of our male youth clients described what his pet means to him this way: "He keeps me grounded, helps me control my temper because if I do something wrong, my pet will be alone. His temperament changes when I am sick so I will admit more that I need to seek help". Indeed, it is this positive effect on human health, both physical and emotional, for which human–animal relationships have demonstrated across socioeconomic levels, and these benefits appear to be even more significant among marginalized pet owners.

Pet Loss

Pet loss, from death, relinquishment, loss, runaway or removal can have profound negative effects on highly attached youth. Loss of animal companions has been identified to be significant negative experiences among homeless pet owners, and is associated with guilt, depression, and anger (Lem 2012; Lem et al. 2013; Slatter et al. 2012). In our study, the majority of youth (88.7 %) who had lost pets agreed that they felt depressed following the loss of their pet and 63.5 % of youth felt angry. Almost half reported that they blamed themselves for the loss (45.1 %). Almost half (46.2 %) agreed that the loss of their pet had made their life harder and over one-third (34.6 %; $n = 18$) of respondents reported using alcohol and/or drugs to cope with the loss of their pet. One male youth in our study said that upon the death of his dog "it made me more of a beast", another male youth described his experience this way: "I had a dog on the street in Montreal...he got ran over by a car while I was sleeping...I didn't get any more dogs after that...I missed him a lot...he was a good dog...I didn't want to have that loss again because it was so hard...I got depressed after" (Lem 2012).

Level of pet attachment has been shown to predict both the severity of grieving symptoms as well as the length of the grieving process among the general population (Wrobel and Dye 2003). Indeed, even among those pet owners who have social support, mourning a pet's loss is not always legitimized by society, and so it is not surprising that high levels of grief from pet loss have also been found to be associated with low social support and additional life stressors (Gosse and Barnes 1994; Sable 2013). Although the occurrences of grief symptoms are higher for females than males, Wrobel and Dye (2003) point out that this does not necessarily reflect the intensity of the individual's experiences. Doka and Marten (2010) describe the pattern of grief more correlated with (but not determined by) the male gender as "instrumental" whereby individuals work through and experience grief in a more cognitive and task-driven manner, expressing less emotion. Individuals who experience this pattern of grief are less likely to reach out for help, and however are still in need of validation and support (Doka and Martin 2010). Social expectations of males' expression of grief play a factor in their experience and expression of grief which may be further exacerbated among already emotionally isolated street-involved youth. Similarly, Risley-Curtiss et al. (2013) found that social workers were less likely to treat people of colour for animal loss, which may be attributed to the misperception that they are less attached to their animal companions (Risley-Curtiss et al. 2013).

It is important to recognize that pet loss can take many forms, not just death of the pet. Grief and/or guilt may be associated with a pet running away, getting lost or stolen, or removed during arrest/incarceration. Similarly, interventions with at-risk or incarcerated youth in which they are paired with shelter dogs may result in similar negative experiences associated with pet loss. Introducing such a relationship and then removing the dog after completion of the programme could be yet another loss for youth for whom many have experienced trauma and abandonment, and warrants further investigation. Acceptance and understanding of human–animal relationships in social work practice may be critical in being able to support highly attached youth through pet loss.

Social Capital and Bonding

Social capital "refers to the social networks, norms and trust that enable people to act together effectively in the pursuit of shared objectives" (Putnam 1995). Research has demonstrated that companion animals contribute to social capital and sense of community, providing increased opportunities for social connection, exercise, helpfulness and reciprocity, and well-being (McNicholas and Collis 2000; Wood et al. 2005, 2007; Wood 2011). Human–animal relationships and therefore dog ownership may be considered social bonds that are important aspects of conventional society, and woven into our social fabric. Bruno et al. (2012) found that gender, conformist aspirations of family, and the type of maltreatment youth had experienced were factors in early conception among street-involved youth, and suggest that youth attempt to conform to a conventional family ideal and may "view pregnancy as an opportunity rather than a constraint". This study found that male youth who had experienced physical maltreatment were more likely to father a child, as were those who were in a relationship, supporting that strain and social bonding contribute to early conception and familial aspiration (Bruno et al. 2012). If we consider companion animal ownership among street-involved youth through the lens of strain and social bonding theory, parallels can be drawn. Either through a conventional view of family of which often includes a family dog, or as an animal companion as chosen family with unconditional love and support, it is not surprising that they may seek to create their own sense of family over which they exert more control.

A part of this sense of family for street-involved youth, are groups of peers and friends that are often referred to as "street families". Peer support is often their only network these street families develop because of a need for companionship, shared interests and experiences, a sense of belonging, acceptance and security, assistance in navigating street life, pooling of resources, and common interactions in street life, such as panhandling (Smith 2008). Male youth are more likely to establish networks via these street-based ties, and not surprisingly, however, these ties may also often expose youth to deviant behaviours including substance abuse (Wenzel et al. 2012). Still, street families are typically self-supportive and are often seen as an adaptive response to a harsh environment with high rates of victimization for which street families offer protection (Smith 2008). For homeless youth, family has been defined as "people you can count on and trust" and among street families, youth often recreate traditional familial roles often associated with gender, with males seen as making the decisions, enforcing rules, and providing security and protection (Smith 2008). In my experience, dogs often have significant roles within street families, and dog ownership is supported through the street family. It is not uncommon for a dog to have multiple owners within the family and shared responsibility for taking care of the dog. For example, if a youth is arrested, the dog will be cared for by another member of the street family. If the dog has puppies, these puppies are often adopted by other members of the street family. It is another shared connection that increases social bonding. Among the 89 pet-owning youth interviewed 19.1 % obtained their pet from a street friend or street family member (Lem 2012). Viewed through the lens of social bonding theory, street families and dog ownership may be seen as attempts to establish a sense of family and social convention within the street-life environment. Companion animals further contribute to social capital on the street among their owners, extended street family, and community.

Panhandling

For many street-involved youth, panhandling is a survival strategy and their higher visibility and accessibility exposes them to greater risk of both physical and sexual victimization (Tyler and Beal 2010). Panhandling for cash meets youth's immediate day-to-day needs and is often done in small youth groups (O'Grady and Gaetz 2007). Street-involved youth are largely excluded from employment within the formal job market, given their lack of education, skills, unstable housing and health, and other necessary factors for success. Opportunities for youth subsistence are few, and therefore are often limited to an informal and street-level economy including panhandling, the sex trade, drug dealing/running, gang, and other illegal activities (e.g. shoplifting, pawning stolen property, etc.). It can therefore be challenging for these youth to earn income within the "space, place, and identity" of the street environment (O'Grady and Gaetz 2007). According to a 2007 study from California, over 20 % of homeless and previously homeless youth ($n = 207$) reported making money from panhandling (Bernstein and Foster 2008). However, because of increased public exposure and interactions, panhandling by homeless youth as a primary source of income has been found to be strongly related to youth's perception of social stigma and self-blame (Kidd 2006). Street-involved youth often face public scrutiny for "using a dog" to panhandle, as it may be assumed by some that youth exploit dogs to increase income earned from panhandling. However, dogs may be both social and economic capital, in that panhandling with a dog may increase social interaction with members of the public, as well as the amount of cash or other goods received such as dog food (Irvine et al. 2012). As Irvine (2012) describes, donations of food provided homeless pet owners with "enabled resistance to stigmatizing confrontations". While male youth have described earning more when panning with their dog, this extrinsic reason was not the primary purpose for youth to own a dog, rather they have them because of a love of animals, youth often believe that they are giving the animal a better life and for companionship (Lem 2012).

For those youth who own animals, having nowhere to safely and consistently leave their animal companion while they are at work is a significant barrier to seeking and maintaining conventional employment (Lem et al. 2013). As one male youth describes,

> When you have a dog and you're living on the street, you can't go to work because you have to look after the dog. …Trying to find a friend that's actually constant to look after your dog while you're at work, I mean, when you're living on the streets you can't find anybody that's actually reliable…I found one guy that lasted a week and then he just disappeared and I was never able to find him for my next shift, I ended up losing my job…

Panhandling may be one of the few income-earning activities that youth can participate in with their animal companion.

Gangs and Dogs

Gang culture and structure varies greatly by country and even within countries, states, or municipalities, and by culture. However, youth who are gang-involved are a unique subset of the street-involved youth population with high rates of delinquency, substance abuse, victimization, and illegal activity (Matsuda et al. 2012; Sanders 2012). Not surprisingly, gang membership is a predominantly male activity (Chettleburgh 2002), and risk factors for gang involvement include the cumulative impact of individual and family characteristics, school engagement, peer group, and community conditions (Howell and Egley 2005). For example, youth who had backgrounds of poverty, social exclusion, racism, dysfunctional families, exposure to violence (e.g. cultural violence, bullying, and family violence), addictions, and leaving school at an early age were found to be at higher risk of being gang-involved. Mental illness, including depression, anxiety disorders and post-traumatic stress disorder, are also common among gang-involved youth (Kelly 2011).

Dog ownership among gang-involved youth is not universal, and there are strong cultural, ethnic, and religious influences that impact interaction, attachment, and perceived roles of animals in general (Risley-Curtiss et al. 2006). For example, Risley-Curtiss et al. (2011) interviewed 12 male companion animal owners and found that participants from indigenous culture reported placing a higher value on animals and demonstrated a greater respect of animals than that of the larger U.S. society, whereas participants who immigrated from nations where the roles of animals were primarily utilitarian, such as sources of food and protection, reported having to learn how animals are treated in American culture (Risley-Curtiss et al. 2011). Nevertheless, Barnes et al. (2006) found that ownership of "vicious" dogs may be a marker for social deviance and, as the authors suggest, a "vicious" dog "is by definition a socially deviant animal" (Barnes et al. 2006). This interpretation of animals as being "socially deviant" should be approached with caution, for it is within the context of our human environment in which this is predicated, not that of the canine. Indeed, there are more human and environmental factors that contribute to aggressive dog incidents, than animal/dog factors themselves. That being said research to date on dogs within gangs shows that dog breed type is a factor in this human–animal relationship, with much of the research coming out of the United Kingdom and United States (Harding 2010; Kalof and Taylor 2007; Maher and Pierpoint 2011).

Dog ownership among gang youth can be interpreted as another form of social capital, as these dogs often confer status, and among some, dogs are considered "weapons" of intimidation and protection. Indeed, use of dogs by gang members for criminal and other illegal purposes, such as dog fighting, has also been reported and bears a larger impact on public safety and society as a whole (Harding 2010; Kalof and Taylor 2007). Despite this, Maher and Pierpoint (2011) found that among 25 gang youth interviewed in South Wales, the most commonly cited role of dogs was for companionship and socialization. Extrinsic roles of dogs were also identified, including security, protection, fighting, and status (Maher and Pierpoint 2011); however, as Kalof and Taylor (2007) point out, "dog fighting and the status it provides among peers are not unique to urban street culture". When asked at a conference I was presenting at why I thought my research did not demonstrate that protection and security were primary reasons for dog ownership among street-involved youth, I replied "I have a German Shepherd, primarily for companionship for my family and children, but do I appreciate and benefit from her large size, keen hearing and deep bark? Absolutely". The existence of roles for dogs beyond those which are intrinsic is not surprising, as extrinsic values were the starting point of canid domestication by humans. Domestication evolved for extrinsic purposes that served us (as well as the ancestral dogs) for scavenging, hunting, and protection and continues to serve us in similar capacities to this day. This domestication process was followed by our genetic manipulation of the dog with artificial selection and neotenization of dogs for traits that would facilitate cohabitation and companionship (Miklosi and Topal 2013).

For male youth on the street or in a gang, status and therefore resources and even survival may be directly related to the display of masculinity within the street or gang context. In some instances, dogs have saved the life of their owner, such as when they have gotten into a fight with another youth or when a "deal goes down wrong"—in speaking about their dog in this context, youth describe their dog as admirable and loyal, and talk about how in return, they want to show that admiration and loyalty back to their dog. Within a safe and anonymous research environment, a more honest narrative about the role of dogs in youth's lives such may be elicited as this narrative from a male gang youth speaking about his dog:

> He was my best friend. Loyal. Companion, when no one else was there. He was my shadow. Always there...that was my way of displaying my good side, you know? By having that dog around me, people could see a better side of me than they usually would.

One Health—Leveraging the Human–Animal Relationship

"Strengths-based" models for youth services and interventions focus on youth's skills and abilities, and are effective in engaging youth because "it is their strengths in overcoming difficulties that mitigate negative outcomes" (Bender et al. 2007). Companion animal ownership among street-involved youth has demonstrated that youth develop many skills and strengths as pet owners, including a sense of responsibility, structure and routine, and pride of ownership (Lem et al. 2013). Similarly, in occupational health and psychosocial rehabilitation fields, companion animal ownership among those with severe mental illness has been described as "a meaningful occupation" that confers non-stigmatizing opportunities for social community integration (Zimolag and Krupa 2009). Companion animal ownership as a productive occupation among those experiencing homelessness provides owners with purpose, responsibility as well as the opportunity for person-level interventions to improve cognitive skills including establishing routine, scheduling, and problem-solving (Slatter et al. 2012).

Animals have been shown to enhance rapport, trust, and safety in therapeutic settings and the body of knowledge on the use of animal-assisted therapy (AAT) in counselling is growing (Chandler 2012; Chandler et al. 2010). Dogs have been shown to improve therapeutic relationships among adolescents in group counselling, providing a calming effect, humour relief, feelings of safety, empathy, and as a motivator to attend (Lange et al. 2006). Providing youth with learning opportunities and resources which focus on strengthening the human–animal relationship may further help youth develop skills that will assist them to integrate into mainstream society. For example, some youth may seek to establish safer and more stable housing for their companion animal, as is demonstrated on this narrative of a male street-involved youth describing his need to find housing for his dog:

> I love him and I get a place for him. Really, like, if it wasn't for him [his dog], I'd be on the streets. That's why I want a place…I don't want him to die. I don't want him to get sick. I want him to eat.

By leveraging the high level of human–animal attachment, service providers can establish rapport with youth through the animal, and this may be more effective than direct interaction between the youth and social worker, especially among youth with insecure attachment. By understanding what the animal means to the youth, we can help uncover the strengths developed through pet ownership and this may be key to engaging street-involved youth in supportive services to aid them in getting off the street.

Motivators for Behaviour Change

Irvine (2013) has described how animals can act as vehicles for redemption among homeless pet owners who "envisioned brighter futures emerging out of their struggles". In this manner, the animal's innocence and dependence served to not only develop the homeless person's sense of responsibility, but also through this commitment and caring for the pet they also positively change their behaviours (such as addictions) and allow them to experience unconditional love without judgement, atonement and salvation (Irvine 2013a).

Among homeless youth, pet owners described putting the needs of their pets before their own needs (e.g. feeding their pet before themselves), how their pets were motivators for taking better care of themselves, making more responsible choices and "staying out of trouble", establishing structure and routine, and provide emotional support, love and safety (Lem et al. 2013; Thompson et al. 2006a). In the interviews with 89 Canadian street-involved youth, almost half of the pet-owning youth (47.2 %) reported that they had decreased their use of drugs and/or alcohol because of their pet, 60.7 % avoided arrest because of their pet, and almost half the youth (46.1 %) agreed that having a pet had saved their life (Lem 2012). In qualitative interviews with street-involved youth, it was the male youth who described decreasing their use of drugs when they became a pet owner (Lem et al. 2013):

> Before, my life was one of like try to make myself more liking the city meaning the drugs, alcohol, all the bad things, the crime. I was in and out of court, I was in and out of jail, life didn't matter to me. Once I got Mackenzie [name of dog] I settled down and my life actually had meaning to it. I haven't gone back to jail yet… it's been at least 2 years since I've actually gone to jail. I don't do heavy drugs anymore.

Veterinary Outreach

As an extension of a strength-based model of service delivery, support in the form of veterinary care is a critical component, as it is not easily accessed due to cost. Lack of basic veterinary care compounds the stress of an already stressful life for street-involved youth who own pets. Irvine et al. (2012) described how veterinary support of homeless pet owners can convey "legitimacy" on the homeless person as an animal caregiver. There are also greater implications for society including animal welfare, criminalization of youth for animal neglect (failing to provide necessary veterinary care), and risk of illegal activity to pay for veterinary care. Of the 89 street-involved youth interviewed in the aforementioned study, it was asked "If your pet was in need of veterinary care would you consider committing a crime to get the money?"—40 % responded "yes" and 13 % responded "Don't know".

Although veterinarians have not traditionally been thought of in social support roles, Community Veterinary Outreach is demonstrating that veterinarians and veterinary care can be a direct link to increased social support and health care delivery for marginalized pet owners. Understanding that many marginalized pet owners will reach out for help for their pet, but not necessarily themselves, we can leverage the desire for veterinary care for their animal companion to engage pet owners in care for themselves through embedded social services and health care workers in our veterinary outreach model. An example of a One Health issue affecting the health of both humans and animals is smoking and exposure to secondhand smoke, respectively. An estimated 70–80 % of homeless adults smoke cigarettes (Tobacco Use and the Homeless 2009). Similarly, it has been found that ~70 % of homeless youth smoke, and Tucker et al. (2014) found that of 292 homeless youth in Los Angeles, youth reported smoking an average of 26.6 days/month and 15 cigarettes/day (Tucker et al. 2014; Wenzel et al. 2010).

Research to date on the risk and effects of environmental tobacco smoke on the health of companion animals has suggested that passive tobacco smoke exposure may lead to an increased risk of developing nasal cancer in long-nosed breeds of dogs (e.g. German Shepherd), lung cancer in short-nosed (e.g. Pug) and middle-nosed breeds (e.g. Husky), and malignant lymphoma and squamous cell carcinoma in cats (Bertone et al. 2002; Knottenbelt et al. 2012; McNiel et al. 2007; Reif et al. 1998; Snyder et al. 2004). Additionally, secondhand smoke exposure has been shown to be associated with atopic dermatitis (Ka et al. 2014) and contribute to airway limitation in dogs (Yamaya et al. 2014). In a large web-based survey of 3293 adult pet owners, Milberger et al. (2009) found that 28.4 % of current smokers ($n = 698$) reported that information on the dangers of secondhand smoke to their pet's health would motivate them to try quitting smoking, 11 % would think about quitting, and 40 % would be interested in receiving information on smoking cessation. Of non-smoking participants who lived with someone who smoked ($n = 531$), 16.4 % reported that they would ask smokers to quit, and 24 % would ask them to not smoke inside (Milberger et al. 2009).

The findings of this study were corroborated at a community level via Community Veterinary Outreach clinics in Toronto, Ontario. In these pilot projects, a nurse practitioner or family physician was embedded into the veterinary outreach clinic serving homeless and vulnerably housed pet owners with free preventive veterinary care, and offered opportunities for clients to discuss their health matters with a human healthcare practitioner, receive information and resources on smoking cessation, and obtain a referral to primary health care while at the veterinary clinic. Veterinarians inquired whether the animal had any environmental exposure to secondhand smoke as part of obtaining the animal's environmental history, and if so and following the veterinary services (e.g. exam, vaccinations, deworming, etc.), the veterinarian educated the owner on the risks of tobacco smoke exposure to their pet's health and offered to connect them with the human healthcare practitioner at the clinic. Over 3 clinics with a total of 71 homeless and vulnerably housed clients, 30 % of clients ($n = 21$) requested information on smoking cessation from the healthcare practitioner, 68 % of clients ($n = 48$) freely engaged with the human health care practitioner regarding their own health matters, and 24 % of clients ($n = 17$) requested referral to primary health care.

Another health issue that marginalized populations experience is low vaccination rates. In one study of the medical charts of 4319 homeless persons from New York City, the influenza vaccination rate was found to be less than 25 %, yet people who are homeless experience high rates of influenza, pneumonia and related deaths (Bucher et al. 2006). In another pilot, Community Veterinary Outreach collaborated with Toronto Public Health to offer an influenza clinic in November of 2014 at one of our veterinary outreach clinics. Of the 35 clients who attended the veterinary outreach clinic, 6 had already received an influenza vaccination (17 %). Of the 29 remaining clients, 17 clients received an influenza vaccination via this collaborative human and veterinary clinic, representing a vaccination rate of 58.6 % among our homeless and vulnerably housed clients. In the fall of 2015, similar results were achieved across Community Veterinary Outreach programs running in 4 communities (Toronto, Hamilton, Kitchener-Waterloo, and Guelph, ON), achieving a flu vaccination rate of 51.4 % among 70 clients attending the veterinary outreach clinics. Leveraging strong human–animal attachment may also include pets as motivators for increased exercise and activity and/or veterinary prescribed exercise for the animal companion (Byers et al. 2014; Kushner et al. 2006).

Indeed, veterinarians may be key community connectors in a One Health model. Below, an outreach nurse describes her experience:

> As a health care provider, I have connected with individuals about health matters, who would have never trusted me before- but by starting with veterinary care for their pet(s), I have engaged [them] in addiction treatment, wound care, housing concerns, and just built trust in using health services again.

Practice Implications

The One Health model proves useful in understanding the context and environment in which human–animal relationships exist and how the health of each sector impacts the other. This model may be effectively used by any health/social/

service professional to better understand and treat the "whole" person rather than the disease or symptoms. In doing so, we move away from the biomedical model of medicine towards the favoured biopsychosocial model. For example, in veterinary medicine, the focus of attention and information typically leans towards the animal, however, equal knowledge of the factors impacting the human owner (e.g. finances, time availability, commitment, sources of support, etc.) as well as the environment (e.g. urban vs. rural, housed vs. homeless) will greatly influence not only diagnostic and treatment options but also compliance and therefore outcome. Similarly, a system-level barrier for homeless pet owners is the lack of pet-friendly shelters and services. In not allowing pets into shelter/services, not only will this fail to engage pet owners in need of support, but even for those accessing the service, front-line workers may not be aware of a human–animal relationship that may heavily influence a client's options, decisions, and motivations for support. In cases of strong human–animal attachment, this relationship can be leveraged using a strength-based approach. Pets are strong motivators for positive health and behaviour change. Knowledge, acceptance, and support of these relationships rather than condemning them will allow those seeking to help reach clients at a deeper personal level to establish rapport, a relationship, and trust.

Future Directions

There is a small but growing body of literature examining the roles of companion animals in the lives of street-involved youth and both the benefits and liabilities of this relationship. However, the role of youth's gender and how this impacts the human–animal relationship has not been explored. Longitudinal studies investigating the trajectory of male youth with animal companions as they move into adulthood, as well as case–control studies examining the effects of pet ownership among male youth, are needed. As a predominantly male activity, further research of the role of dogs in gang youth culture is also warranted. Leveraging these strong human–animal attachments for positive change has been discussed in this chapter, and this is an area of great opportunity in need of research. Incorporation of veterinary medicine into an integrated health and social support model is proving effective to reach difficult to engage companion animal owners in care for themselves through their pet. Within this collaborative service-based context, research investigating the impact of gender on help seeking via their pet is worthy of further investigation.

Conclusion

Street-involved youth face numerous challenges to leading healthy and fulfilling lives, including histories of abuse, neglect, abandonment, substance abuse, and mental health disorders. Add to this system failures, social stigma, criminalization, and overwhelmed social services systems, the future looks bleak for many youth who face becoming chronically homeless as adults. For many street-involved youth, the adults in their lives have failed to provide them with emotional and physical security, and it is often only through the love of an animal that youth have the opportunity to experience unconditional love and acceptance without judgement. Ironically, for some, it is an animal that teaches youth about compassion, empathy, and humanity. A front-line youth worker describes the roles of animals in the lives of youth:

> Unconditional love. I think that they've just been so broken and especially with the horror stories that I've heard over the years and I think one of the bridging gaps back into society is that they've lost all trust with people. They've seen the dark side of humanity and I think that when you have a dog or a cat that just wants to love them for who they are, protect them, give them unconditional love, a hug, a warm body when it's cold.

The study of street-involved youth is challenging, as they are heterogeneous population that are often transient, that has its own unique and shifting culture. Roots of and solutions to youth homelessness are multifaceted and require significant shift in public attitude, policy, and funding. The research on the role of companion animals in the lives of marginalized people is starting to grow and there is increasing awareness of many benefits that homeless people derive from their animal companions. In the time that I have been doing outreach work, I have experienced the gradual shift from the condemnation of impoverished pet owners to growing support, with books like "A Street Cat Named Bob" (Bowen and Jenkins 2012) and "My Dog Always Eats First" (Irvine 2013b), and services including VETSOS (www.vetsos.com) in San Francisco, Pro-Bone-O in Oregon (www.proboneo.org), Pets of the Homeless (www.petsofthehomeless.org/), and Dogs Trust's Hope Project (www.moretodogstrust.org.uk/hope-project/hope-project) in the UK, to name a few. There is still much needed research in this field, such as understanding the role of dogs in the culture of gang-involved youth, and the role gender plays on issues affecting youth homelessness. Yet, despite the numerous risks and challenges these youth face, their companion animal may be the one constant.

Coming back to the question "Should homeless people have pets?" and by extension "Should homeless youth have pets?", it should be clear now that the question is inherently flawed, for we should not be asking whether homeless youth should have pets, but rather "Should we have youth who are unwanted, uncared for, and without a home?". If we help the person, we will help the animal, and quite reciprocally, by helping the animal we can reach the person. Over the years, it has become so clear to me that the human–animal relationship is one of reciprocities and symbioses, and among youth and their pets, often a codependence. In order to support the needs of either human or animal, we need support the relationship in the context in which it exists.

References

2013 National Pet Obesity Awareness Day Survey. (2014). Retrieved January 27, 2015 from http://www.petobesityprevention.org/pet-obesity-fact-risks/

Addis, M. E., & Mahalik, J. R. (2003). Men, masculinity, and the contexts of help seeking. *The American Psychologist, 58*(1), 5–14.

Aydogdu, H., & Cam, M. O. (2013). Comparison of attachment styles, parent attitudes and social supports of normal adolescents and those diagnosed with substance use disorder. *Journal of Psychiatric Nursing, 4*, 137–144.

Barnes, J. E., Boat, B. W., Putnam, F. W., Dates, H. F., & Mahlman, A. R. (2006). Ownership of high-risk ("vicious") dogs as a marker for deviant behaviors: Implications for risk assessment. *Journal of Interpersonal Violence, 21*(12), 1616–1634.

Bender, K., Thompson, S. J., McManus, H., Lantry, J., & Flynn, P. M. (2007). Capacity for survival: Exploring strengths of homeless street youth. *Child & Youth Care Forum, 36*(1), 25–42. doi:10.1007/s10566-006-9029-4.

Bernstein, N., & Foster, L. K. (2008). *Voices from the street: A survey of homeless youth by their peers*. Sacramento, CA: California Research Bureau.

Bertone, E. R., Snyder, L. A., & Moore, A. S. (2002). Environmental tobacco smoke and risk of malignant lymphoma in pet cats. *American Journal of Epidemiology, 156*(3), 268–273. doi: 10.1093/aje/kwf044.

Blazina, C. (2001). Analytic psychology and gender role conflict: The development of the fragile masculine self. *Psychotherapy: River Edge, 38*, 50–59.

Blazina, C., & Watkins, C. E. (2000). Separation/individuation, parental attachment, and male gender role conflict: Attitudes toward the feminine and the fragile masculine self. *Psychology of Men and Masculinity, 1*, 126–132.

Bowen, J., & Jenkins, G. (2012). *A street cat named Bob: How one man and his cat found hope on the streets*. London: Hodder and Stoughton Ltd.

Bowlby, J. (1982). Attachment and loss: Vol. 1. Attachment (2nd ed.). New York: Basic Books (Original Ed. 1969).

Bruno, T. L., Butters, J. E., Erickson, P. G., & Wekerle, C. (2012). Missed conceptions: A gendered extension of early conception among street youth. *Deviant Behavior, 33*(7), 550–565. doi:10.1080/01639625.2011.636698.

Bucher, S. J., Brickner, P. W., & Vincent, R. L. (2006). Influenza like illness among homeless persons. *Emerging Infectious Diseases, 12*, 1162–1163.

Byers, C. G., Wilson, C. C., Stephens, M. B., Goodie, J. L., Netting, F. E., & Olsen, C. H. (2014). Owners and pets exercising together: Canine response to veterinarian-prescribed physical activity. *Anthrozoös, 27*(3), 325–333. doi:10.2752/175303714x14036956449224.

Canadian Observatory on Homelessness. (2012). Canadian definition of homelessness. Retrieved April 9, 2015 from http://www.homelesshub.ca/CHRNhomelessdefinition

Carlson, J. L., Sugano, E., Millstein, S. G., & Auerswald, C. L. (2006). Service utilization and the life cycle of youth homelessness. *Journal of Adolescent Health, 38*(5), 624–627.

Chandler, C. K. (2012). *Animal assisted therapy in counseling* (2nd ed.). New York, NY: Routledge.

Chandler, C. K., Portrie-Bethke, T. L., Minton, C. A. B., Fernando, D. M., & O'Callaghan, D. M. (2010). Matching animal-assisted therapy techniques and intentions with counseling guiding theories. *Journal of Mental Health Counseling, 32*(4), 354–374.

Chettleburgh, M. C. (2002). *Canadian police survey on youth gangs*. Ottawa.

Coates, J., & McKenzie-Mohr, S. (2010). Out of the frying pan, into the fire: Trauma in the lives of homeless youth prior to and during homelessness. *Journal of Sociology and Social Welfare: Special Issue on Homelessness in Canada, 37*(4), 65–96.

Doka, K. J., & Martin, T. L. (2010). *Grieving beyond gender: Understanding the ways men and women mourn*. New York: Routledge.

Evenson, J. (2009). Youth homelessness in Canada: The road to solutions. In J. Evenson (Ed.). Toronto: Raising the Roof.

Gaetz, S. A., Donaldson, J., Richter, T., & Gulliver, T. (2013). *The state of homelessness in Canada 2013*. Toronto: Homeless Hub Press.

Gaetz, S., Gulliver, T., & Richter, T. (2014). *The state of homelessness in Canada: 2014*. Toronto: Homeless Hub Press.

Gaetz, S., O'Grady, B., & Buccieri, K. (2010). *Surviving crime and violence street youth and victimization in Toronto*. Toronto: Justice for Children and Youth and Homeless Hub Press.

Garrett, S. B., Higa, D. H., Phares, M. M., Peterson, P. L., Wells, E. A., & Baer, J. S. (2008). Homeless youths' perceptions of services and transitions to stable housing. *Evaluation and Program Planning, 31*(4), 436–444.

Gosse, G. H., & Barnes, M. J. (1994). Human grief resulting from the death of a pet. *Anthrozoös, 7*(2), 103–112. doi:10.2752/089279394787001970.

Government of Canada. (2006). *Street Youth in Canada: Findings from enhanced surveillance of Canadian Street Youth, 1999–2003* (Vol. March, 2006). Canada: Public Health Agency of Canada.

Harding, S. (2010). Status dog's and gangs. *Safer Communities, 9*(1), 30–35.

Heath, S. E., Voeks, S. K., & Glickman, L. T. (2000). A study of pet rescue in two disasters. *International Journal of Mass Emergencies and Disasters, 18*(3), 361–381.

Henry, M., Cortes, A., Shivji, A., & Buck, K. (2014). *The 2014 Annual Homeless Assessment Report (AHAR) to Congress—Part 1*.

Howell, J. C., & Egley, A. (2005). Moving risk factors into developmental theories of gang membership. *Youth Violence and Juvenile Justice, 3*(4), 334–354. doi:10.1177/1541204005278679.

Irvine, L. (2013a). Animals as lifechangers and lifesavers: Pets in the redemption narratives of homeless people. *Journal of Contemporary Ethnography, 42*(1), 3–30. doi:10.1177/0891241612456550.

Irvine, L. (2013b). *My dog always eats first: Homeless people and their animals*. Boulder, Colorado: Lynne Rienner Publishers.

Irvine, L., Kahl, K. N., & Smith, J. M. (2012). Confrontations and donations: Encounters between homeless pet owners and the public. *The Sociological Quarterly, 53*(1), 25–43. doi:10.1111/j.1533-8525.2011.01224.x.

Johnson, T. P., Garrity, T. F., & Stallones, L. (1992). Psychometric evaluation of the Lexington attachment to pets scale (LAPS). *Anthrozoös, 5*(3), 160–175.

Ka, D., Marignac, G., Desquilbet, L., Freyburger, L., Hubert, B., Garelik, D., et al. (2014). Association between passive smoking and atopic dermatitis in dogs. *Food and Chemical Toxicology Food and Chemical Toxicology, 66*(5), 329–333.

Kalof, L., & Taylor, C. (2007). The discourse of dog fighting. *Humanity & Society, 31*(4), 319–333.

Kelly, K. (2011). Life course of youth gang members. Retrieved January 28, 2015 from http://www.crimepreventionottawa.ca/uploads/files/initiative/life_course_of_youth_gang_members-_final-october_21-2011_.pdf

Kelly, K., & Caputo, T. (2007). Health and street/homeless youth. *Journal of Health Psychology, 12*(5), 726–736. doi:10.1177/1359105307080594.

Kidd, S. A. (2006). Youth homelessness and social stigma. *Journal of Youth and Adolescence, 36*(3), 291–299. doi:10.1007/s10964-006-9100-3.

Kidd, S. (2013). Mental health and youth homelessness: A critical review. In S. Gaetz, B. O'Grady, K. Buccieri, J. Karabanow, & A. Marsolais (Eds.), *Youth homelessness in Canada: Implications for policy and practice* (p. 217). Canada: Canadian Homelessness Research Network Press.

Kidd, S. A., & Carroll, M. R. (2007). Coping and suicidality among homeless youth. *Journal of Adolescence, 30*(2), 283–296. doi:10.1016/j.adolescence.2006.03.002.

Kidd, S. A., & Davidson, L. (2007). "You have to adapt because you have no other choice": The stories of strength and resilience of 208 homeless youth in New York City and Toronto. *Journal of Community Psychology, 35*(2), 219–238.

Kidd, A. H., & Kidd, R. M. (1994). Benefits and liabilities of pets for the homeless. *Psychological Reports, 74*(3, Pt 1), 715–722.

Kidd, S. A., & Kral, M. J. (2002). Suicide and prostitution among street youth: A qualitative analysis. *Adolescence, 37*(146), 411–430.

Kidd, S., & Shahar, G. (2008). Resilience in homeless youth: The key role of self-esteem. *American Journal of Orthopsychiatry, 78*(2), 163–172.

Knottenbelt, C. M., Hammond, J., Mellor, D., Bawazeer, S., & Watson, D. G. (2012). Nicotine hair concentrations in dogs exposed to environmental tobacco smoke: A pilot study. *Journal of Small Animal Practice, 53*(11), 623–626.

Krüsi, A., Fast, D., Small, W., Wood, E., & Kerr, T. (2010). Social and structural barriers to housing among street-involved youth who use illicit drugs. *Health and Social Care in the Community, 18*(3), 282–288.

Kurdek, L. A. (2009). Pet dogs as attachment figures for adult owners. *Journal of Family Psychology, 23*(4), 439–446. doi:10.1037/a0014979.

Kushner, R. F., Blatner, D. J., Jewell, D. E., & Rudloff, K. (2006). The PPET study: People and pets exercising together. *Obesity, 14*(10), 1762–1770. doi:10.1038/oby.2006.203.

Lange, A. M., Cox, J. A., Bernert, D. J., & Jenkins, C. D. (2006). Is counseling going to the dogs? An exploratory study related to the inclusion of an animal in group counseling with adolescents. *Journal of Creativity in Mental Health, 2*(2), 17–31. doi:10.1300/J456v02n02_03.

Lem, M. (2012). Effects of pet ownership on street-involved youth in Ontario (M.Sc., Department of Population Medicine, University of Guelph, Guelph, ON). Retrieved from http://www.google.ca/url?sa=t&rct=j&q=&esrc=s&frm=1&source=web&cd=1&ved=0CC8QFjAA&url=http%3A%2F%2Fdspace.lib.uoguelph.ca%2Fxmlui%2Fbitstream%2Fhandle%2F10214%2F3600%2FLem%2520Thesis%2520FINAL.pdf%3Fsequence%3D6&ei=XyMuUuPUBJD5rAG22ICQCQ&usg=AFQjCNHzij6pXLlzMwDvhwCgQNH6lWNZow&bvm=bv.51773540,d.aWM

Lem, M., Coe, J., Haley, D., Stone, E., & O'Grady, W. (2013). Effects of companion animal ownership among Canadian street-involved youth: A qualitative analysis. *Journal of Sociology and Social Welfare: Special Issue on Redefining Social Welfare Connections across Species, XI*(4), 285–304.

Lem, M., Coe, J., Haley, D., Stone, E., & O'Grady, W. (2016) The protective association between pet ownership and depression among street-involved youth: A cross-sectional study. *Anthrozoös*, 29(1):123–136.

Leonard, H. A., & Scammon, D. L. (2007). No pet left behind: Accommodating pets in emergency planning. *Journal of Public Policy & Marketing, 26*(1), 49–53.

Leong, F. T. L., & Zachar, P. (1999). Gender and opinions about mental illness as predictors of attitudes toward seeking professional psychological help. *British Journal of Guidance and Counselling, 27*(1), 123–132.

Mahalik, J. R., Locke, B. D., Ludlow, L. H., Diemer, M. A., Scott, R. P. J., Gottfried, M., et al. (2003). Development of the conformity to masculine norms inventory. *Psychology of Men and Masculinity, 4*, 3–25.

Maher, J., & Pierpoint, H. (2011). Friends, status symbols and weapons: The use of dogs by youth groups and youth gangs. *Crime, law and social change, 55*(5), 405–420.

Matsuda, K. N., Esbensen, F.-A., & Carson, D. C. (2012). Putting the "gang" in "eurogang": Characteristics of delinquent youth groups by different definitional approaches. In F.-A. Esbensen & C. Maxson (Eds.), *Youth gangs in international perspective: Results from the eurogang program of research* (pp. 17–33). New York: Springer.

McNicholas, J., & Collis, G. M. (2000). Dogs as catalysts for social interactions: Robustness of the effect. *British Journal of Psychology, 91*(Pt 1), 61–70.

McNiel, E. A., Carmella, S. G., Heath, L. A., Bliss, R. L., Le, K.-A., & Hecht, S. S. (2007). Urinary biomarkers to assess exposure of cats to environmental tobacco smoke. *American Journal of Veterinary Research, 68*(4), 349–353.

Miklosi, A., & Topal, J. (2013). What does it take to become 'best friends'? Evolutionary changes in canine social competence. *Trends in Cognitive Science, 17*(6), 287–294. doi:10.1016/j.tics.2013.04.005.

Milberger, S. M., Davis, R. M., & Holm, A. L. (2009). Pet owners' attitudes and behaviours related to smoking and second-hand smoke: A pilot study. *Tobacco Control, 18*(2), 156–158.
O'Grady, B., & Gaetz, S. (2007). Homelessness, gender and subsistence: The case of Toronto street youth. *Journal of Youth Studies, 7*(4), 397–416. doi:10.1080/1367626042000315194.
O'Neil, J. (2008). Summarizing 25 years of research on men's gender role conflict using the gender role conflict scale. *The Counseling Psychologist, 36*(3), 358–445.
O'Neil, J. M. (2015). *Men's gender role conflict psychological costs, consequences, and an agenda for change*. Washington, D.C.: American Psychological Association.
O'Neil, J. M., Good, G. E., & Holmes, S. (1995). Fifteen years of theory and research on men's gender role conflict: New paradigms for empirical research. In R. Levant & W. Pollack (Eds.), *The new psychology of men*. New York: Basic Books.
Putnam, R. D. (1995). Tuning in, tuning out: The strange disappearance of social capital in America. *PS: Political Science & Politics, 28*, 664–683.
Reif, J. S., Bruns, C., & Lower, K. S. (1998). Cancer of the nasal cavity and paranasal sinuses and exposure to environmental tobacco smoke in pet dogs. *American Journal of Epidemiology, 147*(5), 488–492.
Rew, L. (2000). Friends and pets as companions: Strategies for coping with loneliness among homeless youth. *Journal of Child & Adolescent Psychiatric Nursing, 13*(3), 125–132.
Rew, L., Taylor-Seehafer, M., Thomas, N. Y., & Yockey, R. D. (2001). Correlates of resilience in homeless adolescents. *Journal of Nursing Scholarship, 33*(1), 33–40.
Rhoades, H., Winetrobe, H., & Rice, E. (2014). Pet ownership among homeless youth: Associations with mental health, service utilization and housing status. *Child Psychiatry and Human Development,*. doi:10.1007/s10578-014-0463-5.
Risley-Curtiss, C., Holley, L. C., & Kodiene, S. (2011). "They're there for you": Men's relationships with companion animals. *Families in Society, 92*(4), 412–418.
Risley-Curtiss, C., Holley, L. C., & Wolf, S. (2006). The animal–human bond and ethnic diversity. *Social Work, 51*(3), 257–268.
Risley-Curtiss, C., Rogge, M. E., & Kawam, E. (2013). Factors affecting social workers' inclusion of animals in practice. *Social Work, 58*(2), 153–161. doi:10.1093/sw/swt009.
Rukmana, D. (2010). Gender differences in the residential origins of the homeless: Identification of areas with high risk of homelessness. *Planning Practice and Research, 25*(1), 95–116. doi:10.1080/02697451003625422.
Saade, R., & Winkelman, C. (2002). Short- and long-term homelessness and adolescents' self-esteem, depression, locus of control and social supports. *Australian Journal of Social Issues, 37*(4), 431–445.
Sable, P. (2013). The pet connection: An attachment perspective. *Clinical Social Work Journal, 41*(1), 93–99. doi:10.1007/s10615-012-0405-2.
Sanders, B. (2012). Gang youth, substance use patterns, and drug normalization. *Journal of Youth Studies, 15*(8), 978–994. doi:10.1080/13676261.2012.685707.
Singer, R. S., Hart, L. A., & Zasloff, R. L. (1995). Dilemmas associated with rehousing homeless people who have companion animals. *Psychological Reports, 77*(3 Pt 1), 851–857.
Slatter, J., Lloyd, C., & King, R. (2012). Homelessness and companion animals: More than just a pet? *The British Journal of Occupational Therapy, 75*(8), 377–383. doi:10.4276/030802212x13433105374350.
Smith, H. (2008). Searching for kinship: The creation of street families among homeless youth. *American Behavioral Scientist, 51*(6), 756–771.
Snyder, L. A., Bertone, E. R., Jakowski, R. M., Dooner, M. S., Jennings-Ritchie, J., & Moore, A. S. (2004). p53 expression and environmental tobacco smoke exposure in feline oral squamous cell carcinoma. *Veterinary Pathology, 41*, 209–214.
Staats, S., Miller, D., Carnot, M. J., Rada, K., & Turnes, J. (1996). The Miller-Rada commitment to pets scale. *Anthrozoös, 9*, 88–94.
Taylor, H., Williams, P., & Gray, D. (2004). Homelessness and dog ownership: An investigation into animal empathy, attachment, crime, drug use, health and public opinion. *Anthrozoös, 17*(4), 353–368.

Thompson, S. J., McManus, H., Lantry, J., Windsor, L., & Flynn, P. (2006a). Insights from the street: Perceptions of services and providers by homeless young adults. *Organizational Learning, 29*(1), 34–43. doi:10.1016/j.evalprogplan.2005.09.001.

Thompson, S. J., McManus, H., Lantry, J., Windsor, L., & Flynn, P. (2006b). Insights from the street: Perceptions of services and providers by homeless young adults. *Evaluation and Program Planning, 29*(1), 34–43. doi:10.1016/j.evalprogplan.2005.09.001.

Thompson, S. J., McManus, H., & Voss, T. (2006c). Posttraumatic stress disorder and substance abuse among youth who are homeless: Treatment issues and implications. *Brief Treatment and Crisis Intervention, 6*(3), 206–217.

Thompson, S. J., Ryan, T. N., Montgomery, K. L., Lippman, A. D. P., Bender, K., & Ferguson, K. (2013). Perceptions of resiliency and coping: Homeless young adults speak out. *Youth & Society,*. doi:10.1177/0044118X13477427.

Tobacco Use and the Homeless. (2009). Retrieved January 28, 2015, 2014 from http://www.nationalhomeless.org/factsheets/tobacco.pdf

Tucker, J., Edelen, M., Ellickson, P., & Klein, D. (2011). Running away from home: A longitudinal study of adolescent risk factors and young adult outcomes. *Journal of Youth and Adolescence, 40*(5), 507–518. doi:10.1007/s10964-010-9571-0.

Tucker, J. S., Shadel, W. G., Golinelli, D., & Ewing, B. (2014). Alternative tobacco product use and smoking cessation among homeless youth in Los Angeles County. *Nicotine & Tobacco Research,*. doi:10.1093/ntr/ntu133.

Tyler, K. A., Akinyemi, S. L., & Kort-Butler, L. A. (2012). Correlates of service utilization among homeless youth. *Children and Youth Services Review, 34*(7), 1344–1350. doi:10.1016/j.childyouth.2012.03.010.

Tyler, K. A., & Beal, M. R. (2010). The high-risk environment of homeless young adults: Consequences for physical and sexual victimization. *Violence and Victims, 25*(1), 101–115.

van Helden, P. D., van Helden, L. S., & Hoal, E. G. (2013). One world, one health. Humans, animals and the environment are inextricably linked—A fact that needs to be remembered and exploited in our modern approach to health. *EMBO Reports, 14*(6), 497–501. doi:10.1038/embor.2013.61.

Vaughn Heineman, T. (2010). Relationships beget relationships: Why understanding attachment theory is critical to program design for homeless youth. *California Homeless Youth Project.* Sacramento, CA: CA Research Bureau & CA State Library.

Wenzel, S., Holloway, I., Golinelli, D., Ewing, B., Bowman, R., & Tucker, J. (2012). Social networks of homeless youth in emerging adulthood. *Journal of Youth and Adolescence, 41*(5), 561–571. doi:10.1007/s10964-011-9709-8.

Wenzel, S. L., Tucker, J. S., Golinelli, D., Green, H. D., & Zhou, A. (2010). Personal network correlates of alcohol, cigarette, and marijuana use among homeless youth. *Drug and Alcohol Dependence, 112*(1–2), 140–149. doi:10.1016/j.drugalcdep.2010.06.004.

Wood, L. J. (2011). *Community benefits of human–animal interactions…The ripple effect.* Baltimore, MD, USA: Paul H Brookes Publishing.

Wood, L., Giles-Corti, B., & Bulsara, M. (2005). The pet connection: Pets as a conduit for social capital? *Social Science & Medicine, 61*(6), 1159–1173. doi:10.1016/j.socscimed.2005.01.017.

Wood, L. J., Giles-Corti, B., Bulsara, M. K., & Bosch, D. A. (2007). More than a furry companion: The ripple effect of companion animals on neighborhood interactions and sense of community. *Society & Animals, 15*(1), 43–56. doi:10.1163/156853007X169333ER.

Wrobel, T. A., & Dye, A. L. (2003). Grieving pet death: Normative, gender, and attachment issues. *Journal of Death and Dying, 47*(4), 385–393.

Yamaya, Y., Sugiya, H., & Watari, T. (2014). Tobacco exposure increased airway limitation in dogs with chronic cough. *Veterinary Record, 174*(1), 18.

Zilcha-Mano, S., Mikulincer, M., & Shaver, P. R. (2012). Pets as safe havens and secure bases: The moderating role of pet attachment orientations. *Journal of Research in Personality, 46*(5), 571–580. doi:10.1016/j.jrp.2012.06.005.

Zimolag, U., & Krupa, T. (2009). Pet ownership as a meaningful community occupation for people with serious mental illness. *The American Journal of Occupational Therapy, 63*(2), 126–137.

Chapter 5
A Boy's Best Friend: Using Human–Animal Interaction with At-Risk Teen Boys

Jessica Thomas

Introduction

According to the Office of Juvenile Justice and Delinquency Prevention the number of juvenile cases handled in a single year has increased nearly 50 % in the last two decades, where cases involving males now represent well over two-thirds of all delinquency cases nationwide (Sickmund 2009). Additionally, once incarcerated, 50–77 % of these young offenders are being identified as having Conduct Disorder (Fazel et al. 2008; Stahlberg et al. 2010), a disorder known for its higher prevalence in males, disregard for others, lacking prosocial emotions and poorer prognosis (American Psychiatric Association 2013). Combined, this steady increase in delinquency cases and high prevalence of serious pathology, demonstrates a real need for innovate proactive interventions to perhaps inhibit escalation into serious crime, by intervening at the emotional level for these boys. While imperative, such goals are difficult to attain; a report commissioned by the United States Surgeon General (2001) for example, found that nearly half of all violence prevention programs and strategies evaluated, were ineffectual or even damaging to the youth they proposed to assist. Compounding this conundrum of "what we have isn't working," quite often just simply engaging these at-risk youth, particularly the teen boys, can be complex if not outright difficult for clinicians due to barriers caused by previous negative interactions with adults and resulting generalized mistrust. As such, there is a need for something uniquely different.

J. Thomas (✉)
The Chicago School of Professional Psychology, Los Angeles, California, United States
e-mail: jxkthomas@gmail.com

C. Blazina and L.R. Kogan (eds.), *Men and Their Dogs*,
DOI 10.1007/978-3-319-30097-9_5

Purpose of the Study

The study presented in this chapter will explore the use of human–animal interaction (HAI), specifically interactions with a shelter dog, as a unique means of intervening with at-risk teen boys, holding immense promise in fostering their emotional and intrapersonal growth as evidenced by the resulting highly significant findings. These interactions with dogs appear to offer the boys something they had perhaps not fully attained through human interactions; a relationship devoid of judgment, lacking social pretenses or gender-based assumptions, and offered by the dogs free of any emotional coercion or expectations for the boys. Further, these positive quantitative outcomes are part of larger results formally collected during an eight month study which was conducted by the author (see Thomas 2014) and reflect changes and significant intrapersonal growth that occurred in as little as three weeks for the male participants.

Definitions: When we discuss intrapersonal growth, we are specifically speaking about improving a distinct part of these boys' overall emotional intelligence. Using Bar-On's model of Emotional and Social Intelligence (2006), we understand the larger construct of emotional intelligence as made up of several overlapping social and emotional competencies or skills which can work in concert to influence how effectively someone understands or relates emotionally and ultimately adapts or copes with daily stressors. The intrapersonal dimension, like the others which make up overall emotional intelligence, can be honed or developed, is subject to growth if fostered and can be reliably measured. Further, according to Bar-On and Parker (2000) this dynamic intrapersonal dimension is made up of various related abilities or skills such as; accurately perceiving, understanding and accepting oneself (self-regard), recognizing and understanding one's own feelings (emotional self-awareness), effectively and constructively expressing one's feelings, thoughts and beliefs (assertiveness), freedom from emotional dependency with the ability to be self-directed in thought or behavior (independence), as well as striving to realize and achieve one's personal goals (self-actualization).

Combined these abilities, if fostered, could therefore result in true intrapersonal growth. Which, for the purposes of this chapter, simply represent the measured development or growth of these five distinct intrapersonal abilities. The outcome of which, may reflect a young person who is seen as more introspective and self-directive as well as more able to understand, express and effectively communicate their needs and feelings to others. But how does one develop into such an emotionally aware and self-reflective individual, particularly as an at-risk teen who is simultaneously dealing with very real psychosocial stressors and risk factors such as poor school performance or drop out, low parental nurturance and monitoring, and living in high crime neighborhoods? Further, how can interacting with a dog possibly help these boys transcend the effects of poor attachment models and constricted masculine role expectations, enhance development of these skills in themselves and in turn, perhaps better engage with other people?

To truly understand the use of HAI as such an intervention with the teen boys, it will be important to first briefly examine the historical use of the human–animal bond, particularly with children—while such application may seem novel, it is certainly not new. After presenting the research findings, the application of a theoretical context using Bowlby's Attachment Theory (1969, 1973, 1988) will be explored in an effort to provide a potential framework for how the efficacy of HAI within the study, may be understood specifically for the at-risk teen boys.

Animals and Children from Past to Present

With more than 12,000 years of known cohabitation, the human–animal relationship has held meaning for centuries (Schaefer 2002). While initially driven by survival, ancient and historical examples of the perceived positive influence of HAIs on human mental and physical health are plentiful (see Serpell 2010). Further, HAI researchers have suggested a particularly special bond with children (Melson 2001; Melson and Fine 2011). Ancient examples of the bond with boys in particular have for example, been noted and documented by both researchers and anthropologists alike. Whereby, some of the earliest known evidence of this bond and the domestication of dogs, was unearthed by archeologists (Davis and Valla 1978) in Northern Israel as the striking image of a small 12,000 year old skeleton of what many believe to be a boy, who was buried with his puppy.

With children, the documented influence of this affectionate bond becomes particularly apparent during the late seventeenth century, where companion animals were believed to enhance a child's socialization. Writers such as John Lock (1699, as cited in Serpell 2010) touted the use of animals as a means of enhancing a child's emotional growth and increased understanding of responsibility by caring for another living being. This idea of children learning more socially acceptable means of interacting through compassion and sensitivity was also seen during the Victorian era. In fact, in their efforts to strive for virtuous morality, the children of the Victorian era were encouraged to care for animals so that they could learn more about their own 'beastly qualities' (Grier 1999). By seeking to minimize these qualities in themselves, the children were believed be better able to strive for "kindness all around" (Sigourney 1838 as cited in Grier 1999). This idea of learning what it is to be a virtuous human from interactions with an animal is truly profound and will be revisited as we progress toward the results of the study, which in essence, supports this notion.

In more recent history, the formal therapeutic use of HAI with children can be easily traced back to Levinson (1969). Dr. Levinson stumbled upon the benefits of using his dog, Jingles, with a particularly difficult child client and ultimately began documenting the benefits. In his research, Levinson (1969, 1978) discussed his theory that animals may serve as transitional attachment objects in therapy, to which the young patients he worked with may identify with, project onto and ultimately emotionally bond with due to the nonthreatening, unconditional emotional companionship they offered. This attachment, he proposed, may then be expanded to include humans. Not so dissimilar to the use of companion animals during the Victorian era as a means of fostering those idyllic prosocial behaviors for children, here Levinson suggested that relational interactions with animals may come to inform ideal relationships with other humans and even with themselves. Whereby, acting as a seemingly model relationship, Levinson believed that interaction with the animal offers a child the opportunity, "to move away from his egocentric view of the world and can recognize his common humanity with others. Treated with adequate love and respect he will come to love and respect himself and then extend those feelings to others as he recognizes that they are like him" (Levinson 1978, p. 1036). Further, through the human–animal bond developed with a companion animal, Levinson proposed several positive impacts on personality development for the child; promoting self-confidence, efficacy and self-control as well as fostering nurturing qualities such as compassion and empathy (Levinson 1978). Whereby, this proposed development is remarkably similar to the exact abilities and skills afore-described as making up the intrapersonal dimension of emotional intelligence.

Moving into the present, several contemporary HAI researchers have surveyed the immense significance of animals in the lives of children (Fawcett and Gullone 2001; Melson 2001, 2003; Melson and Fine 2010), and frequently call for more empirical exploration of the benefits of those interactions. Such empirical research is necessary to provide much needed support for the formal application of HAI as a viable and effective intervention, rather than simple novelty, particularly for young populations which may be difficult to reach utilizing traditional therapeutic means. As of this publication for example, only three such published studies are known to this author to exist involving the use of HAI with juvenile offenders. While varying in methodological rigor, these studies (Harbolt and Ward 2001; Cournoyer and Uttley 2007; Davis 2007), each involving the use of HAI with young male offenders, have, however, found that the interactions provide excellent opportunities for emotional and intrapersonal growth for the boys. While employing largely qualitative measures and not proactive in their intervention, the positive results of these studies provide important information regarding the possible efficacy of HAI, if perhaps applied prior to these boys' first criminal offense. While equally as scant, a few recent studies have also begun to examine the interaction as it relates to faucets of emotional intelligence for youth. For example, researchers in Vienna (Burger et al. 2009; Turner et al. 2009; Stetina 2011) have specifically demonstrated measured increases in both emotional recognition and regulation, two important emotional intelligence abilities, when utilizing HAI in structured groups for youth of varied ages. While scarce, such studies also inform the research presented in this chapter, whereby, HAI has yet to be examined as a proactive intervention with at-risk teen boys by enhancing their intrapersonal functioning and abilities. As such, the effect involvement in a formal HAI program had on the measured intrapersonal functioning of identified at-risk teen boys was explored and presented here.

Research Question and Hypothesis

From this we arrive at our larger overarching research question and resulting hypothesis to be tested, that is; what effect does involvement in a formal HAI program have on the intrapersonal abilities of identified at-risk teen boys? More specifically, will there be an increase in intrapersonal functioning as measured by the Intrapersonal Scale on the Emotional Quotient Inventory: Youth Version (EQ-i: YV; Bar-On and Parker 2000) from pre to post-HAI intervention?

Hypothesis 1: There will be a change in intrapersonal functioning, as measured by the Intrapersonal Scale of the EQ-i:YV, from pre-intervention testing to post-intervention testing.

Methods

Participants: As part of a larger study (Thomas 2014), this researcher collected data from all consenting participants involved in a formal HAI program during a single year. This data was ultimately collected across five, three week HAI class cycles. Presented here, we will focus specifically on the male ($N = 21$) participants, aged 13–18 years old, and their measured intrapersonal functioning. Information was gathered from the participants via a created self-report demographic questionnaire. Based on demographic data gathered from the sample (Table 5.1), the mean age of the male participants was 16.33 years old (SD = 1.35). Further, most of the participants ($n = 14$) reported being in the continuation high school system for up to six months, with just over one-third (33.3 %) reporting this educational placement for six months to two years. Neither racial nor ethnic data was collected from the participants.

Table 5.1 Descriptive statistics and frequency distribution of male participants ($n = 21$)

	M	SD	Frequency	Percent
Age of participant (years)	16.33	1.35		
13 years old			1	4.8
14 years old			2	9.5
15 years old			1	4.8
16 years old			5	23.8
17 years old			9	42.9
18 years old			3	14.3
Length of time in continuation high school				
0–6 months			14	66.7
6 months–1 year			3	14.3
1–2 years			4	19.0

Program Description: All of the study participants were involved in a formal HAI program called k9 Connection, a program which targets at-risk youth from various continuation high schools and alternative educational or residential placements in the greater Los Angeles area. The youth were referred to the program by school personnel and/or volunteered to participate but each class was limited to no greater than eight students and eight dogs. Each of the five separate HAI class cycles met on-site at their school or host site, two hours a day, five days per week for the three weeks (totaling approximately 30 intervention hours for each boy). During that time each student was paired with a shelter dog and tasked with training the dog to increase their prospective adoptability from the shelter. As such, for the first of the two hours the students trained the dogs (e.g., obedience, agility, tricks) as a part of a group led by a trainer and in the second hour the youth along with their dogs, attended a group led by program facilitators. At the end of each of the three week class cycles, a graduation was held to allow the youth to demonstrate the training and goals achieved in a ceremony for their peers and teachers or invited supportive others. During these graduation ceremonies each participant also made a speech reflecting on their time in the program and with their dog. Each dog was then placed up for adoption, and ultimately adopted through their respective shelter or rescue group.

Measures: A brief self-report demographic questionnaire was created by the author to gather demographic characteristics of the youth (e.g., age, gender, length of time in continuation high school system) and adequately describe the sample.

Data regarding the boys' intrapersonal abilities was assessed utilizing the Emotional Quotient Inventory: Youth Version (EQ-i: YV; Bar-On and Parker 2000) a 60 item self-report instrument which has been empirically validated and is widely used to measure emotional intelligence across various scales for youth aged 7–18 years old. One such scale, the Intrapersonal Scale, which is a composite of several afore described intrapersonal skills (self-regard, emotional self-awareness, assertiveness, independence, and self-actualization), was utilized here to measure intrapersonal functioning. When assessing the intrapersonal construct, participants were presented with questions such as, "I can easily describe my feelings" or "when I get angry, I act without thinking" and asked to respond by selecting the most appropriate response, using a 4-point Likert scale ranging from "very seldom true of me" to "very often true of me."

Test-makers of the EQ-i:YV (Bar-On and Parker 2000) report acceptable validity and reliability for the measure, whereby, the Intrapersonal Scale on the assessment maintains internal consistency estimates of reliability from 0.81 for males age 13–15 years old and 0.83 for males age 16–18 years old. Additionally, test-retest reliability coefficient, for the Intrapersonal Scale, for an interim of 3 weeks, is reported by the test-makers to be 0.84. Further, the EQ-i:YV requires only a 4th grade reading level, is ideal for repeat administration to assess effectiveness of interventions over time and may be administered in groups. As such, the data discussed here will reflect the intrapersonal scores obtained from the male participants before beginning the HAI program and again upon completion, three weeks later; utilizing the Intrapersonal Scale score on the EQ-i:YV.

Procedures: As part of IRB approval for the larger study (Thomas 2014), permission to conduct the study was obtained and data was collected during an interval of one year, spanning five k9 Connection class cycles. Prior to beginning each class cycle, signed Informed Consent and Minor Assent forms were collected from each prospective participant. After this was secured, the first pre-HAI intervention administration of the EQ-i:YV (Bar-On and Parker 2000) and the demographic questionnaire were given in a group setting by the author. At the end of the three week class, the EQ-i:YV (Bar-On and Parker 2000) was re-administered in a group setting by the author, resulting in the participants post-HAI intervention scores. This procedure was repeated for each of the five class cycles during the data collection interval.

Data Preparation and Statistics: Random assignment to the treatment group was not feasible given referral and voluntary participation in the program. Additionally, the use of a control or comparison group, while attempted, was not possible for this study. As such, the current study was carried out utilizing a quasi-experimental, within subject, repeated measure (pre/post) design. All data collected was coded and analyzed utilizing The Statistical Package for the Social Sciences (SPSS-20).

Prior to running any inferential statistics, scores were tested and confirmed for normality and validity for all observations and data collected in the larger study, as is a perquisite assumption for the use of a paired-samples *t*-test analysis. This information is beyond the scope of this chapter but can be found elsewhere (see Thomas 2014). Following confirmation of normality for all observations of the variables assessed as part of the larger study and exploratory data analyses of demographic data collected, paired-samples *t*-tests were then utilized to determine whether the difference between the mean scores collected from pre to post-HAI intervention assessment, indicated a statistically significant difference resulting from the intervention. Specifically for this chapter, the paired-samples *t*-test analysis was used to determine whether the difference between the mean Intrapersonal Scale scores collected from pre-HAI intervention (pretest) to post-HAI intervention (posttest) indicate a statistically significant difference. Additionally, effect size was calculated to determine the effect or magnitude of the measured change.

Results

A paired-samples *t*-test was conducted to compare overall intrapersonal functioning before and after participation in the formal HAI program (Table 5.2). The results of this test found for a significant increase in overall intrapersonal functioning from the Intrapersonal pretest summary score ($M = 98.71$, SD = 14.44) to the Intrapersonal posttest summary score ($M = 108.61$, SD = 13.61) $t\ (20) = -4.24$, $p = 0.000$. These results suggest that participation in the formal HAI program significantly increased intrapersonal functioning for the at-risk teen boys, as measured by the EQ-i:YV (Bar-On and Parker 2000). Further, with an effect size

Table 5.2 Results from t-test assessing intrapersonal functioning ($n = 21$)

	M	SD	t	d	p
Pretest intrapersonal score	98.71	14.44	−4.24	0.92	0.000
Posttest intrapersonal score	108.61	13.61			

($d = 0.92$) calculated as "large" using Cohen's guidelines (1969), the increase represents a difference of nearly one full standard deviation, on average, for the male teen participants.

Discussion

In support of the hypothesis, the author was able to measure the effect, involvement in a formal HAI program had on the intrapersonal abilities of identified at-risk teen boys. In doing so, it was found that a highly significant and meaningful improvement in intrapersonal functioning was made after the three week group HAI intervention. These findings, in combination with the larger results, expand previous research using HAI as an effective intervention with at-risk youth, particularly at-risk teen boys.

Anecdotal Themes: As previously discussed, the intrapersonal construct of emotional intelligence is made up of various related abilities or skills (self-regard, emotional self-awareness, assertiveness, independence, and self-actualization), which aide in self-expression and awareness. While not a mixed methods study, per se, stunning examples of these developing skills were frequently noted as themes by this author in observing the boys and dogs, whereby, they truly support the measured highly significant change in intrapersonal functioning presented in this chapter. As such, the noted expressions of the participants, during their graduation speeches, are offered informally to further substantiate, support and further the discussion of the quantitative results.

Self-Regard and Emotional Self-Awareness: For example, several of the boys noted mutual growth and insightfully identified aspects of themselves in their partnered dogs. Here for instance, one of the boys shares how proud he is of his dog, but in doing so demonstrates intrapersonal skills such as self-regard and emotional self-awareness as he likens the dogs' process to his own, so much so that it becomes easy to forget if he is speaking about the dog or about his own progress:

> Stitch[1] is my best bud and [he] has made so much progress; he's practically a different dog now. When we started k9 together Stitch was too much of a handful, doing stuff his way and running around as he pleased, ignoring commands. Now he can't wait to learn a new trick…he is a great listener…he's been taught so much during this program and I'm so proud of him for overcoming his anxious behavior. He was a lot like a younger me

[1]Names of the dogs have been changed to further protect the confidentiality of the boys that worked with them.

> when he began, with huge attention problems and was so anxious around others, probably preferring people to dogs; and during this program he's made a huge leap in recovery.

Assertiveness and Self-actualization: Other intrapersonal themes noted were that of both assertiveness and self-actualization skills, where the boys would remark on having to learn to effectively express themselves with their dog to aide in achieving the goals they had for them, harnessing that developing emotional self-awareness. Frequently they described how this involved developing and practicing patience, a complex emotion which involves not only regulation but inhibition and delayed gratification. One boy beautifully illustrates this as he described his work and progress in working with his dog, Palmer.

> At first Palmer was just getting to know me and was treat motivated; now he listens to commands without treats! The first time we worked on tunnels he was terrified of going in until I had to stick my head in the other end to help him through…now he goes happily. Patience is a huge necessity for training anything…no one starts off perfect but they can work to be perfect.

Independence: Building on this even further, some of the boys also made remarks which indicated the addition of the intrapersonal skill of independence. This theme was frequently noted in conjunction with the others, where it appeared that through the enhanced emotional self-awareness, learned assertive expression and strive to achieve goals with the dogs these boys could also develop the confidence to be self-directed. One boy truly illustrates each of these noted themes as he shared about his dog, Doogie, and the progress they made:

> He has a very independent mindset but also has a very sweet puppy-like attitude. When he came to me he didn't even know how to sit on command or even look at me. Now he can jump hurdles and come on command. I got to be very excited for this dog. I see myself in his eyes and know he will find a forever home. One of my favorite days…was when I shouted out with joy because Doogie finally sat on command! I had been trying to teach him to sit for days and he finally did it. Doogie is a great dog…because Doogie is more like a brother than a dog [and he] helped me through all of this giving me the confidence I needed.

Providing further support for the presented significant quantitative results, these anecdotes are offered to, in effect, provide a more personal illustration of the intrapersonal growth and functioning that the teen boys experienced following the HAI intervention. In combination with the presented quantitative results it seems evident that in working with the dogs, these boys not only developed their capacity to understand, accept and express themselves emotionally but also reflect and integrate that understanding into goal-directed behavior—an astonishing feat in just three weeks.

Attachment Theory: To truly understand how such a significant change could occur with these teen boys, the application of a theoretical context may prove useful. Using contemporary psychoanalytic perspectives such as Bowlby's Attachment Theory (1969, 1988), we understand that a child, in response to their caregiver's availability, consistency and responsivity to their needs, comes to develop a way to view the world as well as a way of viewing themselves. These resulting internal working models, Bowlby (1973) proposed, then come to influence the processing of important socially relevant information as well as how the child may come to engage in future relationships. Such that, when the child's caregiver is unavailable or inconsistent in responding to those needs, an insecure attachment and thus insecure framework for viewing future relationships can emerge. It stands to reason then, that by spending a disproportionate amount of time being concerned about their safety or mistrusting their environment, that these at-risk youth may then grow up lacking the full development of their self-reflective capacity (Ansbro 2008), hindering their ability to grow intrapersonally and both think and reflect on their own feelings. This emotional underdevelopment may also in turn greatly affect their ability to self-regulate, leading to the reactive or aggressive behaviors seen in many of the youth who are at greatest risk of escalation into crime. While typically focused on human caregivers as attachment figures, what if animals, or dogs as seen in the current study, could aide in fostering this underdevelopment through the attachment or bond they develop—particularly if those human attachment relationships have perhaps been unfulfilling?

While attachment research has historically focused on human caregivers as attachment figures, HAI researchers have begun to discuss the applicability of such models to relational interactions with animals, just as Levinson proposed decades ago. Researchers have found that meaningful results can, for example, be obtained when applying a human attachment model and essential attachment characteristics such as proximity maintenance, secure base and safe haven to animal relationships. In fact, in doing so we now understand that not only can pets be perceived with features or qualities of traditionally "human-only" attachment figures, but that they can also be perceived as a consistent source of attachment security or relational support (Beck and Madresh 2008; Kurdek 2009). Similarly, within self psychology, the relationship with a companion animal has been classified as serving a "self object" function for owners, which may provide for their self-cohesion, self-esteem, calm, soothing, and acceptance needs not unlike an empathic mother during childhood (Brown 2007). Here, animals were seen as able to support and enhance the complex emotional needs of their human, with even greater efficacy as that of a human–human interaction.

Finally, with children, just as Levinson proposed, animals may hold immense opportunities as transitional attachment objects, frequently seen as "living security blankets" (Triebenbacher 1998, p. 192). Originally discussed by Winnicott (1953) such objects serve as supplemental attachment figures to assist the child in transitioning between self and the outside world and adapt to the needs of that child much like a "good enough mother." For children, animals may therefore provide opportunities for mutual love and affection as well as a comfort, security, satisfaction, protection and security particularly if adult attachment relationships have been unsatisfying or strained. As such, it stands to reason that if a child has unfulfilling human attachment models, perhaps integration of the use of animals via HAI may assist in supporting enhanced emotional growth and intrapersonal development.

Although relatively stable across a lifetime, attachment style is not necessarily fixed (Bowlby 1973, 1988). Whereby an individual's actual attachment orientation has actually been found to change based on both context and experience (Pietromonaco et al. 2002) and activation of a congruent attachment orientation may occur following real or imagined encounters with others (Mikulincer and Shaver 2001). Further, we understand that exposure to factors or relationships which challenge maladaptive internal representations, such as the HAI with the dogs in the current research, can in fact, act as a corrective experience. In fact, researchers propose that exposure to these corrective experiences may alter the resulting maladaptive functioning (Shorey and Snyder 2006). In so doing the teen boy is afforded an opportunity to re-experience the relational interaction differently, in an effort to perhaps correct, challenge and repair those previous internal working models. Applied here, the interactions with the dogs may then have provided the teen boys an opportunity to engage in a bonded relationship which served to foster their emotional growth, activated a congruent attachment orientation and perhaps challenged maladaptive working models about relationships with others.

Gender Socialization and Emotional Intelligence: Research has demonstrated that insecure attachment promotes mistrust, poor sociability and externalizing behavioral problems (Thompson 1999; Fearon et al. 2010) as well as being linked to an overly hostile cognitive attributional style in aggressive youth (Dodge 2006). Further compounding this for adolescent males, we understand that adherence to traditionally masculine ideology, such as restricting emotionality and affection, has also been linked to psychological or emotional distress as well as ineffectual anger management and conduct problems (Blazina et al. 2005; Watts and Borders 2005). Such restricted emotionality would therefore appear to negatively impact the development of various emotional intelligence competencies for young boys, particularly, the intrapersonal abilities measured in the current study, but how might this happen?

Schemas about gender are particularly prevalent in development, coming to shape how an individual, as a male or female, comes to think about and assimilate into their sense of self a particular subset of behaviors or attitudes. Such schemas built upon insecure attachment relationships and model relationships, however, may then also be distorted or extremely polarized. Where gender polarization specifically, is believed to create mutually exclusive scripts for males and females (Bem 1993). That is, that men cannot have similar qualities as women; if a woman is to be nurturing, submissive and emotionally expressive, then a man must be the opposite—exuding power, demanding control and restricting their emotionality. Such polarization and extreme adherence to constricted traditional male gender roles can, however, be in conflict with what these boys actually want intrinsically, that is, to be emotionally expressive and engage in a relationship where they are free from fear or emotional distress. This gender role conflict can be harmful in its rigidity and restriction (O'Neil 2008) and has been found to cause significant and measurable stress; for example, a situation is viewed as requiring behavior more aligned with feminine and thus "unmanly" attributes, such as open emotional expression (Eisler and Skidmore 1987). Strikingly, however, dogs know nothing about such emotional and cognitive processes or socially created gender roles and expectations. As such, these very pretenses about masculinity, relational interactions and gender roles appear to be absent or greatly minimized for the boys in the interactions with their dogs allowing them to explore, practice and ultimately develop such intrapersonal skills in a more 'gender role neutral' context. Such a corrective emotional experience, where these skills can be practiced relationally within the safe context of the HAI with the dogs, thus appears to provide a very real milieu for exacting highly significant intrapersonal growth and emotional development for these teen boys.

Limitations

While the findings from this study are highly significant and meaningful, limitations are present. The use of self and teacher referred youth, who voluntarily participated in the k9 Connection program, may have resulted in an unintentional selection bias of the teen participants. As such, their willingness and motivation to participate in the HAI program may have positively inflated outcomes. The small, male-only sample size of this study may also limit application of the findings to larger at-risk youth populations; however, given the identification of the large effect size, this limitation was minimized. Additionally, the findings of the larger study (Thomas 2014) reflect significant results collected from both at-risk teen male and female participants. Nevertheless, additional data collection using larger sample sizes would be recommended in the future to further minimize the likelihood of spurious findings.

In addition to limitation due to sample size, the current study did not collect any information regarding race or ethnicity. While done purposefully to minimize any potential defenses, collecting this information in future studies may allow for increased generalizability of findings to specifically identified racial or ethnic groups. Whereby, examining the presence of any varied effects by race or ethnicity may also provide useful information for the specific application of using HAI with diverse at-risk youth.

The lacking comparison or control group for the current study also represents a limitation. Despite efforts to include a wait-listed control group for the current study, there was simply not an adequate number of controls available and willing to complete both the pre and post assessments without participation in the program. As such, it is difficult to rule out any possible misattribution of the findings to the effect of meeting with the dog versus the effect of meeting with the human facilitators or even their peers, five times a week, two hours a day, for three weeks. Incorporation of a comparison or control group for future studies may provide further value to the current findings by seeking to control for these outside influences.

Finally, the current findings represent a change that was noted after only three weeks of intervention, but longitudinal data was not collected to measure if the change held up over time. While the HAI intervention may seem short in duration, the actual number of intervention hours for the three weeks total approximately 30 hours across 15 sessions, which is analogous to the average number of sessions attended within a large study of leading evidenced-based therapy models (Hansen et al. 2002). Unlike leading evidenced-based models, data regarding maintenance of treatment gains over time was not able to be collected in the current study, however. As such, incorporation of additional follow-up measurement for future studies would be beneficial in minimizing this limitation and adding value to the current findings by determining if and to what extent the treatment gains measured here, were maintained over time.

Conclusions and Future Directions

With the growing increase in delinquency cases, high prevalence of serious pathology for young incarcerated males and lack of effective prevention programs nationwide there is a real need for innovate proactive interventions. Such interventions are needed in the hopes of perhaps inhibiting escalation into serious crime, by intervening at the emotional level with at-risk teen boys. As evidenced by the outcomes of current study the use of HAI with at-risk teen boys could in fact be such an intervention. The use of HAI as an intervention, as implemented here with shelter dogs, may offer these boys a unique opportunity to reexperience an intimate relational interaction differently, challenging and combating previous maladaptive internal working models and allowing for emotional growth within the attachment bond developed with a dog. Free from fear or judgment about relational expectations or constricted gender-based social pretenses, these boys appear to be able to practice intrapersonal skills with the dogs, who ask for very little in return.

This idea that interactions with dogs may, in effect, teach these boys what it is to be effectively human is astonishing. As a result of the HAI, we see that the boys were better able to be emotionally self-aware, recognizing and understanding their feelings as well as effectively and assertively expressing those feelings more freely. Further we see that they were also able to accurately perceive and accept themselves, holding increased self-regard while striving to realize and actualize goals. Such self-reflection and emotional awareness are truly and undoubtedly central to our human nature—but here, this emotional growth was learned, in effect, from interactions with dogs.

With thousands of years of interactions with animals, the field of HAI is, however, very much still in its infancy. Similarly, while the relational interactions with animals appear to hold immense promise with children in particular, there is need for more empirical studies. As such, the research conducted and presented here demonstrates highly significant results with very respectable effect size, where it appears that working with the dogs in the formal HAI program meaningfully improved the measured intrapersonal functioning for the boys in the study. While positive, limitations certainly exist for the research presented, however, as replication of the study using a larger sample, comparison/control group and perhaps a longitudinal design may further demonstrate the significance by decreasing the likelihood of spurious findings and minimize the effect any extraneous factors had, on the results. As such, further study is absolutely necessary in an effort to continue to build the much needed empirical base for the use of HAI across populations, and especially for at-risk teen boys.

References

American Psychiatric Association. (2013). *Diagnostic and statistical manual of mental disorders: DSM-5*. Washington, DC: Author.

Ansbro, M. (2008). Using attachment theory with offenders. *Probation Journal, 55*, 231–244.

Bar-On, R. (2006). The Bar-On model of emotional-social intelligence (ESI). *Psicothema, 18*, 13–25.

Bar-On, R., & Parker, J. D. A. (2000). *Bar-On emotional quotient inventory: Youth version (EQ-i: YV) technical manual*. North Tonawanda, NY: Multi-Health Systems.

Beck, L., & Madresh, E. A. (2008). Romantic partners and four-legged friends: An extension of attachment theory to relationships with pets. *Anthrozoos, 21*, 43–56.

Bem, S. L. (1993). *The lenses of gender: Transforming the debate on sexual equality*. New Haven, CT: Yale University Press.

Blazina, C., Pisecco, S., & O'Neil, J. M. (2005). An adaptation of the gender role conflict scale for adolescents: Psychometric issues and correlates with psychological distress. *Psychology of Men & Masculinity, 6*, 39–45.

Bowlby, J. (1969). *Attachment and loss: Attachment* (Vol. 1). New York: Basic Books.

Bowlby, J. (1973). *Attachment and loss: Separation* (Vol. 2). New York: Basic Books.

Bowlby, J. (1988). *A secure base: Clinical applications of attachment theory*. London: Routledge.

Burger, E., Stetina, B. U., Turner, K., Lederman-Maman, T., Handlos, U., & Kryspin-Exner, I. (2009). Changes in emotion regulation and recognition in adolescents: Improvements during animal-assisted training. *Journal of Veterinary Behavior, 4*, 92–93.

Brown, S. E. (2007). Companion animals as selfobjects. *Anthrozoos, 20*, 329–343.

Cohen, J. (1969). *Statistical power analysis for the behavioral sciences*. San Diego, CA: Academic Press.

Cournoyer, G. P., & Uttley, C. M. (2007). Cisco's kid's: A pet assisted therapy intervention program. *Journal of Emotional Abuse, 7*, 117–126.

Davis, K. (2007). *Perspectives of youth in animal centered correctional vocational program: A qualitative evaluation of project pooch*. Paper presented at the National Technology Assessment Conference on Animal Assisted Programs for Youth at Risk, Baltimore, MD.

Davis, S. J. M., & Valla, F. R. (1978). Evidence for domestication of the dog 12,000 years ago in the Natufian of Israel. *Nature, 276*, 608–610.

Dodge, K. A. (2006). Translational science in action: Hostile attributional style and the development of aggressive behavior problems. *Developmental Psychopathology, 18*, 791–814.

Eisler, R. M., & Skidmore, J. R. (1987). Masculine gender role stress: Scale development and component factors in the appraisal of stressful situations. *Behavior Modification, 11*, 123–136.

Fearon, R. P., Bakermans-Kranenburg, M. J., Van IJzendoorn, M. H., Lapsley, A. M., & Roisman, G. I. (2010). The significance of insecure attachment and disorganization in the development of children's externalizing behavior: A meta-analytic study. *Child Development, 81*, 435–456.

Fawcett, N. R., & Gullone, E. (2001). Cute cuddly and a whole lot more? A call for empirical investigation into the therapeutic benefits for human–animal interaction for children. *Behaviour Change, 18*, 124–133.

Fazel, S., Doll, H., & Langstrom, N. (2008). Mental disorders among adolescents in juvenile detention and correctional facilities: A systematic review and metaregression analysis of 25 surveys. *The Journal of the American Academy of Child and Adolescent Psychiatry, 47*, 1010–1019.

Grier, K. C. (1999) Childhood socialization and companion animals: United States, 1820–1870. *Animals and Society, 7*, 95–120.

Hansen, N. B., Lambert, M. J., & Foreman, E. M. (2002). The psychotherapy dose-response effect and it's implications for treatment delivery services. *Clinical Psychology: Science and Practice, 9*, 329–343.

Harbolt, T., & Ward, T. H. (2001). Teaming incarcerated youth with shelter dogs for a second chance. *Animals and Society, 9*, 177–182.

Kurdek, L. A. (2009). Pet dogs as attachment figures for adult owners. *Journal of Family Psychology, 23*, 439–449.

Levinson, B. M. (1969). *Pet-oriented child psychotherapy*. Springfield, IL: Charles C. Thomas.

Levinson, B. M. (1978). Pets and personality development. *Psychological Reports, 42*, 1031–1038.

Melson, G. F. (2001). *Why the wild things are: Animals in the lives of children*. Cambridge, MA: Harvard University Press.

Melson, G. F. (2003). Child development and the human-companion animal bond. *American Behavioral Scientist, 47*, 31–39.

Melson, G. F., & Fine, A. H. (2011). Handbook on animal-assisted therapy: Theoretical foundations and guidelines for practice. In A. H. Fine (Ed.), *Animals in the lives of children* (3rd ed., pp. 223–245). San Diego, CA: Academic Press.

Mikulincer, M., & Shaver, P. R. (2001). Attachment theory and intergroup bias: Evidence that priming the secure base schema attenuates negative reactions to out-groups. *Journal of Personality and Social Psychology, 81*, 97–115.

O'Neil, J. M. (2008). Summarizing 25 years of research on men's gender role conflict using the gender role conflict scale: New research paradigms and clinical implications. *The Counseling Psychologist, 36*, 358–445.

Pietromonaco, P. R., Laurenceau, J., & Barrett, L. F. (2002). Change in relationship knowledge representations. In A. L. Vangelisti, H. T. Reis, & M. A. Fitzpatrick (Eds.), *Stability and change in relationships. Advances in personal relationships* (pp. 5–34). New York: Cambridge University Press.

Schafer, K. (2002). Human animal interactions as a therapeutic intervention. *Counseling and Human Development, 34*, 1–18.

Serpell, J. A. (2010). Animal-assisted interventions in historical perspective. In A. H. Fine (Ed.), *Handbook on animal-assisted therapy: Theoretical foundations and guidelines for practice* (3rd ed., pp. 17–32). San Diego, CA: Academic Press.

Shorey, H. S., & Snyder, C. R. (2006). The role of adult attachment styles in psychopathology and psychotherapy outcomes. *Review of General Psychology, 10*, 1–20.

Sickmund, M. (2009). *Delinquency cases in juvenile court, 2005*. Washington, DC: Office of Juvenile Justice and Delinquency Prevention, U.S. Department of Justice.

Stahlberg, O., Anckarsater, H., & Nilsson, T. (2010). Mental health problems in youth committed to juvenile institutions: Prevalences and treatment needs. *The European Journal of Child and Adolescent Psychiatry, 19*, 893–903.

Stetina, B. U., Turner, K., Burger, E., Glenk, L. M., McElheney, J. C., Handlos, U., et al. (2011). Learning emotion recognition from canines? Two for the road. *Journal of Veterinary Behavior, 6*, 108–114.

Thomas, J. (2014). *Human animal interaction as an intervention with at-risk youth: Assessing the change in cognitions, emotional intelligence and empathy*. (Doctoral dissertation). Retrieved from ProQuest/UMI Dissertation and Theses. (Accession order No. AAT 3599245).

Thompson, R. (1999). Early attachment and later development. In J. Cassidy & P. R. Shaver (Eds.), *The handbook of attachment: Theory, research and clinical applications* (pp. 265–286). New York, NY: Guilford Press.

Turner, K., Stetina, B. U., Burger, E., Lederman-Mama, T., Handlos, U., & Kryspin-Exner, I. (2009). Enhancing emotional regulation and recognition among first graders through animal-assisted group training. *Journal of Veterinary Behavior, 4*, 93–94.
Triebenbacher, S. L. (1998). Pets as transitional objects: Their role in children's emotional development. *Psychological Reports, 82*, 191–200.
U.S. Surgeon General. (2001). *Youth violence: A report of the surgeon general*. Rockville, MD: Office of the Surgeon General, U.S. Department of Health and Human Services.
Watts, R. H, Jr, & Borders, D. L. (2005). Boys' perceptions of the male role: Understanding gender role conflict in adolescent males. *The Journal of Men's Studies, 13*, 267–280.
Winnicott, D. W. (1953). Transitional objects and transitional phenomena. *International Journal of Psychoanalysis, 34*, 89–97.

Chapter 6
Healing Bonds: Animal Assisted Interventions with Adjudicated Male Youth

Amy Johnson and Laura Bruneau

"Rook taught me how to stay calm and relaxed. He also taught me how to have time to wait for things and don't rush. Most important, he showed me how to love." This powerful statement came from Devon, an adjudicated male youth while reflecting on his time with Rook, a German Shepherd/Border Collie mix. Devon participated in Teacher's Pet, an Animal Assisted Intervention (AAI) nonprofit program. The program simultaneously helps youth and hard-to-adopt shelter dogs by providing a safe, therapeutic environment for learning together. This program serves various types of youth, including (a) adjudicated youth serving time at a residential detention center; (b) youth with emotional impairments enrolled at local, alternative schools; and (c) youth from the community participating at a dog training summer camp. Further information on the program can be found on the website: teacherspetmi.org.

The Teacher's Pet program builds upon the symbiotic relationship between the youth and the dog. By training hard-to-adopt shelter dogs, the youth give and receive unconditional love, as well as carry out something selfless, positive, and meaningful. This bonding experience allows the youth to improve in the areas of (a) empathy, (b) patience, (c) impulse control, (d) perseverance, and (e) hope. While learning these skills, the young men and women positively impact the quality of life for shelter dogs, offering an improved likelihood of adoption. This innovative program emerged from theory and research, specifically looking at similar prison and youth intervention programs across the United States and Canada.

A. Johnson (✉)
Oakland University School of Nursing, Rochester, MI, USA
e-mail: johnson2@oakland.edu

L. Bruneau
Department of Counselor Education, Adams State University, Alamosa, CO, USA

C. Blazina and L.R. Kogan (eds.), *Men and Their Dogs*,
DOI 10.1007/978-3-319-30097-9_6

People who have experienced the power of the human–animal bond can personally attest to its effectiveness. The rich, anecdotal stories shared in the next section offer a context for understanding this particular AAI program, as well as highlighting how animals can impact young men and their developing masculinity. Note that we have changed all names to protect the youth's identity and the remainder of the chapter focuses on the experiences of adjudicated boys within the Teacher's Pet program.

Devon

Devon's quote appeared above. Where Devon comes from, dogs are property. Dogs wear heavy chains around their necks, are over-exercised, left outside, fed gunpowder, and trained to fight for large sums of money. For Devon, life at home and school was stressful and unsuccessful. While serving his time in a detention facility, Devon participated in the Teacher's Pet program as a way to escape the daily tedium. Devon had a rough exterior and a controlled affect; he did not seem as excited about working with the shelter dogs as the other boys, nor did his assigned dog, Rook. Rook read Devon's disinterest, and he responded similarly—unfocused and uninterested.

Devon took to the challenge of training Rook. Rather than ruminate about his current situation, Devon thought about Rook and how to help him. While involved in the program, Devon's affect was noticeably different as he smiled widely every time he walked into the kennel area. Sometimes, Devon would just sit quietly with Rook and brush his fur. Rook was also different as he stopped barking and jumping and became a focused, well-mannered dog.

Dustin

Dustin was an angry and aggressive teen with symptoms of Reactive Attachment Disorder. Everyone Dustin had ever loved had abandoned him, leaving him to cling to gang life—a place in which he felt he belonged. Throughout his time with the Teacher's Pet program, he was polite and attentive, absorbing as much information about dog behavior and dog training as he could. At school and in the unit, however, he was always on restriction for disruptive behavior and fighting. Dustin worked with Coco, a stubborn, strong-willed, Pit bull mix. Coco had anger issues of her own and tried to start fights with the other dogs. Dustin was conscientious about this and kept her safe from the other dogs when training.

Coco was a quick study and one day, Dustin wanted to show off a trick. He asked Coco to sit and stay. While she was sitting, he put a piece of string cheese between his lips. She shifted her weight in anticipation of a treat, and he held out his hand in a stay command. After a couple of seconds, he tapped the right side of his chest with his right hand, and she vertically leaped to his face and grasped the cheese from his lips. Dustin developed this command on his own, forcing himself to temper his frustration and aggressive body language to teach Coco impulse control and patience. Because the two were alike, Dustin understood Coco and knew how to teach her. Dustin, who learned early in life to distrust others, ultimately found a special connection with Coco.

Nico

At 16 years of age, Nico had spent nearly three years in detention facilities. He had extreme difficulty interacting with peers and staff. As a child, Nico was molested by a friend of the family. Later, Nico was sexually assaulted by a staff member at another facility. Nico was quick to form new relationships; however, these relationships ended as quickly as they started, leaving him devastated and further hesitant of trusting others. As a result, Nico learned to rely on himself, resulting in aloof, insolent behavior toward others. As he learned about communicating with dogs and how to verbalize what he wanted, he was able to reflect on his interacting with people.

Nico took these new insights and applied it to other relationships, such as the youth in his unit. For example, he was surprised to find that when he modified his verbal and nonverbal language, the feedback he received from others was much more positive. Nico was excited and proud of the changes he saw in his relationships. The more he practiced this with his peers and staff, the better and more consistent was the feedback. His ability to demonstrate self-awareness and how he came across to others was a huge step toward a healthier emotional well-being. Like Devon, Nico expressed some powerful insights as a result of the program, "saying goodbye to someone you loved didn't mean that your world had to fall apart."

Summary of Cases

To merely tell a troubled youth to be more patient or to have more empathy is futile. These are not elements to address cognitively, but experientially. For one to foster empathy, one has to experience empathy. These case studies highlight the benefit of pairing adjudicated male youth with shelter dogs. Doing so increased the opportunity for Devon, Dustin, and Nico in getting what they needed most.

For example, Devon's coping strategies were not benefiting him in previous relationships. Like most youth in his social position, being sensitive or showing empathy is dangerous. Putting down this guard can result in being taken advantage of or being injured. However, without the ability to understand or share the feelings of another person, the capacity to steal, violate, or injure another increase. Developing empathy, or a genuine care for others, can provide an element of hope and help adjudicated youth to acclimate to healthier social groups and generally improve relationships with others.

Adjudicated youth often come from an environment of dysfunction, resulting in a variety of faulty thinking patterns. These youth may be quick to misinterpret the tone of voice, body language, and others' reactions to them. Or, the youth might assume all relationships must mirror those in their past. Both Dustin and Nico are great examples of this tendency. By training a shelter dog, the youth are able to work through these faulty thinking patterns. For example, when using a lure and reward technique in training, the youth can elicit certain responses from the dog. Based on the feedback from the dog (e.g., he performs the command, recoils in fear, ignores the trainer), the youth can modify the way they request the command. For example, the youth can alter body language and tone of voice, or simply try again.

The purpose of this chapter is to discuss the needs of adjudicated male youth and to propose how a program, such as Teacher's Pet, can be a useful adjunct in treatment. This chapter provides an inside look at the AAI program designed for troubled adolescents, who are often considered a difficult population to treat. In addition to this discussion, theoretical underpinnings of AAI will be examined within the context of working therapeutically with this population. Finally, preliminary research on the AAI program will be presented and discussed.

Adjudicated Male Youth

Devon, Dustin, and Nico's stories are typical of young males in correction facilities. A study of 898 youth residing in a large, temporary detention center in Cook County, Chicago indicated that 92.5 % of these youth had experienced one or more traumas in their lifetime. An example of trauma is seeing someone seriously injured or killed. Furthermore, more males (93.2 %) than females (84.0 %) reported at least one traumatic experience (Abram et al. 2004). Being traumatized inhibits the ability to trust and to feel safe. As a result of not having these basic needs met, these youth tend to have poor emotion regulation strategies and a punitive style of dealing with others (Hirsh and Kang 2015). Adjudicated youth typically present with diagnosable mental health disorders, such as substance use and conduct disorders (Grisso 2008; Teplin et al. 2002) as well as a host of health problems and psychosocial issues (Forrest et al. 2000). Unfortunately, only half of the juvenile justice facilities provide mental health counseling beyond substance use treatment (Young et al. 2007).

Adolescent male youth are trying to assert themselves as men, but find themselves trapped on the precipice of childhood. The conditions in which the masculine self develops has profound consequences on the emotional well-being of young men (Blazina 2001). Adjudicated youth are often without positive male role models to teach them how to be men. Or, many of these young men have a father figure who displays antisocial behavior (Farrington et al. 2001). As a result, the emerging masculinity of these young men is based on societal norms expressed in their culture, communities, and within the media. Young men are left to emulate the men they admire, often those in the entertainment industry who idolize money, sex, and drugs. These youth gravitate toward those who will make them feel that they belong, often associated with gang life, as every person needs to feel a sense of love and belonging (Glasser 1998).

It seems contradictory for men to be told to act one way, and then punished for doing so—as seen so clearly in the earlier case illustrations of Devon, Dustin, and Nico. As David and Brannon (1976) described decades ago, young men are warned against being a "sissy" and told to be strong, brave, and powerful. As young men are trying to fit in within a set of societal norms and expectations, they are often confronted with conflicting expectations within their multiple social identities (Hirsh and King 2015). The higher the conflict between expectations of men and who they want to be, the greater the difficulty in identifying feelings, self-disclosing to others, and navigating interpersonal relationships. However, how U.S. culture perceives men and emotions are significantly changing as men are increasingly being *allowed* to show emotions and vulnerability—these mixed messages about gender are the heart of Gender Role Conflict (GRC; O'Neil 2015). GRC is a state in which stereotypical, socialized gender roles have negative consequences for self and others, overall resulting in a restriction of human potential (O'Neil 2015). Negative consequences of GRC can lead to (a) gender role devaluation, e.g., negative critiques of oneself or others when diverging from stereotypical gender roles; (b) gender role restrictions, e.g., confining oneself or others to restrictive gender roles; and (c) gender role violations, e.g., harming self or others because of stereotypical gender roles (O'Neil 2015).

For example, some of the boys in the Teacher's Pet program will state that they cannot be *soft*. Being soft or empathic is physically and emotionally dangerous as this leaves them vulnerable to ridicule, bullying, and violence. However, many of these youth desire to be *soft*. This conflict between behavior and desire is a prime example of GRC, in which boys restrict themselves to traditional gender roles and negatively self-evaluate for wanting to be different. As a further case illustration, there have been several incidences in the program where a video or group discussion highlights shelter dogs being mistreated, euthanized, or unwanted. These instances may cause a young man to well up with tears, hit a desk, or walk off to a corner. However, by showing physical signs of sadness (e.g., eyes filling with tears, turning red, or voice cracking); the youth exposes himself to later ridicule.

For these behaviors to *leak out*, the environment must be perceived as safe. These instances provide valuable teaching moments for the Teacher's Pet facilitators to discuss feelings and behaviors openly and immediately. In most cases, the other youth have supported each other with remarks like "it's okay, man" or by showing their own feelings of sadness. These raw and honest moments allow the boys to deeply and safely experience their emotions, furthering their own emotional connections with each other. There are other times, however, when the youth do not feel safe emoting in front of others and will request time alone with their dogs. The youth are able to take their dogs further away within the room or yard, allowing for some needed privacy. Being in the dog's presence is therapeutic, and the youth enjoy having a chance to talk to their dogs.

A particular occurrence at Teacher's Pet highlights the importance of being able to communicate with the dog. One of the juvenile justice centers is a low security, open facility in a rural area. Mick, a youth in the unit, was training an Akita mix named Moto. As typically seen with the pairings in Teacher's Pet, Mick and Moto were much alike as both were headstrong and resistant. Moto was kenneled at a boarding facility about a mile down a dirt road. One cold afternoon, Moto scaled the fence of his kennel. The kennel staff was able to spot him from a distance, but could not catch him. However, they were finally able to leash him when he arrived on the juvenile justice center campus and was sitting in the very spot where he received training!

When the Teacher's Pet facilitators informed Mick about Moto running away (Mick also had a history of running away), Mick was not fazed in the least. He stated that Moto simply knew where to go because of conversations the two of them had during training sessions. During these conversations, Mick would tell Moto they both had to work on their behaviors so they could go home. If Moto were ever to feel unsafe, he should go to *their* safe place. Whether it was coincidence or not that Moto ended up in this spot is irrelevant. From a therapeutic standpoint, this incident gave valuable insight into Mick's inner world as this is not something that would naturally come up in individual or group counseling sessions.

Current programming in residential juvenile justice centers include peer-to-peer culture programs; individual, group, and family therapy; and academic curriculum. In some cases, the youth are punitively treated or mistreated. However, these harsh punishments do not reform troubled teens. Instead, healthy and restorative relationships guide positive change. Through these nurturing, responsive, and empathic relationships in psychotherapy, one can develop new working models of the self (Brendtro et al. 2009). Authors have posited that these changes can also be achieved through interactions with a therapy animal as bonding with an animal can be a catalyst for attachment and psychological and emotional growth (Geist 2011; Parish-Plass 2008).

Animal Assisted Intervention (AAI)

AAI is the umbrella term for various modalities such as Animal Assisted Therapy, Animal Assisted Activities, and Animal Assisted Education. By definition, Animal Assisted Therapy is a "goal-directed intervention is designed to promote improvement in physical, social, emotional and/or cognitive functioning of the person(s) involved and in which a specially trained animal-handler team is an integral part" (Animal Assisted Interventions International 2013). Research findings indicate that even short-term exposure to a dog has been shown to reduce cortisol (Polheber and Matchock 2014). The reduction of cortisol reduces blood pressure, heart rate, and ultimately minimizes the symptoms of stress and anxiety. Without excessive stress, the person can be more receptive to healing (Leftkowitz et al. 2005).

Adding an AAI to the psychotherapy process can hasten the therapeutic relationship between the counselor and client. For example, if a client sees a dog that is calm and happy around the psychotherapist, the client might also feel they can trust the psychotherapist. As a result, there is increased rapport between the client and psychotherapist. Fawcett and Gullone (2001) found that youth with conduct disorders could form a positive bond with the psychotherapist in the presence of a therapy animal as the psychotherapist was considered to be more gentle and kind.

When considering the theoretical underpinnings of AAI in the therapeutic process, there are a few large, overarching ideas frequently cited in the literature. The biophilia hypothesis (Wilson 1993) is one of the most well-known theories to support humans' inherent interest in nature (Berget and Braastad 2008). This hypothesis identifies an instinctive connection between human beings and other living things, referred to as biophilia (Wilson 1993), which can explain why people want to rescue hurt animals or take care of houseplants. From an evolutionary standpoint, humans are attuned to nature and desire a relationship with animals and nature (Fawcett and Gullone 2001). Friendly animals convey a sense of safety (Melson and Fine 2010), allowing a healing presence in animals.

Theoretical Framework for AAI

While AAI is largely considered a useful adjunct to the therapeutic process, there is little to no unified theoretical framework for explaining how the process works (Geist 2011). While AAI can be integrated into the techniques and tenets of most conventional counseling and psychotherapy theories, a blend of humanistic counseling theories and attachment theory have grounded the practice of the AAI discussed in this chapter.

Humanistic counseling theories, which include Person-Centered Therapy, Existential Therapy, and Gestalt Therapy, posit that the client innately self-actualizes. As Fritz Perls noted, "every individual, every plant, every animal has only one inborn goal—to actualize itself as it is" (1969, p. 33). In Person-Centered therapy, the client is the expert on himself. The client directs counseling and resolves his issues (Rogers 1961) through the gentle guidance of the psychotherapist. Through being genuine and having unconditional positive regard for the client, the counselor expresses empathy (Raskin and Rogers 2005) and creates a safe environment.

There is an anonymous quotation within the field of AAI, "All dogs have read Carl Rogers." Indeed, counselors could learn about how to be present from observing the nonjudgmental interactions between dogs and humans. As dogs are highly skilled at reading body language in both dogs and humans (Hare and Tomasello 2005), dogs are a natural and effective fit for AAI's and can hasten the bonding process. Dogs possess the instinctual characteristics of showing warmth, being genuine, and having unconditional positive regard. Furthermore, Rogers (1961) believed that the need for love and acceptance is paramount. Many adjudicated youth have faced tremendous obstacles in their lives and did so with few, if any, consistent support figures. A child's self-concept is molded by his early interaction with others and the external messages he receives (Raskin and Rogers 2005). Through the unique relationship with an animal, adjudicated youth are given a new opportunity to relate to another being.

Like Person-centered therapy, Existential therapy proposes self-actualization in people. Existential therapy delves into human nature (May and Yalom 2005), while focusing on key therapeutic issues, e.g., death, freedom, isolation, and meaninglessness. These constructs are clearly relevant for the adjudicated youth and shelter dogs. Addressing the dogs' experience with these topics allows the youth to process the constructs in an objective manner, creating a deeper impact. For example, as the youth begin to see changes in the dogs as a result of the training program; this instills a sense of hope, responsibility, and purpose.

Gestalt therapy also stresses a warm, genuine, and active counseling relationship. This present-based approach allows clients to try new things, making use of experiments within the counseling session to increase awareness (Yontef and Jacobs 2005). From this approach, working with the dogs allows the youth to immediately explore boundaries and contact styles. The youth are able to practice prosocial skills, reinterpret body language, alter verbal communication, and learn to trust in a safe, nurturing environment.

Attachment theory is perhaps the foundation for AAI (Geist 2011; Zilcha-Mano et al. 2011). Bowlby (1979) posited that attachment is rooted in the mental representation of the parent–child relationship. Attachment theory helps us to understand how a child perceives, interprets, acts, and reacts to experiences within other relationships (Parish-Plass 2008). Positive attachments with *good enough* caregivers (Winnicott 1971) lay the groundwork for healthy feelings of self-worth, adaptive emotion regulation skills, and favorable psychosocial functioning. In contrast, without consistency, love, and attunement from the primary caregiver, children can form insecure, anxious, and avoidant attachments. As primary caregivers are the most important and relevant relationships for a child, children can later recreate the same types of behaviors, thoughts, and beliefs in other relationships. When attachment figures compromise feelings of safety and security in young children, negative models of self and others develop, and emotional problems and maladaptive behaviors are more likely to coexist (Zilcha-Mano et al. 2011). In particular, victims of trauma, abuse, or neglect commonly suffer from insecure attachment with their caregivers, leading to delinquent behaviors (Hoeve et al. 2012), and negative externalizing behaviors (Fearon et al. 2010).

Levinson (1969) believed that an animal companion is naturally an object of attachment—an attachment that is more appropriate than an inanimate or symbolic one. For example, the animal companion can provide reciprocity in the relationship that is crucial for attunement and bonding, and ultimately empathy. Furthermore, bonds with animal companions meet the prerequisites of an attachment bond

(Zilcha-Mano et al. 2011), including (a) proximity seeking, (b) safe haven, (c) secure base, and (d) separation distress (Ainsworth 1991; Bowlby 1982; Hazan and Zeifman 1994). Humans feel an emotional closeness to their animal companions that is often stronger than their bonds with family members; for boys in particular, animals can play a variety of roles, including siblings, friends, and teachers (Fine et al. 2011). Animal companions provide a safe space to share and explore feelings and emotions and losing an animal companion triggers distress and a significant grieving process (Zilcha-Mano et al. 2011).

The deep connection between people and animals provides a unique therapeutic opportunity to practice new behaviors. As previously noted, adjudicated youth may have difficulty empathizing with others, often relying on aggression and coercion within relationships (Feshbach et al. 1983). Furthermore, these youth may show deficits in emotional language expression and the ability to identify emotions in others' facial expressions in others, which inhibits positive perceptions of situations and creates false filters (Geist 2011). Promoting a secure attachment with a dog through an AAI program can help with developing emotional regulation skills that can also be transferable to other relationships and situations. Adjudicated youth may experience gains in empathy toward their human counterparts as the dog serves as a transitional object from which to explore healthier human relationships (Krueger and Serpell 2010).

Furthermore, feeling loved unconditionally is linked to positive self-esteem. A youth who feels the love and acceptance from an animal may believe they are worthy of love. One example of how attachment with an animal can positively impact self-esteem is Colin, another youth in the Teacher's Pet program. With an alcoholic father and chronically depressed mother, Colin spent much time home alone. His father was abusive, and his mother typically locked herself in her room. Colin dressed all in black, wore black eyeliner and nail polish, and grew his hair so that his face hid beneath the lacquered spikes. Colin talked about wanting to harm himself, to "shrivel up and die." As a child, Colin recounted loving a dog. Later, as a student trainer in the program, the dogs showed a lot of love and affection to Colin, suggesting he had a gift in relating to dogs. After only a few weeks in the program, Colin stated, "You know, I always thought I was this horrible, worthless kid. After working with these dogs, I realize that I am not."

The Teacher's Pet Program

Arluke (2007) selected five AAI programs that treated at-risk and incarcerated adolescents, including two obedience dog programs. From his review, he provided some suggestions as to how an AAI, such as Teacher's Pet, makes an impact on these clients. For example, youth are both curious and excited about working with animals, *hooking* them onto the idea of AAI. Youth tend to feel secure and accepted by both the animal and the psychotherapy staff, and as a result, the youth form close relationships with the animal and staff. Through the training component, youth feel empowered but also have to learn to be patient and accept when they make mistakes. Finally, working with animals allow for perspective taking, or for the youth to consider how others might experience situations (Arluke 2007). These propositions provide a foundation for the success of the Teacher's Pet program.

Additionally, a program such as Teacher's Pet can also help break down barriers that practitioners often face with this population. These barriers are often exacerbated by the fact that many of the youth are court mandated for individual, family, or group counseling. As described earlier, integrating an animal into the counseling process may increase the rapport building process between psychotherapists and clients. Likewise, the youth can see how the staff and facilitators interact with the dogs and are then able to generalize these positive reactions to their relationships with staff and facilitators. Furthermore, this intervention allows for staff and facilitators to develop a new frame of reference for working with this population. Staff and psychotherapists may view adolescents in juvenile justice centers as a demanding population to treat. Troubled youth often have long histories of negative experiences with adults throughout their lives, making the therapeutic connection difficult to establish. For example, a staff member might initially view a resident as willful, antagonistic, or disrespectful. This same staff member might view the resident in a new light once the youth is lying on the ground with his dog, embracing the dog, and calling him "Schmoopy!" When the perception of the youth has changed, or the *blinders* have been removed, the staff can interact with the resident in a different and gentler way.

It is important to note that an AAI such as Animal Assisted Therapy (AAT) uses a trained animal under the direction of a facilitator. Animals are not simply present in room (Chassman and Kinney 2011), but intentionally integrated into the therapeutic process and are seen as a treatment partner (Parish-Plass 2013). In the case of Teacher's Pet, however, shelter dogs are incorporated into the treatment program rather than relying on trained dogs. All dogs go through a health examination, a temperament test, and screened for aggression toward human and other dogs. Utilizing rescued, shelter dogs increases the opportunity for bonding as the youth feel a connection to the dogs. The dogs, for example, are locked up, unwanted, behaviorally challenged, and may have ended up on the street or may have been abused or neglected. As such the youth identify with the dogs, often verbalizing the commonalities between them. The youth then project their emotions and cognitions on the dogs, providing further insight into the youth. The previous story of Mick and Moto is a great example of this benefit. Bringing in dogs with similar histories and tendencies can pave the way for insight, unconditional love, and mutual respect.

Perry (2006) described a neurobiological relationship between humans and dogs are similar to that of an adult and a baby or toddler, noting the importance of mirror neurons. Integrating dogs into therapy may calm and soothe clients and help them both engage and relate to the therapeutic process. Dogs' facial expressions are very similar to those of humans (Coren 2001), furthering the bonding experience. Dogs may be the best animal for helping those with social deficits, and may also be promising for working with maltreated children (Brooks 2006; Perry 2006; van der Kolk 2014). Indeed, the way dogs and humans related on a neurobiological level may be the described *magic* of AAI. Working with behaviorally challenged, unwanted, abandoned shelter dogs can be an effective way to evoke and cultivate empathic feelings as well as improve impulse control, manage anger, and foster necessary prosocial skills in adjudicated youth.

Program Details

In the Teacher's Pet program, student trainers can consist of adjudicated males and females, in addition to mixed-gender students with emotional impairments, as well as young men and women from the community. Teacher's Pet consists of both a didactic component (canine education) as well as an experiential component (dog training). The main focus of the canine education is for these student trainers to learn foundational information about canine communication and positive reinforcement training. Understanding others, as well as other species, is paramount to living in harmony with others. Understanding also facilitates a bond. If the student trainer can understand why a dog is behaving in a certain way, the trainer can translate this knowledge into their interactions with humans.

During the canine education program, the student trainers first learn safety information by identifying body language in dogs (e.g., ears back means the dog is fearful, head high and ears up means the dog is very alert or hackles raised; ears forward and wrinkled muzzle identifies the dog as being ready to attack, etc.). The student trainers need to recognize when a dog is uncomfortable, aggressive, or hyper-aroused in order to know how to handle that situation. In these situations, if the dog can be redirected with a treat or verbal command, it would fall under arousal rather than aggression. The facilitators use video footage, pictures, and real dogs throughout the curriculum to teach these concepts. In addition to learning about identifying particular emotions in dogs, the student trainers learn how to help calm the dog. As often as possible, concepts are connected to the dogs' feelings and how these feelings match the student trainers' experiences.

Other topics within the curriculum include responsible animal companion ownership and humane treatment of animals (e.g., dog fighting, puppy mills, animal testing, animal cruelty around the world, and animals harmed in the entertainment industry). These topics are purposeful in that they emphasize the larger world around the student trainers. For example, many of the young men in the program have had experience training dogs, such as Pit bulls, for fighting, including feeding the dogs gunpowder, attaching chains around the neck to thicken the neck muscles, and running the dogs on treadmills for hours at a time. The canine education component addresses the history of Pit bulls, highlighting how the breed's strengths have been exploited by humans due to greed, and emphasizing the innate loving nature of the Pit bull type breeds. Student trainers often express gratitude for gaining new perspectives about the world around them. A journal entry from one of the male student trainers captures this new perspective, "I used to think it was weird to get real close to dogs the way people do, but now I see dogs are just like us."

Focusing on the experiential component of the curriculum, student trainers use small treats to lure dogs into various postures (e.g., sit, down, heel, take a bow, etc.). Once the trainer obtains the desired action, the trainer lets the dog know it is correct by saying "Yes!" and feeds the dog the treat. This cycle repeats until the dog can perform the action with a word or hand signal alone. Harsh corrections like yelling or coercing is never used as this would suggest to the youth that they can get what they want by using force or negative behavior. Lure and reward-based training has also been shown to increase the bond between human and canine (Greenebaum 2010). Overall, the training is focused on the safety of dogs, obeying commands, and helping the dogs become more suitable for adoption.

The student trainers then work hard to prepare the dog for adoption. Each youth works with two dogs during a 10-week session (each dog for five consecutive weeks), teaching the dogs basic commands and obedience training. With the help of the shelter manager, the dogs eventually are matched with an adoptive family. At the completion of each five-week session, the student trainers write a letter to the adoptive family telling them about the dog. This letter advises the new family on how to best care for their potential family member. The adoptive family is also encouraged to write a letter back to the student trainer explaining how the dog fits into their home and any news involving the dog.

The 10-week program culminates with a graduation ceremony. This ceremony provides a sense of closure for the student trainers and a chance to work through any feelings of sadness or grief. As the youth get quite attached to their dogs, many of them resist working with a new dog because of feelings of loss. For many of the youth, painful memories of abandonment or loss in their personal lives are still very raw. Working through a separation process with their dog can be a catalyst for processing their previous experiences of loss and changing their schemas about the loss. The graduation ceremony provides a medium to talk about the dog's progress and how the student trainers were able to make a difference in the dog's life. As described by one of the male student trainers, "I enjoyed being able to help save them, even though it was extremely sad for me to leave them, I knew it was the right thing to do, and that I helped give them the ability to be adopted." Student trainers and their families do not have the option of adopting the dogs as it would change the dynamic of the student trainer-dog team. Doing so would also contradict the overall purpose of the program in that the youth are selflessly giving to the shelter animal.

During the 10-week training program, there is always a staff member present and the psychotherapists will also watch the student trainers and dogs in action. There are many benefits to observing the student trainer-dog team. For example, the youth feel pride in their work and are often excited to share what they are doing with the psychotherapists and staff. Additionally, the psychotherapist can use specific examples from the training experience as a part of the therapeutic process or can encourage the youth to make analogies about their work with the dogs.

In conclusion, the Teacher's Pet program works best when there is collaboration between the psychotherapists, staff, and student trainers.

Researching the Impact of AAT with Incarcerated Youth

Teacher's Pet was the focus of a randomized control trial, supported by the Eunice Kennedy Shriver National Institute of Child Health & Human Development and Mars-WALTHAM® (Seivert et al. 2015). An article with specific results to the study has been submitted for publication (Seivert et al. 2015). The sample included 138 incarcerated youth from two detention centers. Approximately 70 % of the youth in the study were male and were on average, 15.7 years of age. Forty-six percent identified as White/Caucasian and 44 % identified as Black/African American. Participating in the Teacher's Pet program was expected to increase empathy and decrease internalizing and externalizing behavior problems.

All participants attended the 1 h canine education classes twice per week for ten weeks. Youth in the experimental group trained two dogs for 1 h, two times per week, over the course of ten weeks. Control group participants walked a variety of dogs for the same time and duration. The control group did not participate in the dog training component, which was identified as the active ingredient of the intervention as training would instill a sense of responsibility for the animal as well as a greater awareness of the dogs' needs (Seivert et al. 2015).

The Interpersonal Reactivity Index (IRI; Davis 1980), a self-report measure, was used to assess Empathic Concern and Perspective Taking and the Achenbach System of Empirically Based Assessment (ASEBA; Achenbach 2009) was used to assess Internalizing and Externalizing behaviors, per youth and staff report. Participants completed the forms before and after the intervention. Additionally, coding of exit interviews with each participant was used to provide context for the quantitative data.

Contrary to the research hypothesis, participants in both the experimental and control groups had increased Empathic Concern ($p < 0.001$) as well as increased Internalizing Behavior, per youth ($p < 0.001$) and staff report ($p = 0.023$). The researchers concluded that the time spent with the dogs appeared to increase empathy in the youth, regardless of treatment group (Seivert et al. 2015). As both groups had direct contact with the animals, perhaps simply spending time with the dogs was enough to increase levels of empathic concern. Furthermore, the dog walking intervention may have provided more time for the youth to bond with the dogs as the dog training time was more structured than the dog walking time. Although the dog training component was initially considered to be the active ingredient of the intervention, perhaps engaging with the dog was the active ingredient (Seivert et al. 2015).

Additionally, the canine education component of the program could have impacted levels of empathy across the two groups. For example, those youth in the control group would have learned about the benefits of getting the dogs out of the kennel, allowing the dogs to engage in physical activity and spend time with a variety of different people. Furthermore, the classroom discussions often centered on putting oneself in another being's shoes, or *paws*. Questions like, "What must it be like to be a dog in the shelter?" or "How do you think the dog felt when his family left him behind?" were a central part of the group discussions and may have influenced the levels of empathy. A study by Ascione (1992) supports this potential explanation as a humane education curriculum, without animal contact, increased empathy in children.

The themes that emerged from examining the exit interviews supported the increase in empathy for both groups. The youth in the control group were aware that they were a part of the overall training for the animal. Instead of only working with one or two dogs, like the treatment group, these youth described making a bigger difference by caring for more dogs. It is also important to note that approximately 30 % of the study participants were female. Therefore, it is possible that the inclusion of females lead to greater mean scores on the Interpersonal Reactivity Index (Davis 1980) as women tend to show higher levels of empathy than men (Mestre, Samper, Frias and Tur 2009).

When considering the increase in internalizing behaviors in both groups, this could be attributed to the participants gaining greater emotional awareness throughout the Teacher's Pet program (Seivert et al. 2015). Upon reviewing the themes from the exit interviews, the youth expressed sadness and loss about not having contact with the dogs. Being in the program may stir up unmet needs and unresolved psychological issues for the youth, which may be heightened while saying goodbye to the animal. Furthermore, during the canine education component the participants may have become more in tune with their emotions as they learned about how to identify emotions and learn about animal abuse (Seivert et al. 2015). These discussions were connected to their current situation, life at home, and offenses that brought them into the juvenile justice system. Likewise, Hanselman (2001) identified an increase in depressive symptoms in youth involved in an AAI, focused on anger management. In conclusion, the combination of time spent with dogs (with or without dog training) and participation in the canine education component could have increased empathy for these participants and the increase in internalizing behaviors could be due to the youth gaining emotional awareness as a result of the AAI (Seivert et al. 2015).

Discussion

The aim of the study by Seivert et al. 2015) was to examine the effectiveness of the Teacher's Pet program on increasing empathy and decreasing internalizing and externalizing behaviors in incarcerated youth. This study had an adequate sample size, control group, random group assignment, and multi-informant outcome measures, which meets the methodological rigor as noted by Krueger and Serpell (2010). In the best possible situation, the control group would have had no exposure to the dogs or the canine education curriculum. Additionally, having a 6-month or 1-year follow-up on these youth would have provided valuable information; however, with the transient nature of many of these youth, that often proves to be very difficult.

Based on the research findings, youth who participate in the program may develop greater levels of empathy, which can lead to lower levels of recidivism and a higher quality of life for the youth (Seivert et al. 2015). Thus, there is empirical evidence to support the overall mission of the program. Furthermore, the benefit for the animals, as obedience training increases the likelihood of adoption, is an important component of the Teacher's Pet program. The dogs learned valuable skills such as patience, impulse control, and developed appropriate in-home behaviors. The interaction with the dogs, whether training or walking, was beneficial as the dogs gained mental and emotional stimulation during the shelter stay. Indeed, the shelter staff often commented on the improvement of the physical, mental, and emotional health of the dogs as a result of participating in the research study.

Although the results were unexpected, the findings do present an interesting discussion and help to open the door for further research on AAI. As previously mentioned, emerging themes from the exit interviews provided an in-depth perspective on the youths' experience with the Teacher's Pet program. Initial coding of these sources provided four emerging themes from the dog training component, including: (a) patience, (b) perseverance, (c) hope, and (d) desire to contribute (Johnson et al. 2015).

Patience correlates with impulse control, which is a significant problem for youth in detention facilities. Acting first and thinking next is common practice. The youth are committed to seeing the dogs through the training program, but will often have to wait for the dogs to catch on to what is being asked of them. At the end of the program, youth were more able to stay on task and expressed less aggravation when waiting for the dogs to catch on. As one resident stated,

> The main thing is just to continue with my patience, I say that a lot 'cause I used to have a really bad patience problem. I used to get frustrated so easily, and it just teaches you to take a minute to yourself.

The student trainers often express difficulty in sticking with something, particularly when it becomes difficult or frustrating. This behavior repeats in most situations, from completing homework assignments, keeping a job, or following through on chores or tasks. The process of getting a dog, who cannot grasp the concept of "lay down," to actually lie down, can be arduous. However, the student trainers described feeling proud, as if they accomplished something significant. This sense of *perseverance* has the potential to scaffold into future events. For example, if they can follow through with this task and it works and feels good to them, the likelihood of following through on another task increases. As one resident described,

> Some dogs you have to put all your effort into it. You can't give up. You never can give up. You just have to keep going, and some dogs won't even reach the goal that you have strived for. Long as you tried. It's better to try and fail, than to not try at all.

One of the main tasks of psychotherapy is to help instill hope within clients. As Rollo May said, "the purpose of psychotherapy is to set people free" (1981, p. 19). Adjudicated youth often feel that they are the product of their environment. When these student trainers see a dog with a similar history change his behavior, and as a result, have an improved quality of life through adoption, this results in a sense of *hope* for the youth. In this situation, the youth might believe that the same thing can happen to them, changing the filter from which the youth views the self and the world. This sentiment was expressed numerous times, including one student trainer who expressed, "No matter what bad things you have done in the past you are still going to have that happy feeling like I just accomplished something and it will help you in life too." Another student trainer succinctly stated, "I learned that if dogs can change, so can I."

The *desire to contribute* comes from a shift in state of mind. As a result of working with the dogs, the youth are no longer confined to the parameters of their internal working models but can see the changes happening around them. This shift in perspective allows the youth to feel excited about the future and possibilities and wanting to be a part of the change. Furthermore, shouldering the responsibility of improving the quality of life and potential adoptability of the dogs provides the youth with an opportunity to engage in positive, age-appropriate activities that will impact the dog, the adopting family, and community at large. Adler (1938) referred to this as having social interest, which is a central precursor to wellness and emotional health. As a student trainer described,

> Well my second dog, that I just graduated, I am going to miss her a lot. I trained her good, she went straight to a home after she graduated. It just makes me want to help out more... as soon as I leave [the detention facility] I'm going to volunteer.

Conclusion

The purpose of research is to ask questions and test hypotheses; but the real value of psychotherapy research is to consider how results inform practice. The preliminary findings of the aforementioned research study have already impacted how the Teacher's Pet program is implemented. Most importantly, the Teacher's Pet staff are considering alternative ways to promote bonding between the youth and the dogs. Contrary to the initial hypothesis, time spent with the dog during dog training may not be the essential element for the bonding process to occur. As those in the dog walking group liked having more unstructured times with the dogs, this piece may be integrated into the overall program. For example, the detention center facilities could have the dogs on site more frequently and for longer periods of time. During this time, the youth could be responsible for their overall care and well-being.

Second, the Teacher's Pet facilitators are reading the youths' journals more frequently and responding to them directly. This strategy is intended to open doors for more communication between the staff and youth. Facilitators are also attending weekly team meetings to discuss the behaviors and needs of the youth.

During the team meetings, the Teacher's Pet facilitators can share how the youth are performing in the dog training program. Often, this is new information for the juvenile detention center staff and psychotherapists. Likewise, the Teacher's Pet facilitators learn more about the student trainers and as a result, change the curriculum to better meet their needs. For example, if the youth are struggling with perspective taking or experiencing feelings of loss, other lesson plans may be introduced to provide support and facilitate psychological insight for the youth.

Another programmatic change would be to have the detention center staff, and psychotherapists visit the youth and dogs more frequently. Doing so would allow the student trainers to show off the dog's progress, which could result in more intrinsic motivation for their efforts and hard work. This would also benefit the staff and psychotherapists as they would be able to integrate this information into the youth's care and treatment as well as have an opportunity to see the residents in a different light.

Additionally, the program has been expanded to include a mentorship component for youth who have already completed the 10-week canine curriculum and dog training program. Once the student trainers have graduated, they are eligible to participate as a mentor to new members of the Teacher's Pet program. The mentorship program is designed to further enhance the desire to contribute. Finally, as many of the youth in the program have expressed an interest in continuing with dog training, Teacher's Pet has started a crowd funding site to raise money for the graduates. These funds will go to youth scholarships for further education in dog training programs.

This program also has implications for the meaning of the human–animal bond in the boys' lives. Boys need opportunities to show their soft, vulnerable side. Through developing a loving relationship with a shelter dog, the young men in the program are able to break down their internal walls as they give and share love with another being, opening up their full potential to living authentically. Men who are able to show this type of vulnerability can make better sons, partners, and community members. Hopefully, the young men who participate in the Teacher's Pet program will take their insights and new ways of interacting with the world and apply it to their life outside of the juvenile justice system.

References

Abram, K. M., Teplin, L. A., Charles, D. R., Longworth, S. L., McClelland, G. M., & Dulcan, M. K. (2004). Posttraumatic stress disorder and trauma in youth in juvenile detention. *Archives of General Psychiatry, 61*(4), 403–410. doi:10.1001/archpsyc.61.4.403.

Achenbach, T. M. (2009). *The Achenbach system of empirically based assessment (ASEBA): Development, findings, theory, and applications*. Burlington, VT: University of Vermont Research Center for Children, Youth and Families.

Adler, A. (1938). *Social interest: A challenge to mankind* (J. Linton & R. Vaughan, Trans.). London: Faber and Faber Ltd.

Ainsworth, M. D. S. (1991). Attachments and other affectional bonds across the life cycle. In C. M. Parkes, J. Stevenson-Hinde, & P. Marris (Eds.), *Attachment across the life cycle* (pp. 33–51). London: Tavistock Publications.

Animal Assisted Interventions International. (2013). *Animal assisted interventions*. Retrieved from http://www.animalassistedintervention.org/AnimalAssistedIntervention.aspx

Arluke, A. (2007). *Animal assisted activities for at-risk and incarcerated children and young adults: An introductory ethnography on five programs*. Unpublished paper presented at the National Technology Assessment Workshop on Animal Assisted Programs for Youth at Risk, Baltimore, MD.

Ascione, F. R. (1992). Enhancing children's attitudes about the human treatment of animals: Generalization to human-directed empathy. *Anthrozoös, 5*, 176–191.

Berget, B., & Braastad, B. O. (2008). Theoretical framework for animal-assisted interventions: Implications for practice. *Therapeutic Communities, 29*, 323–337. doi:10.1186/1745-0179-4-9.

Blazina, C. (2001). Analytic psychology and gender role conflict: The development of the fragile masculine self. Psychotherapy: Theory. *Research, Practice, and Training, 38*, 50–59.

Bowlby, J. (1979). *The making and breaking of affectional bonds*. New York, NY: Tavistock Publications.

Bowlby, J. (1982). Attachment and loss: Retrospect and prospect. *American Journal of Orthopsychiatry*, *52*, 664–678. 10.1111/j.1939-0025.1982.tb01456.x

Brendtro, L., Mitchell, M., & McCall, H. (2009). *Deep brain learning: Pathways to potential with challenging youth*. Albion, MI: Starr Commonwealth.

Brooks, S. M. (2006). Animal-assisted psychotherapy and equine-assisted psychotherapy. In N. Boyd-Webb (Ed.). *Working with traumatized youth in child welfare* (pp. 196–218). New York, NY: Guilford Press.

Chassman, L., & Kinney, E. (2011, February). *Integrating dogs into your professional practice*. Workshop Presented at Animal-assisted Therapy Programs of Colorado, Denver, CO.

Coren, S. (2001). *How to speak dog: mastering the art of dog-human communication*. New York: NY: Simon and Schuster.

David, D. S., & Brannon, R. (1976). *The forty-nine percent majority: The male sex role*. Reading, MA: Addison-Wesley.

Davis, M. H. (1980). A multidimensional approach to individual differences in empathy. *JSAS Catalog of Selected Documents in Psychology, 10*, 85.

Farrington, D. P., Jolliffe, D., Loeber, R., Stouthamer-Loeber, M., & Kalb, L. M. (2001). The concentration of offenders in families, and family criminality in the prediction of boys' delinquency. *Journal of Adolescence, 24*, 579–596.

Fawcett, N. R., & Gullone, E. (2001). Cute and cuddly and a whole lot more? A call for empirical investigation into the therapeutic benefits of human-animal interaction for children. *Behaviour Change, 18*, 124–133. doi:10.1375/bech.18.2.124.

Fearon, R. P., Bakermans-Kranenburg, M. J., vanIJzendoorn, M. H., Lapsley, A., & Roisman, G. I. (2010). The significance of insecure attachment and disorganization in the development of children's externalizing behavior: A meta-analytic study. *Child Development, 81*, 435–456.

Feshbach, N., Feshbach, S., Fauvre, M., & Ballard-Campbell, M. (1983). *Learning to care: A curriculum for affective and social development*. Glenview, IL: Scott, Foresman, & Company.

Fine, A. H., Dennis, A. L., & Bowers, C. (2011). Incorporating animal-assisted interventions in therapy with boys at risk. In C. Haen (Ed.), *Engaging boys in treatment: Creative approaches to the therapy process* (pp. 115–133). New York, NY: Routledge.

Forrest, C. B., Tambor, E., Riley, A. W., Ensminger, M. E., & Starfield, B. (2000). The health profile of incarcerated male youths. *Pediatrics, 105*, 286–291.

Geist, T. (2011). Conceptual framework for animal assisted therapy. *Child Adolescent Social Work Journal, 28*, 243–256. doi:10.1007/s10560-011-0231-3.

Glasser, W. (1998). *Choice theory: A new psychology of personal freedom*. New York, NY: HarperCollins.

Greenebaum, J. B. (2010). Training dogs and training humans: Symbolic interaction and dog training. *Anthrozoös, 22*, 129–141.

Grisso, T. (2008). Adolescent offenders with mental disorders. *The Future of Children, 18*, 143–164. doi:10.1353/foc.0.0016.

Hanselman, J. L. (2001). Coping skills interventions with adolescents in anger management using animals in therapy. *Journal of Child and Adolescent Group Therapy, 11*, 159–195. doi: 10.1023/A:1014802324267.

Hare, B., & Tomasello, M. (2005). Human-like social skills in dogs? *Trends in Cognitive Sciences, 9*, 439–444.

Hazan, C., & Zeifman, D. (1994). Sex and the psychological tether. In K. Bartholomew & D. Perlman (Eds.), *Attachment processes in adulthood. Advances in personal relationships* (Vol. 5, pp. 151–177). London: Jessica Kingsley.

Hirsh, J. B., & Kang, S. K. (2015). Mechanisms of identity conflict: Uncertainty, anxiety, and the behavioral inhibition system. *Personality and Social Psychology Review,*. doi:10.1177/1088868315589475.

Hoeve, M., Geert, J. J., Stams, M., Van der Put, C. E., Semon Dubas, J. S., van der Laan, P. H., et al. (2012). A meta-analysis of attachment to parents and delinquency. *Journal of Abnormal Child Psychology, 40*, 771–785. doi:10.1007/s10802-011-9608-1.

Johnson, A., Cano, A., Casey, R., May, D., & Seivert, N. (2015, July). *Findings from an animal assisted intervention with adjudicated youth.* Posted presented at International Society for Anthrozoology, Sarasota Springs, NY.

Krueger, K. A., & Serpell, J. A. (2010). Animal-assisted interventions in mental health: Definitions and theoretical foundations. In A. H. Fine (Ed.), *Handbook on animal-assisted therapy: Theoretical foundations and guidelines for practice* (3rd ed., pp. 33–48). Amsterdam: Elsevier.

Leftkowitz, C., Paharia, I., Prout, M., Debiak, D., & Bleiberg, J. (2005). Animal-assisted therapy for prolonged exposure: A treatment for survivors of sexual assault suffering from posttraumatic stress disorder. *Society and Animals, 13*, 275–295.

Levinson, B. (1969). *Pet-oriented child psychotherapy*. Springfield, IL: Charles C. Thomas.

May, R. (1981). *Freedom and destiny*. New York, NY: W. W. Norton & Company, Inc.

May, R., & Yalom, I. (2005). Existential psychotherapy. In R. J. Corsini & D. Wedding (Eds.), *Current psychotherapies* (7th ed., pp. 269–298). Belmont, CA: Brooks/Cole.

Melson, G. F., & Fine, A. H. (2010). Animals in the lives of children. In A. H. Fine (Ed.), *Handbook on animal-assisted therapy: Theoretical foundations and guidelines for practice* (3rd ed., pp. 207–226). San Diego, CA: Academic Press. doi:10.1016/B978-012369484-3/50019-0

Mestre, M. V., Samper, P., Frias, M. D., & Tur, A. M. (2009). Are women more empathetic than men? A longitudinal study in adolescence. *The Spanish Journal of Psychology, 12*, 76–83.

O'Neil, J. M. (2015). *Men's gender role conflict: Psychological costs, consequences, and an agenda for change*. Washington, DC: American Psychological Association.

Parish-Plass, N. (2008). Animal-assisted therapy with children suffering from insecure attachment due to abuse and neglect: A method to lower the risk of intergenerational abuse? *Clinical Child Psychology and Psychiatry, 13*, 7–30.

Parish-Plass, N. (2013). *Animal-assisted psychotherapy: Theory, issues, and practice.* West Lafayette, IN: Purdue University Press.

Perls, F. (1969). *Gestalt therapy verbatim.* Lafayette, CA: Real Person Press.

Perry, B. D. (2006). Applying principles of neurodevelopment to clinical work with maltreated and traumatized children. In N. B. Webb (Ed.), *Working with traumatized youth in child welfare*. New York, NY: The Guilford Press.

Polheber, J. P., & Matchock, R. L. (2014). The presence of a dog attenuates cortisol and heart rate in the Trier social stress test compared to human friends. *Journal of Behavioral Medicine, 37*, 860–867.

Raskin, N. J., & Rogers, C. R. (2005). Person-centered therapy. In R. J. Corsini & D. Wedding (Eds.), *Current psychotherapies* (7th ed., pp. 130–165). Belmont, CA: Brooks/Cole.

Rogers, C. (1961). *On becoming a person*. Boston, MA: Houghton Mifflin.

Seivert, N. P, Cano, A., Casey, R. T., Johnson, A., & May, D. K. (2015). Animal-assisted therapy for incarcerated youth: A randomized-controlled trial. Manuscript submitted for publication.

Teplin, L. A., Abram, K. M., McClelland, G. M., Dulcan, M. K., & Mericle, A. A. (2002). Psychiatric disorders in youth in juvenile detention. *Archives of General Psychiatry, 59*, 1133–1143.

van der Kolk, B. (2014). *The body keeps the score: Brain, mind and body in the healing of trauma*. New York, NY: Penguin Group.

Wilson, E. O. (1993). Biophilia and the conservation ethic. In S. R. Kellert & E. O. Wilson (Eds.), *The biophilia hypothesis* (pp. 31–41). Washington, DC: Island Press.

Winnicott, D. W. (1971). *Playing and reality*. London: Tavistock Publications.

Yontef, G., & Jacobs, L. (2005). Gestalt therapy. In R. J. Corsini & D. Wedding (Eds.), *Current psychotherapies* (7th ed., pp. 299–336). Belmont, CA: Brooks/ Cole.

Young, D. W., Dembo, R., & Henderson, C. E. (2007). A national survey of substance abuse treatment for juvenile offenders. *Journal of Substance Abuse Treatment, 32*, 255–266. doi:10.1016/j.jsat.2006.12.018.

Zilcha-Mano, S., Mikulincer, M., & Shaver, P. (2011). Animal companion in the therapy room: An attachment perspective on animal assisted therapy. *Attachment and Human Development, 13*, 541–561. doi:10.1080/14616734.2011.608987.

Chapter 7
Lifetime Bonds: At-Risk Youth and At-Risk Dogs Helping One Another

Cynthia L. Bathurst and Lisa Lunghofer

Lifetime Bonds, one of Safe Humane Chicago's flagship programs, provides opportunities for at-risk youth—particularly teenage males—and at-risk dogs, particularly dogs impounded as victims of cruelty and neglect, to help one another. In this chapter, we describe the program, beginning with background information on Safe Humane Chicago. Next, we provide an overview of the issues faced by incarcerated teens and then describe research on effective interventions with at-risk youth, specifically mentoring, positive youth development, and human–animal interaction. The Lifetime Bonds conceptual framework is described, and the program's successes and challenges are discussed. The chapter concludes with comments and poems written by young men who participated in the program.

Safe Humane Chicago

Safe Humane Chicago's mission is to create safe and humane communities by inspiring positive relationships between people and animals. Its vision is a city in which people and companion animals are free from all forms of violence and live in safe, humane neighborhoods. To accomplish this vision, the organization formed an alliance of nontraditional partners that recognize the connections between animal abuse and interpersonal violence, and the benefits of the

C.L. Bathurst
Safe Humane®, PO Box 7342, Chicago 60680, IL, USA
e-mail: cbathurst@safehumane.org

L. Lunghofer (✉)
Making Good Work, LLC, 330 Chestertown Street, 20878 Gaithersburg, MD, USA
e-mail: llunghofer@makinggoodwork.org

C. Blazina and L.R. Kogan (eds.), *Men and Their Dogs*,
DOI 10.1007/978-3-319-30097-9_7

human–animal bond. Safe Humane Chicago engages that alliance to provide the community with a variety of innovative and collaborative programs focused on humane treatment of people and animals and an improved quality of life. Programs emphasize education, advocacy, and second chances to engage in prosocial activities focused on human–animal interaction.

The fundamental idea that led to Safe Humane Chicago is that community safety and the humane treatment of animals are closely related. Violence toward animals in a community is highly correlated with violence toward people (Vaughn et al. 2009; Luke et al. 1997; Degenhardt 2005). In particular, the Chicago Police Department recognizes that where there are gangs, guns, and drugs, there are also likely to be dog fighting and abused animals. The Safe Humane founders recognized that a campaign to reduce violence against children and companion animals could make a community safer and more humane. Moreover, they understood that positive relationships with animals could help children develop empathy as well as provide comfort in the face of stress and anxiety.

Safe Humane Chicago began as a project of D.A.W.G. (Dog Advisory Work Group), a 501(c)(3) nonprofit incorporated in 2000. D.A.W.G. focused on bringing dog owners and non-dog owners together to educate the community about sharing public spaces wisely. It began as a committee of a neighborhood association in 1998 before expanding its mission beyond neighborhood boundaries to the entire City of Chicago and elsewhere. The focus was on responsible care of companion animals, including the creation of dog-friendly public spaces, public education, and engagement of a broad coalition of stakeholders.

Over time, the organization's founders recognized the growing need to address the violence against animals and children in their city. As a result, programs were developed that focused on the benefits of the human–animal bond and the essential connection between public safety and the humane treatment of both people and animals. Youth engagement programs and advocacy programs for dogs who were victims in cruelty cases were among the first programs offered. As programs were piloted, expanded, and endorsed by a coalition of organizations and agencies, they became the focus of the nonprofit, leading the organization to change its name to Safe Humane in 2013. The first programs were Kids, Animals and Kindness; Youth Leaders; Lifetime Bonds; Court Advocacy; and training for law enforcement professionals. Later, Court Case Dogs® was added, a program that focuses on dogs seized as evidence in abuse investigations or abandoned by prisoners and impounded at Chicago Animal Care and Control (CACC). As part of the Court Case Dogs program, these dogs are socialized, trained, and loved by volunteers; adopted into homes through partner rescues; and offered free behavioral support for life. In 2014 VALOR—Veterans Advancing Lives Of Rescues, a program similar to Lifetime Bonds in which veterans who have posttraumatic stress disorder (PTSD) work with shelter dogs, was piloted. With the impact and success of these programs, Safe Humane Chicago has become a leading resource for education and training about the human–animal bond and its benefits for safer, more humane communities.

Lifetime Bonds and its focus on teaming at-risk youth with at-risk dogs is one of Safe Humane Chicago's most popular programs. The program serves male youth aged 13–18 held in secure detention at the Illinois Youth Center—Chicago (IYCC). Begun in 2009, Lifetime Bonds is a collaboration among IYCC [and the governing Illinois Department of Juvenile Justice (IDJJ)], CACC, and Safe Humane Chicago. In the program, incarcerated male teenagers learn how to care for, socialize, and train shelter dogs from CACC using positive, relationship-based training techniques; and along the way, they develop a sense of accomplishment and empathy for traumatized dogs and hone life skills for themselves. They learn about issues related to animal welfare and safety, including pet overpopulation and dog fighting; societal issues involving personal responsibility and stereotyping; and the many job opportunities available in the pet industry. They develop patience, confidence, and dog-related skills by working with Safe Humane Ambassador Dogs (trained dogs owned by Safe Humane Chicago volunteers who have been assessed and approved for various programs and situations in which dogs represent Safe Humane Chicago) and extend those skills by connecting with and training shelter and Court Case Dogs®. They also are encouraged to draw parallels from their own lives and traumas and their own coping strategies and life situations to those of the dogs and to think and talk about how they are able to build trusting relationships with the dogs because of their pasts. As the review of the literature in the following section suggests, Lifetime Bonds is one of the few programs that provides young incarcerated males with opportunities to develop life skills essential to successfully reentering the community and avoiding future violent and antisocial behavior.

Incarcerated Youth: Risk and Protective Factors

Youth who enter correctional facilities face myriad risk factors that challenge their healthy social and emotional development. Moreover, they have few opportunities while in custody to develop the skills and social competencies necessary to successfully reenter the community and grow into responsible adults. As a result, youth in custody are at greater risk of recidivism than youth who are diverted from detention (Holman and Zidenberg 2006).

The Illinois Juvenile Justice Commission (2011) estimates that more than 50 % of youth released from IDJJ facilities will commit new offenses and return to the juvenile or adult corrections systems. The cost of this failure is extremely high, both in terms of youths' lost potential and the cost to taxpayers. The State of Illinois Auditor General (2010) estimates that it costs almost $87,000 per year, per youth to house juvenile offenders. The Commission's report goes on to say, "There is good news: Young people are capable of tremendous positive change and growth and—with the right support, supervision and services—youth leaving DJJ facilities can become valued assets in our communities" (p. 9). Mentoring programs that seek to minimize risk and enhance protective factors may provide the kind of support youth need to become valued community assets.

Lessons from Mentoring Programs in Community Settings

In a recent comprehensive meta-analysis of youth mentoring programs, DuBois et al. (2011) found modest effects of mentoring programs on positive outcomes for youth. Specifically, youth who are mentored appear to benefit psychologically and socially, and across a range of outcomes, from increases in self-efficacy to better grades to fewer behavioral problems. Programs that specifically address the impact of mentoring on delinquency also report small, but in many cases significant, effects on self-reported delinquency (Joliffe and Farrington 2007; Tolan et al. 2008).

In terms of best practices, programs that offer the most promise provide youth with the opportunity to engage in structured activities and build positive relationships with carefully screened and matched volunteers (Rhodes and DuBois 2008; Rhodes and Lowe 2008). Further, evidence suggests that mentoring activities that are part of a broader program, including education and employment training, are more effective in reducing recidivism (Joliffe and Farrington 2007).

Mentoring Youth in Custody: Challenges, Opportunities, and Research to Date

Mentoring youth in custody presents special challenges. Mentoring programs in juvenile correctional facilities must comply with the facilities' rules and regulations. They also include youth with special educational, mental health, and addiction needs (Bazron et al. 2006). However, mentoring incarcerated youth also presents an opportunity to guide these young people as they make the very difficult transition from the correctional institution back into their community.

In one of a handful of programs designed for youth in custody, Aftercare for the Incarcerated through Mentoring (AIM), youth are assigned a mentor while in the correctional facility and the relationship is sustained for up to a year upon release (Jarjoura 2005). AIM mentors help youth to develop decision-making and problem-solving skills, seek out educational and employment opportunities, and build prosocial bonds in their communities. However, no formal evaluation of the program has been undertaken.

Research on mentoring programs for incarcerated youth is, in fact, very limited, and the few studies that have been done reveal great variation in the definition and application of mentoring and how it is evaluated (Britner et al. 2006; Blechman and Bopp 2005). In one of the few evaluations of a mentoring program for youth in custody, Barnoski (2006) found that mentored youth had lower recidivism rates over a 12-month period following release compared to those with no mentoring, but the effect disappeared at a 36-month follow up. However, methodological limitations, specifically the absence of an experimental design with random assignment to treatment and control groups, suggest that any observed differences, or lack thereof, might be due to spurious or selection effects.

Positive Youth Development: A Conceptual Framework for Helping At-Risk Youth

In addition to a lack of research on whether or not mentoring reduces juvenile offending or reoffending, there is also a critical gap in understanding how mentoring affects positive change for youth. Rhodes' (2002) model posits that mentoring relationships promote social-emotional, cognitive, and identity development, which in turn promotes positive outcomes. While it is important to understand if a mentoring program reduces juvenile offending, it is equally important to understand the program's conceptual framework and the developmental factors it targets to produce positive outcomes. Such an understanding is critical to clearly articulating and advancing evidence-based practice.

Consistent with Rhodes' emphasis on developmental processes, the PYD model offers a robust conceptual framework for mentoring programs, particularly those designed for at-risk youth. The PYD model is rooted in decades of sociological, criminological, and psychological research focused on understanding protective factors that promote resilience and positive outcomes (Butts et al. 2005). Programs based on a PYD framework emphasize youth attachment to supportive adults, civic engagement, and socialization, and provide opportunities to experience a sense of usefulness and belonging. A meta-analysis of 25 PYD programs provided empirical evidence of the impact of these programs on enhancing positive attitudes and behaviors, and reducing delinquency and other problem behaviors (Catalano et al. 1998). Butts et al. (2005) at Chapin Hall argue that "Concentrating on PYD goals in working with young offenders may provide the juvenile justice system with a new and compelling framework for service delivery."

Constructs central to the PYD model are social, emotional, cognitive, behavioral, and moral competencies (Catalano et al. 2002). These competencies are significant for youth development to the extent that they assist youth in integrating their feelings with thinking and action (Catalano et al. 2002). Emotional competence, empathy in particular, can help youth to identify, understand, and share how others are feeling; thus, empathy is central to moral development and serves as an individual protective factor, decreasing risky and delinquent behavior (Jolliffe and Farrington 2004). Accordingly, many studies have examined the role that empathy plays in shaping one's moral development and influencing offending and recidivism. In a meta-analysis examining the relationship between empathy and offending, evidence suggests that young offenders who lack empathy are more likely to offend (Jolliffe and Farrington 2004).

Positive Youth Development and the Role of Human–Animal Interaction

Building on this line of research that indicates empathy is a key protective factor in preventing youth delinquency, recent studies of the human–animal bond shed light on the role that animals may play in building empathy, enhancing youth's moral, cognitive, and identity development, and ultimately reducing recidivism. Scholars working in this field have found that children's relationships with animals can have an important impact on human-directed empathy (Ascione 2001; Ascione and Weber 1996; Daly and Morton 2006). Children's relationships with animals allow them to emotionally invest in another creature's well-being and freely express love and compassion; these experiences are thought to foster positive affect, self-esteem, and self-efficacy (Thompson and Gullone 2003).

Though systematic evaluations of programs promoting human–animal interaction are rare (Ascione 1997) and evaluations of such programs in juvenile correctional facilities rarer still, several qualitative studies suggest the positive effects of animal care on youth in custody. Interviews with participants in Project POOCH, a program established in 1993 in which youth in an Oregon correctional facility train shelter dogs for adoption, found that youth reported improvements in honesty, empathy, nurturing, social growth, understanding, self-confidence, and pride of accomplishment (Deaton 2005).

The Lifetime Bonds Program Model

Based on a PYD framework, Lifetime Bonds offers a critical opportunity to foster prosocial attitudes and behaviors among court-involved male youth. Unlike the traditional juvenile justice system approach that focuses on youth deficits and seeks control as a primary goal, Lifetime Bonds focuses on the role that adult mentors and animals play in enhancing young men's empathy and self-esteem, shaping cognitive and identity development and their capacity for self-determination, and ultimately increasing the likelihood of successful reentry into their community. The companionship of the dogs during the sessions at IYCC provides positive psychological impact for these young men, who struggle with loneliness and emotional isolation as well as physical isolation. Volunteers consistently comment on the calming effect the dogs have on the young men and the ways in which the dogs motivate the youth to develop problem-solving skills, particularly with respect to helping the dogs learn new cues or tasks.

Lifetime Bonds also aims to help young men learn nonviolent, compassionate ways of interacting. Working with adult volunteers, the youth learn to bond with, socialize, and train shelter dogs, saving their lives, and making them more adoptable. Consistent with PYD principles, Lifetime Bonds focuses on the assets of youth in custody and provides them with opportunities to: (1) form prosocial relationships with caring adults, (2) develop skills, (3) participate in structured activities, and (4) engage in efforts that benefit the community, including receiving emotional satisfaction from contributing to another creature's well-being. The ultimate goal is to provide a model of how to live a life of respect and kindness toward animals and people that also helps the young men thrive in communities beyond their neighborhoods. The program reaches those who can stop the cycle of violence—male youth who are among those most affected by the cycle, some of whom have also contributed to the violence.

In fact, comments often made week after week during the program concern the need for these young people to be "men." "I'm not a kid anymore," said one 15-year-old to a volunteer facilitator. "I have two babies, and I have to do what I do to provide for them—and that probably means I'll have to stay in the gang." What it means to be a man is most often connected to a status founded on being "street tough" and having money. Conversations about dog fighting and breeding dogs for fighting and protection often focus on the payoff in cash and the "respect" (generated by fear) others show to vicious fighters and those accompanied by proven fighters or vicious-looking dogs. Program participants also comment that they feel safer discussing these issues in the program environment than "on the outside" and even sharing their feelings in journals, poetry, rap, and art. One young man drew a very gentle portrait of a dog, commenting to a facilitator who noted the gentleness that he could do it because of the calm he had experienced and achieved in being around the dogs and hearing the facilitators' love and concern for dogs.

The population served in the IYCC program is primarily African–American and Hispanic/Latino, and most of the youth are from low-income families who live in the south and west sides of Chicago, communities most impacted by violence (including abuse of both people and animals) and lack of resources for their human family members and companion animals. A minority but significant number of the youth at IYCC are from low-income families who live outside the city of Chicago, in Chicago suburbs and Illinois counties west of Cook.

All youth at IYCC have a record of arrests and justice involvement. Some two-thirds to three-fourths have a diagnosis of some mental health or developmental issue and substance abuse. Excluding those with substance abuse issues, about half of the young men have mental health or developmental issues (Illinois Models for Change Behavioral Health Assessment Team 2010). A few would have been arrested for animal abuse, but many will admit to have engaged in or seen animal abuse.

Lifetime Bonds has two phases. Phase I involves a small-group format while young men are at IYCC, and Phase II, following release from IYCC, uses a team format in which young men work with adult mentors in community-based internships. Figure 7.1 provides an overview of the Lifetime Bonds conceptual framework. Figure 7.2 is a brief overview of the curriculum. A more detailed curriculum and supporting materials may be obtained by emailing getconnected@safehumane.org.

Lifetime Bonds Phase I: Inside the Illinois Youth Center—Chicago

In Phase I, the program is provided by a dedicated group of 10–15 adult volunteers, including mentors, dog handlers, and trainers. To date, the majority of these volunteers are women between the ages of 25 and 65; the men who are the minority of volunteers are in the same age range. This 12-week program involves weekly, 90-min sessions during which young men work with in small groups with adult mentors and first with trained ambassador dogs and then with shelter dogs. Sessions are

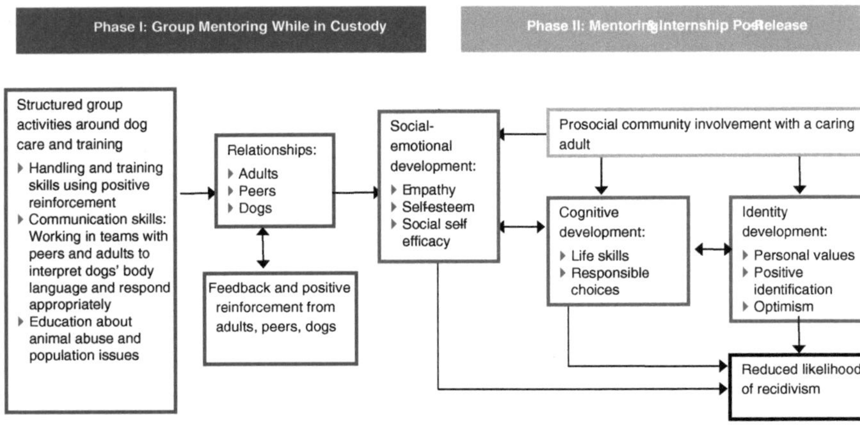

Fig. 7.1 Lifetime bonds conceptual framework

led by the Lifetime Bonds Facilitator who is assisted by dog handlers and other facilitators. The first three or four classes are spent connecting the youth to trained dogs (Safe Humane Ambassador Dogs), learning how to train dogs with positive, relationship-based methods, learning "safe humane" messages about companion animals, and helping the youth connect those messages to their own interactions with other people. In the remaining classes, the youth work mainly with Safe Humane Court Case Dogs or other shelter dogs, allowing youth and dogs to help and learn from each other. The facilitators are trained to listen and encourage comments, questions, journal-writing, rapping, drawing. Following a discussion of the benefits of positive, healthy relationships with one of the facilitators, a 17-year-old came back to the next class with a journal entry that included 5 short-term goals for himself (Fig. 7.3).

Key Phase I objectives include: (1) teaching young men dog handling and training skills using only positive, relationship-based reinforcement and making the connection to building healthy relationships with others; (2) helping the young men learn and practice communication skills by interpreting dogs' body language and responding appropriately and compassionately and making the connection to communication and coping strategies in other relationships; (3) developing the young men's sense of social responsibility by educating them about animal abuse and population issues and making the connection to accountability and caring for others who depend on them; (4) allowing the youth to give back to the community by saving dogs from euthanasia and making them more adoptable and then enjoying the feelings of making positive differences in their own and others' lives; and (5) educating the young men about animal-related careers through guest speakers (dog trainers, dog business owners, dog groomers, dog masseuses, and dog agility instructors, among others). The session with the canine masseuse is especially noteworthy for the young men, as they learn to understand the importance of touch as a connection and a calming tool as well as a stimulus. The field trip to CACC drives home the societal point about homelessness and responsible animal care and always results in comments about compassion and empathy (usually expressed as "sympathy" from the young men).

SAFE HUMANE CHICAGO

Lifetime Bonds Curriculum Template
Illinois Youth Center Chicago (IYCC)

Week 0: Recruitment
Goal/Educational Theme: Understanding the Safe Humane Chicago Lifetime Bonds program. Recruit a maximum of 12 to 15 youth for a session in which 10-15 volunteers are available; invite "graduates" who are still at IYCC and interested in continuing to join next session for advanced programming. Interested youth complete a simple application with help from volunteers.

Week 1
Goal/Educational Theme: Respect, positive reinforcement, compassionate regulation in dog training. Connect with dogs as individuals: understand that each dog is a unique being, a unique personality; begin learning positive reinforcement, compassionate regulation in training, and basic training concepts. Facilitate connection to all types of relationships.

Week 2
Goal/Educational Theme: The human-animal bond. Focus on humane and responsible pet care. Connect with dogs as individuals; learn humane, responsible care giving of dogs. Facilitate connection to all types of relationships.

Week 3
Goal/Educational Theme: Hygiene and Grooming; dog grooming as a job, profession or business. Learn how to make a dog feel good about grooming; learn tools of the grooming trade. Understand the importance of touch and massage. Invite groomer or dog massage therapist. Effectively implement problem solving with individual dogs.

Week 4: field trip to city animal shelter (if possible)
Goal/Educational Theme: Need for spay/neuter, focusing on homeless and abused pets and respect for life; the life of shelter animals; what we can do to help (such as socialization and training for shelter and court case dogs and adopting animals from shelters). Learn about spaying/neutering animals and the connection to animal homelessness.

Week 5
Goal/Educational Theme: Shelter dogs. Learn about (and address) typical feelings and behaviors of shelter dogs: shy, fearful, excited and anxious. Review field trip to CACC, spay/neuter, and life of homeless animals.

Week 6
Goal/Educational Theme: Dog-breed stereotyping, fears and facts about pit bull type dogs. Understand negative impacts of dog-breed stereotypes/breed labeling. Discuss stereotyping and prejudices applied to youth.

Week 7
Goal/Educational Theme: Animal abuse and dog fighting. Understanding animal abuse; educate about dog fighting and the negative impacts it has on the community. Discuss what we in the program can do about animal abuse and dog fighting.

Week 8
Goal/Educational Theme: Job opportunities with animals, particularly dogs. Learn about the many job opportunities working with animals (provide lists and discuss jobs that the volunteers may have). Invite dog massage therapist or groomer if not previously a guest.

Week 9: field trip to agility center (if possible)
Goal/Educational Theme: Positive, fun, beneficial activities you can do with dogs. Learn about positive activities you can do with dogs such as agility, nose work, and obedience and get introduced to them with Ambassador Dogs, practicing the skills themselves.

Week 10
Goal/Educational Theme: Preparing for graduation. Decided what two special skills each youth will do with assigned dog and practice pre-graduation run through. Discuss comments that would be usefully shared with the audience by each youth.

Last Week: Graduation
Goal/Educational Theme: Graduation, called the "dog show." Celebrate the boys' and the dogs' skills and knowledge while educating the IYCC population about the program and Safe Humane messages. Complete the end-of-session questionnaire.

Fig. 7.2 Lifetime bonds curriculum overview

Lifetime Bonds Phase II: Internships in the Community

In Phase II, upon release from custody, the young men are provided a 6-month internship with Safe Humane Chicago's Court Case Dogs program, during which they work one-on-one with a mentor and trainers to socialize and advocate for dogs who are victims in animal cruelty cases, coming full circle from juvenile offenders to productive community members actively defending innocent victims

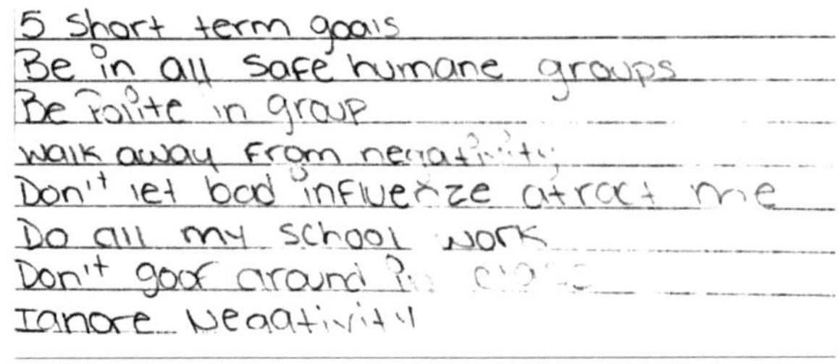

Fig. 7.3 Lifetime bonds participant's journal entry: short-term goals

of violence, abuse, and neglect. The internship allows youth to build on the prosocial skills they learned in the program at IYCC and further support their successful reentry into the community. Each youth begins the internship by participating in three consecutive dog training classes with Safe Humane volunteers at CACC. Following those trainings, each youth helps to develop a set of learning objectives for working with the dogs and is paid a stipend of $10.12 per hour plus transportation costs for 12 weeks. They are also provided with necessary equipment (e.g., dog collars, leashes, treats) and a shirt and badge to be worn while at CACC. Upon successful completion of the session, each youth is eligible to participate in another 12-week session with a new and more demanding set of goals. Those who complete 6 months of interning are helped with finding job opportunities in the growing pet industry, should the young man be interested.

Lifetime Bonds: Challenges and Successes

The key challenge for Lifetime Bonds is offering enough sessions to accommodate the interest shown by the youth at IYCC. The demand for the program exceeds Safe Humane Chicago's capacity to provide it, particularly because it is essential to ensure a program ratio of no more than two youth per dog and mentor. The volunteer approval process is lengthy and the state budget constraints limit the number of background checks that can be performed and have significantly extended the amount of time required to complete them.

There are also challenges engaging the youth in Phase II of Lifetime Bonds. Approximately, 10 % of the youth who have been released from IYCC contact Safe Humane Chicago about internships. Safe Humane Chicago has provided internships for 21 of these young men since 2012. A key finding is the importance of connecting interns with social workers who are assigned to help the youth during their reentry in order to encourage and facilitate their continuing participation in the program. Social workers are able to establish a relationship with the young men, providing the support they need to avoid the people and situations that precipitated their entry into IYCC and choose more prosocial pursuits. They also offer practical assistance getting the youth to the program, as many of the young men live a long distance from CACC. Without the encouragement of the social worker, many of these young men drop out of the program to pursue activities—some of which may not be prosocial—in their own neighborhoods. Six young men dropped out of Phase II or completed only one 3-month session for positive reasons, having gotten a job or begun a college education. One strategy being explored to address this challenge is offering more Lifetime Bonds activities in the neighborhoods of youth who participate in Phase I at IYCC.

Despite the challenges, since September 2009, the numbers show positive impact and success: 23 three-month sessions of Lifetime Bonds at IYCC have served 270 youth. Of these youth, less than 20 % have come back into the justice system following release from IYCC. This compares to a 50 % recidivism rate estimated by the Illinois Juvenile Justice Commission (2011) for youth released from IYCC. These young men have helped some 290 shelter dogs become more adoptable, increasing their chances of finding permanent homes. To date, all of the dogs who participated in the program have been adopted.

Comments from volunteers, program staff, and the young men reflect the impact of the program. One volunteer observed: "It's amazing to watch the boys from when they first come in. They're very straight-faced and quiet. They're not quite sure why they're doing this. And then as the weeks go by you see smiles and them actually warming up to us and the dogs. By the end of the sessions they are very comfortable with us, they tell us about their personal lives." Another volunteer commented, "It feels like a miracle seeing young men initially so defensive and angry become so caring and humane toward dogs that have been rescued/abused. These men open up and share their feelings about the dogs. The dog-human bond is transformative." Yet another: "It's amazing when you bring the two [young men and animals] together, this nonjudgmental, silent bond happens between the two. It's amazing what animals do."

The Lifetime Bonds program manager emphasizes the importance of giving young men opportunities to show compassion: "It's so important if we're ever going to help animals to help people. It's been amazing to see each of these boys as individuals and their capacity and potential for compassion and learning. They're just starving for it." In fact, IYCC staff note that "This is one of the few programs for which we don't need security." Indeed, the dogs provide an opportunity for young men to show affection and simply to touch, something that is especially significant because young men at the detention center are discouraged from physical contact with anyone. "When they can actually touch the dogs, put their hands on them, it's pretty powerful," observed a volunteer. "Being a man" while in the class with the dogs, facilitators, and fellow classmates means working as a team with all of them and sharing insights, questions, help, and just hanging out quietly with the dogs in small groups.

The parallels between the experiences of the dogs and the young men are also important to the success of the program. As one of the young men said, "You take a throw-away boy and a throw-away dog, and you put us together. We help them; they get adopted and find homes. We get out and have better skills and feel like we've accomplished something." The field trip the youth take to CACC is often a turning point for the young men. During the trip, the youth have the opportunity to see the shelter dogs in cages, and they immediately identify with the fact that the dogs are behind bars. They say, "Hey, we understand what you're going through" and "I got it, man." One youth said, "They feel just like people in jail feel. They don't want to be in cages. I never knew there were so many dogs that were abandoned. The population of abandoned dogs is really large. If everyone came together we could change that." Another commented, "They feel worse than zoo animals, just being in a cage looking at each other." In commenting on the youth's reaction to the trip to CACC, the Safe Humane Chicago Executive Director said, "It's very touching because not only are the boys showing empathy but they're also talking about respect for life and freedom."

As the young men develop relationships with the dogs, they also have opportunities to just have fun with them. At a recent Lifetime Bonds graduation ceremony attended by the entire population at IYCC, Devon, one of the program's graduates, performed a break dance while Chico, a Safe Humane Ambassador Dog, performed his version of the dance, both taking a bow together at the end of the performance.

The success of the program is due in large measure to the commitment of Safe Humane Chicago volunteers to the program and the youth they work with: between 2010 and mid-2015, 70 volunteers led by a dog trainer and program facilitator staffed approximately 50 classes and field trips for a total of some 1100 h per year.

The success and popularity of the program among youth and youth service providers are clear and reflected in requests for more neighborhood programming. With the generous support of a grant from the Kenneth A. Scott Charitable Trust, in 2015 Lifetime Bonds will be offered in collaboration with Becoming a Man (B.A.M.) program, a dropout and violence prevention program for at-risk male students in grades 7–12. The program will be held at the K.L.E.O. Community Family Life Center, a nonprofit that offers an array of violence prevention programs to children and families living in some of the most isolated and dangerous neighborhoods in Chicago. Ninety percent of students who participate in B.A.M. are low income, and more than 95 % are African American and Hispanic/Latino.

Modeled on the Lifetime Bonds program at IYCC, a 3-month pilot and a 3-month follow-on program will be offered to a total of 15–20 at-risk males recruited from B.A.M. and other programs at K.L.E.O. Center. Objectives include helping the youth to develop a sense of social responsibility, educating them about animal abuse and population issues, providing them with animal-related job skills and allowing them to give back to the community by saving dogs' lives. Youth will work with trained and adoptable rescue dogs or participants' own dogs, depending on the class composition.

Of note, an evaluation of the project will be conducting, including outcome and process components. Although attempts have been made to evaluate Lifetime Bonds at IYCC, significant challenges were encountered with respect to obtaining consent to participate and facilitating the evaluator's access to the secure facility. As a result, pre-post changes in variables of interest such as empathy have not been formally assessed.

The evaluation of the Lifetime Bonds program in collaboration with B.A.M. will examine changes in participants' knowledge with respect to responsible pet ownership, dogs' body language, pet overpopulation, dog fighting, and animal abuse. In addition, standardized measures of positive core values and sense of self from The After-School Initiative's Toolkit for Evaluating Positive Youth Development will be completed by participants prior to and following program participation. A 6-month assessment will also be conducted to understand the extent to which these changes persist over time, something that has not been attempted with IYC Lifetime Bonds graduates because of the challenges accessing them after release from IYC. The evaluation will also include process measures designed to assess the fidelity with which the program is implemented and a qualitative component, including interviews with Lifetime Bonds graduates.

Final Comments from the Young Men

Although not a requirement of the program, some of the young men who have graduated from Lifetime Bonds have written comments and poems, performed raps and skits, and shared art work. Here, we share four pieces that illustrate the profound effect participation in the program had on each of the youth. Justin's written and oral presentation of his thoughts in front of the incarcerated youth, parents, and guardians, staff, and visitors to the Illinois Youth Center Chicago during a "volunteer appreciation" luncheon surprised and delighted the Safe Humane volunteers. Although Justin often asked questions during classes, he did not always volunteer to share comments with the entire class, much less an audience of at least 75 youth and adults.

> … First I would like to thank the volunteers from Safe Humane. Since being in the Safe Humane program, I can honestly say that when I am released I'll do my best to help inform our community about the horrible things that happens to dogs all year long – not even just dogs, all types of animals are given up over some of the craziest, most outrageous things. The other day me and some of my peers went on a trip to the animal control center, and we took a tour around the building; and on the tour one of the volunteers in Safe Humane told us that a cat was given up and brought to the animal control center because it didn't match the owner's couch any more, or the owners are giving up dogs because it poops too much in the grass. And these animals are worth much more than what people in our community and city treat them like. So I would like to thank Safe Humane for sharing that information and wonderful experience with me. It was a good experience for me because I was always the type of kid that thought it was okay and interesting to see a dog chase a cat or see two dogs go at each other or maybe even just mating dogs together so they can have puppies. But once I found out what most of these animals go through from this kind of abuse, I really do owe Safe Humane and the animal control center a big, big apology.…

Another young man decided to write a poem to share with the class what he had been thinking about as a result of the discussions:

Dogs Need Love
By Roma
It's not right how people treat dogs now a days. Yell at them, beat them, keep em in a cage.
I can see it in their eyes. I can feel their rage. How would you like to be yelled at, Beat, Keep in a cage.
Dogs need love.
When I see a dog that has been beaten, I wanna beat up the person that did it. It makes me sad, I cry inside.

OK I'll admit it cuz I'm a man and a man knows real pain just like that dog that has been beaten with belts and chains.
I know some times dogs don't do what you want them to do but think about didn't you have to learn 2.
But at the end of the day. Dogs are sweeter than chocolate dove.
At the end of the day dogs need love.

Dwaun wrote this poem after a field trip that the youth took to Chicago's municipal shelter. This is one of the young men who continues to check in with Lifetime Bonds staff in his life in his community.

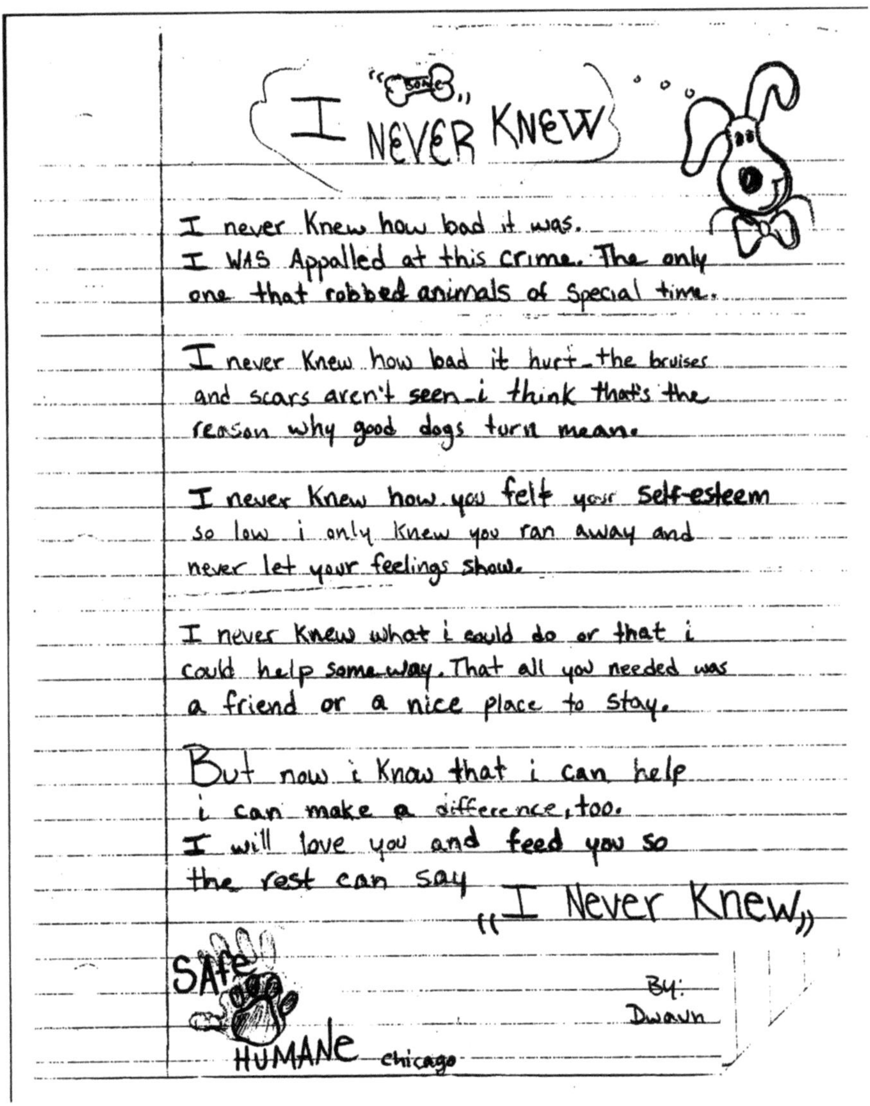
"BONE"
I NEVER KNEW

I never Knew how bad it was.
I WAS Appalled at this crime. The only
one that robbed animals of special time.

I never Knew how bad it hurt the bruises
and scars aren't seen i think that's the
reason why good dogs turn mean.

I never Knew how you felt your self-esteem
so low i only Knew you ran away and
never let your feelings show.

I never Knew what i could do or that i
could help some way. That all you needed was
a friend or a nice place to stay.

But now i Know that i can help
i can make a difference, too.
I will love you and feed you so
the rest can say
"I Never Knew"

By:
Dwaun

SAFE HUMANE chicago

A Lifetime Bonds participant at IYCC, Edward used only the No. 2 pencil allowed at the facility until he was permitted to use in a supervised setting a small number of other pencil weights that the Lifetime Bonds program provided for him. He was one of the young men who completed a Phase II internship and went on to community college.

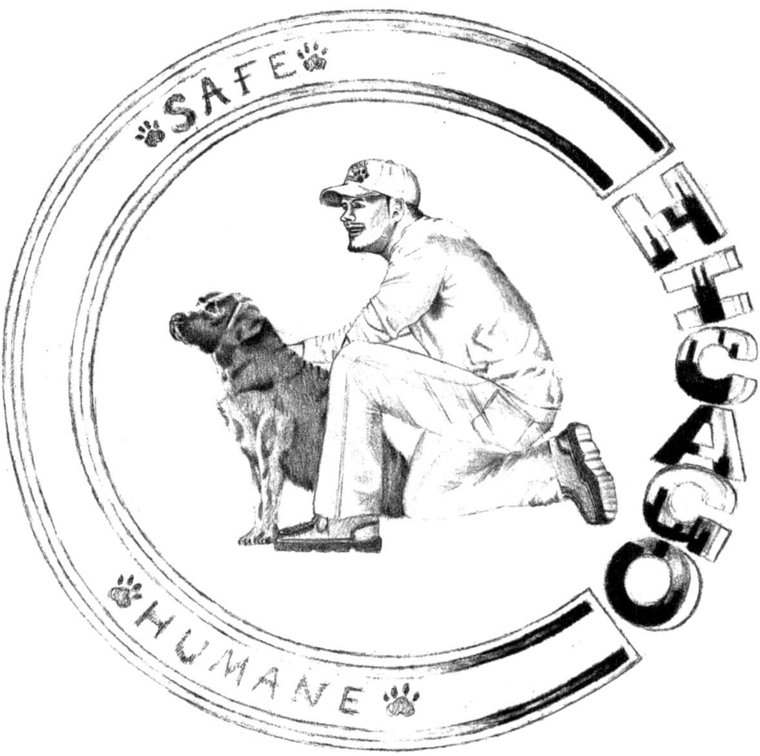

The young men's visual and performing art works reflect their willingness to share their observations and feelings with their incarcerated peers at IYCC. They also demonstrate development of leadership skills, willingness to speak out on behalf of animals, and unabashed pride in connecting with another living being. These young men's words and, in one case, visualization, reflect how deeply their experiences with the dogs changed them and their commitment to sharing their new-found empathy and understanding in an effort to make their communities safer and more humane.

Acknowledgments The authors gratefully acknowledge the contributions of Keri Burchfield, Ph.D. Associate Professor, Department of Sociology, Northern Illinois University, who provided research support and assisted in writing the background section of the chapter.

References

Ascione, F. R. (1997). Humane education research: Evaluating efforts to encourage children's kindness and caring towards animals. *Genetic, Social, and General Psychology Monographs, 123*(1), 59–77.

Ascione, F. R. (2001). Animal abuse and youth violence. *OJJDP: Juvenile Justice Bulletin*, 1–15.

Ascione, F. R., & Weber, C. V. (1996). Children's attitudes about the humane treatment of animals and empathy: One-year follow-up of a school-based intervention. *Anthrozoos, 9*, 188–195.

Barnoski, R. (2006). *Recidivism findings for the Juvenile Rehabilitation Administration's mentoring program: Final report*. Olympia, WA: Washington State Institute for Public Policy.

Bazron, B. J., Brock, L., Read, N., & Segal, A. (2006). *The mentoring tool-kit: Resources for developing programs for incarcerated youth (Unabridged version)*. Washington, D.C.: National Evaluation and Technical Assistance Center for the Education of Children and Youth who are Neglected, Delinquent and At-Risk, U.S. Department of Education.

Blechman, E. A., & Bopp, J. M. (2005). Juvenile offenders. In D. L. DuBois & M. J. Karcher (Eds.), *Handbook of youth mentoring* (pp. 454–466). SAGE: Thousand Oaks, CA.

Britner, P. A., Balcazar, F. E., Blechman, E. A., Blinn-Pike, L., & Larose, S. (2006). Mentoring special youth populations. *Journal of Community Psychology, 34*(6), 747–763.

Butts, J., Mayer, S., & Ruth, G. (2005). *Focusing juvenile justice on positive youth development. Issue Brief #105*. Chapin Hall Center for Children at the University of Chicago, Chicago, IL.

Catalano, R., Berglund, M. L., Ryan, J. A. M., Lonczak, H. S., & Hawkins, J. D. (1998). *Positive youth development in the United States: Research findings on evaluations of positive youth development programs*. Paper submitted to U.S. Department of Health and Human Services, Office of the Assistant Secretary for Planning and Evaluation and National Institute for Child Health and Human Development.

Catalano, R. F., Hawkins, J. D., Berglund, M. L., Pollard, J. A., & Arthur, M. W. (2002). Prevention science and positive youth development: Competitive or cooperative frameworks? *Journal of Adolescent Health, 31*(6), 230–239.

Daly, B., & Morton, L. L. (2006). An investigation of human–animal interactions and empathy as related to pet preference, ownership, attachment, and attitudes in children. *Anthrozoos, 19*, 113–127.

Deaton, C. (2005). Humanizing prisons with animals: A closer look at "cell dogs" and horse programs in correctional institutions. *Journal of Correctional Education, 56*(1), 46–62.

Degenhardt, B. (2005). *Statistical summary of offenders charged with crimes against companion animals*, July 2001–July 2005. Report from the Chicago Police Department.

DuBois, D. L., Portillo, N., Rhodes, J. E., Silverthorn, N., & Valentine, J. C. (2011). How effective are mentoring programs for youth? A systematic assessment of the evidence. *Psychological Science in the Public Interest, 12*, 57–91.

Holman, B., & Zidenberg, J. (2006). *The dangers of detention: The impact of incarcerating youth in detention and other secure facilities*. Washington, D.C.: The Justice Policy Institute.

Illinois Juvenile Justice Commission Youth Reentry Improvement Report. (2011, November).

Illinois Models for Change Report on the Behavioral Health Program for Youth Committed to Illinois Department of Juvenile Justice. (2010).

Jarjoura, R. (2005). *Indiana's juvenile reentry program: Aftercare for Indiana through mentoring (AIM)*. Indianapolis: Aftercare for Indiana through Mentoring.

Jolliffe, D., & Farrington, D. P. (2004). Empathy and offending: A systematic review and meta-analysis. *Aggression and Violent Behavior, 9*, 441–476.

Jolliffe, D., & Harrington, D. P. (2007). Examining the relationship between low empathy and self-reported offending. *Legal and Criminological Psychology, 12*(2), 265–286.

Luke, C., Arluke, A., & Levin, J. (1997). *Cruelty to animals and other crimes*. Report by the Massachusetts SPCA.

Rhodes, J. E. (2002). *Stand by me: The risks and rewards of mentoring today's youth.* Cambridge, MA: Harvard University Press.

Rhodes, J. E., & DuBois, D. L. (2008). Mentoring relationships and programs for youth. *Current Directions in Psychological Science, 17*, 254–258.

Rhodes, J. E., & Lowe, S. R. (2008). Youth mentoring and resilience: Implications for practice. *Child Care in Practice, 14*(1), 9–17.

State of Illinois Auditor General, Department of Juvenile Justice Compliance Examination for the Two Years Ended June 30, 2010.

Thompson, K. L., & Gullone, E. (2003). Promotion of empathy and prosocial behavior in children through humane education. *Australian Psychologist, 38*, 175–182.

Tolan, P., Henry, D., Schoeny, M., & Bass, A. (2008). Mentoring interventions to affect juvenile delinquency and associated problems. *Campbell Systematic Review, 16*, 1–112.

Vaughn, M. G., Fu, Q., DeLisi, M., Beaver, K., Perron, B., Terrell, K., et al. (2009). Correlates of cruelty to animals in the United States: Results from the national epidemiologic survey on alcohol and related conditions. *Journal of Psychiatric Research, 43*, 1213–1218.

Chapter 8
Exploring the Role of Playfulness with Canine Companions in Coping with Stress: How Men Are Impacted by Human–Animal Interaction Through Calling on a Memory of Play

Mary Harlinger and Chris Blazina

Today, animal companions, those nonhumans that by definition are psychologically experienced as a close friend or family member, have become more visible than ever in everyday life (Blazina et al. 2011). According to the Humane Society of the United States (2013), there are approximately 164 million dogs and cats in homes. In research studies, between 87 and 99 % of pet owners defined their pets as being like a friend or family member (Cain 1983; Voith 1985). While the importance of human–animal interaction (HAI) connection may seem like a recent development, animals have long been a valued part of human life as seen through ancient cultures that saw animals as companions, spiritual guides, figures within folklore, or as symbols of luxury (Serpell 2010; Walsh 2009).

By the mid-1980s, veterinary programs began to recognize the importance of the bond by including the concept within curriculum (Hines 2003). The human–animal bond has also become more prominent in social sciences in the twentieth century (Bustad 1987; Levinson 1978). There have been studies to understand the far-reaching physical and emotional wellness benefits of this relationship (see Anderson et al. 1992; Bauman et al. 2000; Friedmann et al. 1980; Knight and Edwards 2008; Morrison 2007; Siegel 1990, 1993; Serpell 1991; Walsh 2009; Wells 2009).

Extending the research further involves understanding the HAI's importance by pairing it with various other contextual factors such as gender (Blazina et al. 2011).

M. Harlinger (✉)
Hampton VAMC, 315 Blair Avenue, Newport News, VA 23607, USA
e-mail: mmharlinger@gmail.com

C. Blazina
College of Education, Department of Counseling and Educational Psychology, MSC 3CEP, New Mexico State University, PO Box 30001, Las Cruces, NM 88003, USA
e-mail: cblazina@nmsu.edu

C. Blazina and L.R. Kogan (eds.), *Men and Their Dogs*,
DOI 10.1007/978-3-319-30097-9_8

The current chapter study focuses upon playful interactions between males and their canine companions and how they can potentially mediate stress. It is argued that in playful encounters, men that may normally feel constricted by traditional gender roles, are instead able to experience and express a more abundant and wider range of emotions and behaviors. Further, the memory of those playful exchanges with a canine companion can be sustained over time and can remain a source of emotional comfort and soothing when called upon.

Attachment Theory

Bowlby (1979, 1999) suggested that much like our nonhuman mammalian counterparts, humans are biologically predisposed toward making connections with others, especially the caregiver. The attachment theory paradigm describes the important relationship between a child and a caretaker as it relates to self-development and interpersonal functioning (see Ainsworth 1982, 1989; Ainsworth et al. 1978; Bartholomew 1990, 1991; Bowlby 1979, 1999). More specifically, a caregiver offers a special type of connection that is exceptionally important, involving qualities that are deemed irreplaceable. While a meaningful tie can be made with a number of friends, teachers, and family members, the place of an attachment figure is unique in a child's life. Bowlby suggested that an attachment figure represents a source of comfort when under distress (safe haven), and one offering encouragement when facing difficult life challenges (safe base). The safe haven concept is especially relevant for this study. Bowlby (1979, 1999) suggested that all mammalian species, both nonhumans and humans alike, are hardwired to seek safety when threatened or in danger. But in the case of human animals, instead of burrowing into a den, the preference is to nuzzle into the arms or care of an attachment figure.

Over time, the attachment figure label that was initially applied to the caregiver–child relationship has been expanded. It now also includes adult romantic relationships (see Hazan and Shaver 1987) and the bond with animal companions (Melson 2002). Bowlby's attachment theory has supplied the theoretical underpinnings for pets' importance in much of the current research literature (Sharkin and Knox 2003). It has been argued that animal companions can also perform the roles of an attachment figure, functioning as a safe base and safe haven (Kobak 2009; Kurdek 2008, 2009). In terms of attachment safety, animal companions provide predictable comfort in stressful times. Dogs may be especially predisposed to act as the attachment figure role (Kobak 2009). They have unique abilities to provide a mutual gaze and read human facial cues and are particularly primed to discern human behavior (Sanders 2003; Müller et al. 2015; Téglás et al. 2012). The reciprocal communication between dog and human, along with routines and instances of play, creates an attachment bond (Horowitz and Bekoff 2007; Sanders 1999, 2003). An animal companion can function as a social support, which may help with handling stress (Margolies 1999).

The tactile experience of canine companions can also be experienced as emotionally soothing. Research supports the idea that blood pressure and heartbeat decrease when petting and stroking animal's fur (Charnetski et al. 2004; DeMello 1999; Nagengast et al. 1997). Research on oxytocin, sometimes referred to as the "bonding-hormone," has been shown to increase in a number of scenarios that involve the presence of dogs (Handlin et al. 2011; Miller et al. 2009; Odendaal and Lehmann 2000; Odendaal and Meintjes 2003). In these moments described above, canine companions are experienced as a safe haven.

The safe haven aspect associated with the presence of a canine companion can be especially pertinent. In a recent study, adults ($n = 192$) reported attachment levels to their romantic significant other and then to their dogs (Beck and Madresh 2008). Participants' ratings between the two types of attachment figures did not correlate; however, attachment figure ratings were significantly higher for animal companions. This suggests that the attachment to a dog is the result of distinct interactions; the human–canine bond is cultivated similar to a human–human relationship where nuanced feelings of closeness can develop. Likewise, Kurdek (2008) found that while college students reported having secure attachment relationships with family and friends, they nevertheless reported their dogs being both a safe haven and safe base. In a related follow-up study, middle-aged dog owners were asked to compare their animal companions to various human companions on attachment-related dimensions (Kurdek 2009). The results found that approximately 45 % of subjects were more likely to turn to their canine companions in times of emotional distress than to their mothers, fathers, brothers, sisters, best friends, and children. There was also an important finding regarding middle-aged men and attachment (Kurdek 2009). While males followed the general trend of the attachment figure findings, they were even more likely to rely on their dogs for emotional support when in distress than any other potential human supporters (Kurdek 2009). The only tie that rivaled the bond between man and dog was one's significant other. These findings support the notion dogs really are "man's best friend." This adage may be especially true for men who feel alone and not at ease revealing personal matters to others. Unfortunately, this solitary state of emotional being can be an all too familiar one for many men, and this can affect forming a secure attachment bonds.

Men, Masculinity, and Psychological Defenses

Attachment theory offers several unique perspectives on styles, strategies, and psychological defenses (see Ainsworth et al. 1978; Bartholomew and Horowitz 1991; Bowlby 1979, 1999; Brennan et al. 1998; Fonagy 2001; Hazan and Shaver 1987; Main 2000; Main and Solomon 1986; Shaver and Mikulincer 2002). Bowlby (1979, 1999) suggested that each individual develops a *working model* or mental representations of self and others. This model is based upon positive and negative experiences of support by initial attachment caregivers. From these memories, one begins to develop an internal working model involving a more systemized view of how one perceives self, others, and the world, which is the basis of attachment bonds (Bowlby 1979, 1999). The working model builds expectations of relationships throughout adolescence and into adulthood (Bowlby 1979, 1999). It is a set of rules guiding thoughts, actions, and feelings in the relational context. That is, the individual will begin forming expected outlooks for the way others will treat them, especially significant others (Ainsworth et al. 1978; Hazan and Shaver 1987).

When an infant experiences consistent positive attachment events, a secure attachment style develops; when there is a chronic occurrence of negative attachment experiences, various types of insecure styles can emerge (see Ainsworth 1982, 1989; Main 2000). The field initially focused on discrete categories of attachment. An individual may believe the world is safe and attuned to one's needs and would be categorized as having secure attachment style, while an individual that views the world as unpredictable in terms of safety and responsiveness or potentially dangerous and rejecting would be categorized as having an anxious or avoidant attachment style, respectively. Later, attachment was conceptualized along a continuum emphasizing how each individual has his or her own unique configuration based upon avoidance and anxiety (see Bartholomew and Horowitz 1991; Brennan et al. 1998). Those with low levels of both are characterized as having a secure attachment style. Those with high levels on either dimension are thought to use particular types of opposing coping strategies: hyperactivation and deactivation of the attachment system (Mikulincer and Shaver 2003). People that rely on hyperactivation attempt to seek constant closeness and emotional support with attachment figures and are very sensitive to any possible signs of or abandonment or rejection. Those that use deactivation strategies suppress or discount the need to seek an attachment figure (Mikulincer and Shaver 2003). People relying on deactivation strategies experience discomfort with closeness, and, therefore, keep an emotional distance from others. The emotional distance is utilized because a desire to appear self-reliant, though much of their striving is actually rooted in counter dependence.

Avoidant styled men and women use deactivating strategies involving distancing from affect, denial of attachment needs, and circumventing emotional involvement and intimacy when under duress (Cassidy 1999). It is suggested, though, that deactivation strategies are particularly relevant for men that struggle with the impact of traditional male socialization (see Blazina and Bartone 2015; Del Giudice 2011; Wexler 2009). In many ways, the avoidant style fits with the traditional male socialization patterns of going-it-alone, constricting emotions, and solving one's own problems. This etiology also theoretically meshes with early childhood issues due to parental separation and empathic misattunement during the disidentification process (Blazina and Bartone 2015; Pollack 1999). Many of these aspects can be operationalized from the perspective of O'Neil's Gender Role Conflict paradigm (O'Neil 1982, 2008; O'Neil et al. 1986).

Gender Role Conflict

O'Neil's research within the Gender Role Conflict paradigm emphasizes the connection between men's gender role strain, psychological distress, and dysfunction (see Chap. 1 for a more extensive review; O'Neil 1982, 2008; O'Neil et al. 1986). Western culture supports men who are overly restricted in emotionality, homophobic, present skewed versions of success and power, and are unyielding in their attempts to balance work and family demands. There is over 40 years of substantiated research linking gender role conflicted men to increases in depression, anxiety, substance use, interpersonal problems, and emotional isolation (O'Neil 2008). Plainly, men who feel constricted by traditional gender roles are adversely impacted by psychological distress and have limited opportunities for intimacy. Gender role conflict emphasizes the restriction of human potential due to stereotypical gender roles.

There have been a few studies connecting gender role conflict to attachment-related issues. College-aged men with separation–individuation issues were found to have poorer parental perceptions (Blazina and Watkins 2000; DeFranc and Mahalik 2002; Fischer 2007; Fischer and Good 1998). Certain aspects of gender role conflict (e.g., higher levels of Success, Power, Competition, Restricted Emotionality, and Restricted Affectionate Behavior Between Men) were found to be significantly related to fearful and avoidant attachment styles (Cachia 2001). Males exhibiting increased gender role conflict also exhibited an avoidant attachment style (Schwartz et al. 2004), and increases in gender role conflict were found to be related to perceptions of the father's own gender role conflict (DeFranc and Mahalik 2002). Further, college-aged men's perceived childhood maternal care, based upon memories of emotional responsiveness and warmth, was a significant predictor of men's adult attachment avoidance (Land et al. 2011). Greater perceived maternal care was related to lower levels of avoidance. This last finding is consistent with Fischer and Good (1998) who found a relationship between male gender role conflict scores and attachment conflicts with mothers.

Exceptions to the Attachment Rule

Although attachment style is theorized as a global orientation operating especially within intimate types of relationships, some researchers believe that a person can make exceptions to their normal internal working model functioning (Mikulincer and Shaver 2003). These exemptions cause the person to think and even act differently to an attachment figure in a contrasting way to one's usual overall attachment style. That is, in some contexts, for example, an insecurely attached person may show behaviors that are consistent with a secure style. This might occur with a new friend, a therapist, or as we suggest for gender role conflicted styled men, with one's canine companion when engaged in play. Further, exceptions to the attachment-related rules can be activated by actual or imagined encounters with supportive or unsupportive people (Mikulincer and Shaver 2001).

Attachment figures provide unique experiences including being a safe haven. Sometimes even the memory of those occurrences can provide moments of solace and are particularly important when one is temporarily separated from the attachment figure or he/she has been lost through old age or death. Even as the child matures into an adult, the recollection of soothing experiences can provide a lasting quality that helps offer comfort when in distress. Bowlby (1979, 1999) argued in the absence of the actual caregiver, the child eventually learns to call on the memory of the soothing qualities for comfort. Likewise, consistent with psychodynamic-orientated theories, calling on the memory of various attachment figures, e.g., the therapist, parent, romantic partner, and even, we argue, one's animal companion may deliver similar results—the temporary soothing of stressful moments. Calling on memories can be an effective because unlike negative affect, positive affect experienced when recalling a positive event does not subside (Pasupathi 2003). Further, there is evidence that as time passes, individuals with a fearful-avoidant attachment style recall positive attachment memories as even more satisfying than they initially report immediately after the event occurred (Pietromonaco and Barrett 1997). It was suggested that this occurs because the positive event disconfirms beliefs about insecure attachment and is consequently intensely valued (Pietromonaco and Barrett 1997). Attachment style can distort emotion associated with an event (Gentzler and Kerns 2006), and perhaps this can be utilized in an adaptive manner by focusing on a secure attachment figure such as a canine companion. However, it is important to consider that there is not only one form of solace. It is argued that an overlooked form of soothing can involve playfulness.

Playfulness

Play is often considered an essential building block of learning for children, it is the way they discover many aspects of the world (Piaget 1972; Samuelsson and Carlsson 2008; Vygotsky 1978). Social play allows one to explore new concepts and experiences without the risk of harsh consequences and teaches cooperative engagement (Bekoff 2001; Lancy and Grove 2011). While play can be difficult to operationalize (Sutton-Smith 2008), focusing on reported internal experience prompts the contextual understanding of the experience (Henricks 2008). This may be particularly important when investigating playfulness in adults, as this has not been widely studied as compared to research on playfulness in children. However, playfulness in children and adults can have similar components; age transforms how playfulness is expressed (Barnett 1991; Guitard et al. 2005). Playfulness in adults might be seen in character traits such as seeking novelty or a circumstance-appropriate lack of inhibition. It could also be seen in situational behaviors like utilizing imagination or trying to dedramatize a difficult situation (Barnett 1991; Guitard et al. 2005; Saunders et al. 1999). More specifically, playfulness might be identified as one exhibiting curiosity, creativity, a sense of humor, and spontaneity (Barnett 2007; Guitard et al. 2005). Playfulness in adults is linked to a better ability to face life challenges because there is a sense of openness to the unknown combined with the ability to frame situations as less overwhelming (Guitard et al. 2005). This can empower adults to feel motivated and able to distance themselves from a problem (Auerhahn and Laub 1987; Lyons 1987; Saunders et al. 1999). Canine companions may be natural playmates because of the innate structure of the human–animal bond.

Playfulness and the Canine Companion

Because canines use play as an avenue to understand the world, the bond in the human–canine relationship can often rely on playfulness (Bekoff 2001). Animals learn social norms, relational standing, and codes of conduct during play (Bekoff and Pierce 2009), which can create context for attachment (Bekoff 2001). Play signals are a form of mutual communication (Bekoff et al. 2002) and can be linked to social intelligence because they are about sharing and appraising intentions (Lancy and Grove 2011). A widely recognized play signal for canines is the play bow. This behavior is ritualized and looks the same across all breeds of dogs because it serves the important purpose of communicating that the canine is about to engage in play (Bekoff and Pierce 2009). For dogs, this communication is crucial because aggressive and playful behaviors may present the same; a bite may be a threat or a summons to play. Signal communication can develop into play routines (Horowitz and Bekoff 2007; Mitchell and Thompson 1990). Play routines inform the players what the game will be and also denote a relational component. An object retrieval routine might be a game of fetch but also shows mutual engagement as seen by looking at the object and back to the playmate (Horowitz and Bekoff 2007; Mitchell and Thompson 1986). One of the most important relational components to play in both human–human and human–animal relationships is contingent activity (Horowitz and Bekoff 2007). This is the turn-taking element of play. For play to be successful, both players must keep the play going by alternating turns. The human must throw the ball to give the canine opportunity to have a turn. The dog must return the ball or else the game is over. Contingent activity shows two partners working together toward the same goal (Bekoff 2001; Horowitz and Bekoff 2007). This partnership creates a pleasurable loop where as one enjoys the moment, feelings of playfulness increase, which creates more satisfaction (Aune and Wong 2002). The cooperation and communication that occur during play strengthens attachment ties and generates shared enjoyment (Aune and Wong 2002; Bekoff 2001; Lancy and Grove 2011; Wood et al. 2005).

HAI, Play, and Psychoanalysis

Placing play within the HAI is aided by various interpretations, many with a contextual psychoanalytic view of the bond's importance (Blazina 2011). Some researchers have argued that the power and value of the human–animal relationship is based on a perceived nonjudgmental emotional support (Allen et al. 2002; Corson et al. 1977). Both Sigmund Freud and his daughter, Anna, wrote of their personal experiences with dogs and how this affiliation taught them about "pure love" relationships (Roth 2005). Although most people may benefit from the support of a pure love relationship, those that have experienced challenging life events may be predisposed to have a special appreciation of the bond. From a self-psychology perspective, an animal companion can be experienced as a resource for enhancing one's emotional or psychological sense of well-being (Brown 2004, 2007). The human–canine bond allows for a sense of social relatedness and belonging. It can serve in a range of roles from companion to child substitute while filling multiple psychological roles, some of which we are not aware of until a loss has occurred (Blazina 2011). The relatedness encompassed within HAI may in turn foster an individual's ability to connect with others in more appropriate ways by increasing self-cohesion and esteem (Brown 2004, 2007). Animal companionship may also serve as a source of emotional sustenance for those who have no or limited connection (both physical and emotional) with people (e.g., Brown 2004, 2007; Sharkin and Bahrick 1990). Likewise, in keeping with Bolwby's attachment theory, the mental representation of the canine companion can even be potentially internalized, acting as a role model to supply a source of soothing (Blazina 2011). In clinician application, Blazina (2011) suggested that when dealing with the loss of an animal companion, part of the work involves helping the client learn to call upon the memory of continued bond for remembrance, comfort, and connection. The use of the technique may ultimately also be used in the context of using a memory of play.

Sadler (1966) noted that play drops pretense and "...gives another courage to be himself" (p. 243). This is of critical importance because insecure attachment styles can utilize coping strategies that obscure one's true experience and self, particularly for men. The canine companion can become a valued attachment figure and play can provide positive attachment experiences. In human–human relationships, play enhances intimacy (Aune and Wong 2002) and this should be applied to human–canine relationships. Animal companions are more than substitutes for humans; they can be consistent attachment figures that are attuned to their human companion and provide mutual communication in both verbal and nonverbal ways (Beck and Madresh 2008; Blazina 2011). While attunement has been a particular focus for the health and welfare of infants and children, (see Bowlby 1979, 1999; Kohut 1984; Stern 2000; Winnicott 1971) this same concept is important for adults. Attunement is a necessary part of vibrant adult relationships that range from friends and romantic partners to the healing power of a therapeutic connection, and we argue, when playing with our animal companions. The power of the HAI may provide increased ability to cope with life (Beck and Madresh 2008).

Method

The research gathered information regarding the nuanced bond between men and their animal companions in the context of play. Specific data was gathered about trait playfulness, perceived stress levels, state playfulness, attachment to canine companion, and gender role conflict. Participants volunteered to take part in this survey by using a link embedded in an online advertisement post on social media sites, Twitter, Facebook, and Craigslist.

Instruments

The survey was formatted so that participants were first given informed consent, a demographic questionnaire, and then were assessed for trait playfulness, perceived stress, and state playfulness. Participants were asked to write a story about a time they had played with their dog and then were reassessed for state playfulness and stress. The survey ended by assessing the attachment to dog and gender role conflict.

Demographic Questionnaire

Participants provided information on age, gender, racial/ethnic identification, educational status, relationship status, and the amount of time they had been with their canine companion.

Short Measure of Adult Playfulness

The Short Measure of Adult Playfulness (SMAP) is an abbreviated self-report measure developed by Proyer in 2012. It contains five items intended to globally assess trait playfulness. The items are positively keyed statements and participants use a 4-point scale to indicate if they (1) strongly disagree to (4) strongly agree with the statement. During scale validation, the alpha coefficients were between 0.83 and 0.99 across the three samples indicating a high internal consistency (Proyer 2012). The test–retest correlation was fair at 0.74 ($p < 0.001$). Upon comparison with the Adult Playfulness Scale and Playfulness Descriptor List (PDL), the SMAP showed congruent validity without being redundant (Proyer 2012).

Playfulness Descriptor List

State playfulness was measured using the PDL developed by Barnett (2007) in a modified format extending playfulness to the relationship with the canine companion. This descriptor list is a self-report measure containing 15 item words (active, adventurous, cheerful, clowns around, energetic, friendly, funny, happy, humorous, impulsive, jokes/teases, outgoing, sociable, spontaneous, unpredictable) associated with the construct of playfulness. The items were developed from focus groups ($n = 649$) identifying correlates of playfulness in self and others; the 15 items had correlations across self-rating and rating of others with differentiation between high and low playfulness that ranged from 0.21 to 0.71 ($p < 0.0001$), indicating high ecological validity (Barnett 2007). This is an asset as playfulness has been a difficult notion to conceptualize for research (Henricks 2008; Sutton-Smith 2008). The alpha coefficients were between 0.73 and 0.87 across the three samples indicating adequate internal consistency. During exploratory factor analysis, the items were associated with four main factor loadings of Gregarious, Uninhibited, Comedic, and Dynamic. Participants will rate themselves using a 10-point Likert scale to indicate they demonstrate the item (1) not at all to (10) a great deal of demonstration with item. An important strength of this measure was that findings were consistent between males and females. The ratings are summed and averaged as a total score. The mean represents the degree of playfulness for the individual as the sum was highly correlated to independent rating ($r = 0.91$; Barnett 2007).

Perceived Stress Scale

Perceived stress was measured using Perceived Stress Scale (PSS-10). It was developed to assess whether respondents find their lives to be unpredictable, uncontrollable, or overloaded (Cohen et al. 1983). The self-report measure contains 10 general questions, which are answered using a 5-point Likert scale ranging from "never" (0) to "very often" (4). During scale validation, the alpha coefficients were between 0.84 and 0.86 across the three samples indicating an adequate internal consistency; the test–retest reliability was high at 0.86 ($p < 0.001$; Cohen et al. 1983). Findings did not show any significant differences between age or sex indicating broad applicability to respondents. The scale is summed for total stress score with four items reverse-scored. Higher scores indicate greater psychological stress (Cohen et al. 1983; Cohen and Janicki-Deverts 2012). Follow-up studies reported high internal reliability at 0.91 ($p < 0.001$; Cohen and Janicki-Deverts 2012).

Description of Play Event

The request for a written description of a play event with a canine companion asked participants to think of a playful time with their dog and describe the interaction. This was intended to activate an autobiographical memory. The autobiographical memory approach allows participants to access personally meaningful memories (He et al. 2011). The use of memory primes cognitive schemas and may impact information processing or emotional arousal (Rowe and Carnelley 2003).

That is, memory recall of an event may impact assessment of behavior (Dudukovic et al. 2004) and remembering a positive event can evoke the positive feelings that were originally felt (Gross 1999; Pasupathi 2003).

Lexington Attachment to Pets Scale

The Lexington Attachment to Pets Scale (LAPS) was developed to assess attachment to animal companion (Johnson et al. 1992). This 23 question self-report measure has positively keyed items with a 4-point scale for participants to indicate if they (1) strongly disagree to (4) strongly agree with the statement. During scale validation, the alpha coefficient was 0.928, indicating a high internal consistency (Johnson et al. 1992). The corrected item-total correlation for each question was 0.50 and above ($p < 0.001$). During principal component analysis, items loaded onto three main factors of: general attachment, people substituting, and animal rights. Correlations between item thresholds were approximately 0.94 ($p < 0.001$). Upon comparison with interviewer rating, the correlation coefficient of the questions to the rating was 0.64 ($p < 0.001$; Johnson et al. 1992).

Gender Role Conflict Scale-Short Form

The Gender Role Conflict Scale-Short Form (GRCS-SF) was developed to assess male gender role conflict (Wester et al. 2012). The original GRCS showed good reliability and validity (O'Neil 2008). This shortened version of the GRCS is a 16-question self-report measure. It has positively keyed items with a 6-point scale for participants to indicate if they (6) strongly agree to (1) strongly disagree with the statement. The GRCS-SF was created by choosing the items that had the strongest loading (>0.60) to four factors (Restricted Emotionality, Success/Power/Competition, Restrictive Affectionate Behavior Between Men, Conflicts Between Work and Family Relations). These factors had coefficient alphas ranging between 0.77 and 0.80, indicating good reliability (Wester et al. 2012). In confirmatory factor analysis, the GRCS-SF factors showed significant correlation with the original GRCS with correlations ranging from 0.90 to 0.96 ($p < 0.001$).

Results

Of a total sample size of 297, there were 168 entries with substantial data from more than one measure and were deleted. This left 129 completed surveys with an all-male sample. Participants mostly reported identifying as non-Hispanic White (82 %) with some level of college education, including trade school, bachelor's, or graduate degree's earned (77 %). Age ranged between 19 and 77, with 71 % being aged 30 and older. A little over half of participants reported being in a romantic relationship (54 %) and having their dog for 5 years or less (54 %). The assumptions of linearity, independence of errors, homoscedasticity, and outliers were met. However, while the data showed a normal distribution among scores, it also showed skewing for playfulness, attachment, and gender role conflict. Playfulness scores were negatively skewed with trait playfulness indicating a skewness of −0.923 (SE = 0.214) and kurtosis of 1.016 (SE = 0.425) and preintervention state playfulness indicating a skewness of −0.165 (SE = 0.214) and kurtosis of −0.912 (SE = 0.425). Attachment also showed negative skewing with a skewness of −0.757 (SE = 0.214) and kurtosis of −0.034 (SE = 0.425). Gender role conflict showed positive skewing with a skewness of 0.265 (SE = 0.214) and kurtosis of −0.104 (SE = 0.425).

Sample Characteristics

Because the majority of the final sample endorsed high levels of playfulness and attachment and reported low gender role conflict, for the sole purpose of reporting this sample bias, the range of possible scores for each measure were divided at the midpoint to create two simulated categories: higher and lower. These categories are reported to give a better understanding of the sample characteristics. For trait playfulness, 86 % of participants scored in the higher range indicating a higher playfulness disposition. For state playfulness before the memory intervention, 81 % of participants scored in the higher range indicating a higher sense of playfulness during the timeframe of completing the survey. For attachment, 94 % of participants reported feelings of attachment in the higher range, suggesting a strong bond with their canine. For gender role conflict, 65 % of participants scored in the lower range indicating low gender role conflict. See Table 8.1 for complete information regarding this analysis.

Table 8.1 Descriptive statistics for characteristics of sample

Scale	Means (SD)	# of items (range per item)	Low range / High range	Frequency* (%)
Short measure of adult playfulness	27.30 (4.88)	5 (1–7)	5–20	18 (14.1)
			21–35	110 (85.9)
Preplayfulness descriptor list**	7.03 (1.58)	15 (1–10)	1–5	23 (19.2)
			7–10	97 (80.8)
Lexington attachment to pets scale	77.48 (10.30)	23 (1–4)	23–57	7 (5.5)
			58–92	121 (94.5)
Gender role conflict scale-SF	52.96 (11.94)	16 (1–6)	16–56	83 (64.8)
			57–96	45 (35.2)

Note *Missing data excluded. **Final score is an average

Does Gender Role Conflict Predict Trait Playfulness, State Playfulness, or Attachment to a Canine Companion?

Separate regression analyses were conducted to evaluate how the sample's characteristics influenced gender role conflict's prediction value. The first regression indicated that gender role conflict did predict trait playfulness, $\beta = -0.221$, $t(126) = -2.540$, $p = 0.012$. The model, with adjusted $R^2 = 0.041$, showed that participants with lower gender role conflict had higher trait playfulness scores. The second regression analyses indicated that gender role conflict did not predict preintervention playfulness, $\beta = -0.120$, $t(126) = -1.361$, $p = 0.176$ nor post-intervention playfulness, $\beta = -0.120$, $t(126) = -1.353$, $p = 0.178$. The models indicated adjusted R^2 values of 0.007 and 0.006, respectively. The last regression analysis indicated that gender role conflict did not predict attachment to a canine companion, $\beta = 0.013$, $t(126) = 0.143$, $p = 0.886$ with adjusted $R^2 = -0.008$.

Does Trait Playfulness Predict Attachment to a Canine Companion? How Do Trait Playfulness, State Playfulness, and Gender Role Conflict Predict Attachment to a Canine Companion?

A regression analysis indicated that trait playfulness, $\beta = 0.270$, $t(126) = 3.149$, $p = 0.002$ was a significant predictor of attachment to canine companion. The model, with adjusted $R^2 = 0.066$, showed that the attachment to canine companion was higher for those with higher trait playfulness scores. A multiple regression indicated that trait and state playfulness and gender role conflict were significantly predictive of pet attachment scores, $F(5, 122) = 7.003$, $p < 0.000$, adjusted $R^2 = 0.191$. Regression coefficients and standard errors can be found in Table 8.2.

Does Trait Playfulness Predict Perceived Stress? Do State Playfulness and Gender Role Conflict Add to the Prediction Model?

Hierarchical regression was used to determine if trait playfulness, post-intervention state playfulness, and then gender role conflict could predict post-intervention perceived stress after controlling for preintervention playfulness and perceived stress. After step 1, with preintervention state playfulness and preintervention perceived stress in the equation, $R^2 = 0.900$, $F(2, 127) = 563.868$, $p < 0.001$. After step 2, with the additions of post-intervention state playfulness and trait playfulness, $R^2 = 0.903$, $F(4, 123) = 284.687$, $p < 0.001$. The addition of these variables

Table 8.2 Summary of multiple regression analysis

Variable	*B*	SE_B	β
Intercept	38.77	7.89	
Trait playfulness	0.39	0.20	0.19
State playfulness	3.99	1.18	0.48
Gender role conflict	0.05	0.07	0.06

Note B = unstandardized regression coefficients; SE_B = standard error of the coefficient; β = standardized coefficient

Table 8.3 Summary of hierarchal multiple regression from trait playfulness, state playfulness, and gender role conflict

Post-intervention stress						
Variable	Model 1		Model 2		Model 3	
	B	β	*B*	β	*B*	β
Constant	3.63		3.00		3.71	
Preperceived stress	0.90**	0.94	0.91**	0.95	0.91**	0.95
Post-state playfulness	−0.25	−0.04	−0.21	−0.03	−0.20	−0.03
Trait playfulness			0.08	0.05	0.08	0.05
Post-state playfulness			−0.26	−0.04	−0.27	−0.04
Gender role conflict					−0.01	−0.02
R^2	0.900		0.903		0.903	
F	563.87**		284.66**		226.56**	
ΔR^2	0.900		0.002		0.000	
ΔF	563.87**		1.44		0.332	

Note B = unstandardized regression coefficients; β = standardized coefficient; $*p < 0.05$; $**p < 0.001$

led to an increase in R^2 (R^2 change = 0.003, $p < 0.001$). After step 3, with the addition of gender role conflict, $R^2 = 0.903$, $F(5, 122) = 226.556$, $p < 0.001$. Adding gender role conflict did not cause a change in R^2 value. See Table 8.3 for full details on each model (below).

Broadly, the only variable that was a significant predictor of post-intervention perceived stress was preintervention stress. Trait playfulness was not a significant predictor and adding post-intervention state playfulness and gender role conflict to the model did not increase the prediction value.

Can State Playfulness and Stress Be Influenced by Recalling a Memory of Playing with Dog?

Using a paired sample T-test, reported levels of playfulness were significantly higher ($M = 7.80$, SD = 1.22) after the use of a play event memory compared to prior to the intervention ($M = 7.18$, SD = 1.18), $t(128) = -9.864$, $p < 0.001$.

Reported levels of perceived stress were not significantly lower (M = 21.41, SD = 8.07) after the intervention as compared to levels prior (M = 21.71, SD = 8.43), $t(127) = 1.253$, $p = 0.213$. Thus, recalling a play memory significantly increased levels of state playfulness but did not produce a significant change in perceived stress levels.

Discussion

The present study is the first to investigate the topic of playfulness as it relates to animal companion attachment and masculine gender role conflict. Joining these topics adds to the contextual understanding of male's bond with canine companions. One of the potential difficulties with this line of inquiry is that adult play is not well-developed in the research literature (Barnett 2007; Guitard et al. 2005). At the same time, this area might serve as an alternative adaptive coping mechanism particularly for men experiencing constricted gender expectations.

Results indicated that using a play memory significantly increased reported levels of playfulness. However, in term of levels of reported stress, while post-stress scores were lower than pretest levels of stress, they did not reach a significant level. The pretest and post-test stress findings may be due to sampling and methodological issues. Our original aim was to explore male playfulness memories, and their ability to increase playfulness and decrease stress among gender role conflicted men. However, our sample was very low on reported levels of gender role conflict and high on trait playfulness, which may in turn affect the results. For instance, levels of stress in low gender role conflicted males are at subclinical levels; therefore, state playfulness brought about by the memory intervention may not lead to further significant reductions. There is also the strength of the intervention to consider. Was the play memory sufficiently developed to alleviate males' stress? If an actual play event occurred in vivo between man and dog, would this exchange have a better chance of not only impacting playfulness but also stress as well? Future research needs to consider these issues when assessing the limits of playful memories in men's lives.

While the study's sample was skewed toward highly playful men with low gender role conflict, the significant increase in state playfulness after recalling a playful memory suggests a complex issue in need of further study. Gender role conflict is often characterized by rigidity (O'Neil 2008) while playfulness is characterized by flexibility (Barnett 2007). Playfulness should be identified and practiced as it relates to the positive social interaction occurring and the meaning that it can provide to a man. The element of play in the male–dog dyad may hold possibilities for some aspects of counseling men, and implementing animal-assisted programs.

Relationships with canines provide a sense of safety that may not be easily found elsewhere in a man's life and so they become important safe havens. An important element to consider is that playfulness in the relationship could be representative of the trust that is established over time with attachment figures

(Ainsworth et al. 1978). The time spent with a dog could be an encounter where gender role constrictions fall away, and the relationship itself takes precedent. Traditional male gender role expectations leave little room for this type of experience, which makes the male–canine relationship even more valuable. When play occurs among male dyads or within a group setting, elements of traditional masculine socialization also tend be present (Messner 1995). This includes competition, posturing, and stigma, all of which turn play into something else—a potentially spoiled opportunity to engage, even reaching toxic levels of play. Play becomes tainted when it loses its spontaneity, flexibility, and mutual communication.

Male socialization practices may even encourage men to alter play among man–dog dyads into a form of competition, a rigid structure, or even a power struggle. Studies suggest that social interactions with humans influence the hormonal states of dogs (Buttner et al. 2015). This is particulary important as humans' disciplinary behavior exhibited toward their dogs has been associated with increased cortisol levels, a stress hormone (Jones and Josephs 2006). Conversely, more positive exchanges with humans (e.g., playing, petting, etc.) have been found to decrease cortisol levels in dogs and led to elevations in oxytocin (Shiverdecker et al. 2013). For example, when examining males and their dogs on agility course/competitions, researchers found that increased levels of cortisol, in the saliva of dog handlers and their dogs (Buttner et al. 2015). There were gender differences; male handlers' dogs experienced greater increases in cortisol than females' handlers' dogs. Likewise, Jones and Josephs (2006) found that following a loss at a dog agility competition, the losing male handlers' testosterone levels predicted increases in their dogs' cortisol levels. The authors suggested that the findings may also be mediated by the trainer's affiliative and/or punitive behaviors toward the dog in this form of play–males stressed by the loss seemed to transfer these reactions to their dog through their behavior. This was especially true if male subjects reported feeling disappointed with their dog's performance on the course. In these moments, play is possibly influenced by male socialization, a pressure to win, and punitive behavior for not doing so. This is a recapitulation of the dark-side of male play: healthy-play becomes toxic-play. The result being the relationship loses out and so does the transformational element of the male–canine bond.

Future research needs to explore healthy and toxic-play found in the male–dog dyad, mediated by male socialization. If the link is substantiated, then there may be a limit to not only the effectiveness of dogs' ability to help overly conflicted men but further, canine companions may be taxed by elevated levels of stress. Research along these lines has direct implications for animal-assisted therapies for males under significant levels of duress. While playfulness should not be seen as panacea for male issues, it may be possible utilizing the bond to learn the difference between healthy-play and toxic-play. The results of our study also indicate that playfulness may offer further understanding into males' gender role conflict. Men with lower gender role conflict were more likely to report being highly playful. This suggests that tapping into men's playfulness may be a beneficial way to address some aspects of male socialization. Additionally, using the bond with a canine companion to activate feelings of attachment while playing could offset the emotional isolation associated with male socialization. The skillset and knowledge of how rigid male gender role behaviors can have a harmful impact on a canine companion may lead to increases in perspective taking and empathy for others. The new perspectives could then be generalized to other contexts replete with toxic-types of play in human dyads that may include male–male friendships and father–son outings involving play and sports. Perhaps playfulness is a quality that can be built upon, a potential skillset to be learned (or relearned) for many males. It is possible that the playfulness found in the relationship with an animal companion could be utilized and then extended into other relationships or areas of functioning. Play is an original way of learning about how to interact with others and could help open relational opportunities in spite gender role conflict restrictions. When in the proper frame, play allows an individual to view exchanges with non-punitive consequences and so lighten the danger that can be felt in interpersonal moments.

A limitation to consider in the present study is that masculine socialization may also prevent men from openly identifying their dogs as a key social support figures. Because of this dynamic, there are likely many positive, adaptive behaviors associated with the canine companions that were not recorded. These could involve turning to someone for support, giving affection as a natural element of a relationship, establishing routines, or receiving unbridled affection. These missed opportunities for more information is a methodological concern for future researchers and could be helped by modifying questionnaires. Animal companions should be among the list of potential attachment figures and social supports. Doing this could provide greater insight into the differences between human relationships and canine relationships and help identify how masculine socialization affects relational functioning.

Another limitation to consider as mentioned was sampling. Another possible issue in this area is participants self-selected to complete the survey. Scores indicated that many participants with low high gender role conflict, were also highly attached to their canine companion, and were highly playful. There is a need for continued data collection in larger and more representative samples including those with varying levels of gender role conflict, attachment to an animal, and playfulness. Possible ways to increase more diverse sampling include conducting research in person, identifying organizations with high populations of men, such as the military or the Veterans Associations, and considering the wording of advertisement. Research methods could include observational, naturalistic, and bio-hormonal formats, which would deepen the context of what is happening during the play interactions. Organizations like the military and the Veterans Associations have already begun to utilize canines as seen in reintegration programs, Battle Buddy programs, and PTSD clinics. The word 'playfulness' may discourage men with higher gender role conflict from participating, so it may be helpful to consider describing the research approaches in a more culturally competent and sensitive manner. Additionally, more research could identify themes of play that occur specifically between men and their canine companion as these may give insight into attachment behaviors.

Nineteenth century British novelist, Samuel Butler (1912), noted that, "The great pleasure of a dog is that you may make a fool of yourself with him and not only will he not scold you, but he will make a fool of himself too" (p. 220). In many men's lives, there are few opportunities to have such an open and life-changing exchange. However, when they do occur, these complex moments are characterized by the release from rigid male gender expectations, and a deepening sense of attachment with an animal companion. The joy of play comprises the full gamut of connecting with what one feels, and the bond with another. These exchanges may help males be happier and healthier men.

References

Ainsworth, M. D. S. (1982). Attachment: Retrospect and prospect. In C. M. Parkes & J. Stevenson-Hinde (Eds.), *The place of attachment in human behavior* (pp. 3–30). New York, NY: Basic Books.

Ainsworth, M. D. S. (1989). Attachments beyond infancy. *American Psychologist, 44*(4), 709–716. doi:10.1037/0003-066X.44.4.709

Ainsworth, M. D. S., Blehar, M. C., Waters, E., & Wall, S. (1978). *Patterns of attachment: A psychological study of the strange situation*. Hillsdale, NJ: Erlbaum.

Allen, K., Blascovich, J., & Mendes, W. B. (2002). Cardiovascular reactivity and the presence of pets, friends, and spouses: The truth about cats and dogs. *Psychosomatic Medicine, 64*(5), 727–739. doi:10.1097/00006842-200209000-00005

Anderson, W., Reid, C., & Jennings, G. (1992). Pet ownership and risk factors for cardiovascular disease. *The Medical Journal of Australia, 157*(5), 298–301.

Auerhahn, N. C., & Laub, D. (1987). Play and playfulness in Holocaust survivors. *The Psychoanalytic Study of the Child, 42*, 45–58. PMID 3438380.

Aune, K. S., & Wong, N. C. H. (2002). Antecedents and consequences of adult play in romantic relationships. *Personal Relationships, 9*(3), 279–286. doi:10.1111/1475-6811.00019

Barnett, L. A. (1991). The playful child: Measurement of a disposition to play. *Play & Culture, 4*(1), 51–74.

Barnett, L. A. (2007). The nature of playfulness in young adults. *Personality and Individual Differences, 43*(4), 949–958. doi:10.1016/j.paid.2007.02.018

Bartholomew, K. (1990). Avoidance of intimacy: An attachment perspective. *Journal of Personal and Social Relationships, 7*(2), 147–178. doi:10.1177/0265407590072001

Bartholomew, K., & Horowitz, L. M. (1991). Attachment styles among young adults: A test of a four-category model. *Journal of Personality and Social Psychology, 61*(2), 226–244. doi:10.1037/0022-3514.61.2.226

Bauman, A., Russell, S., Furber, S., & Dobson, A. (2000). The epidemiology of dog walking: An unmet need for human and canine health. *The Medical Journal of Australia, 175*(11–12), 632–634.

Beck, L., & Madresh, E. A. (2008). Romantic partners and four-legged friends: An extension of attachment theory to relationships with pets. *Anthrozoos: A Multidisciplinary Journal of the Interactions of People & Animals, 21*(1), 43–56. doi:10.2752/089279308X274056

Bekoff, M. (2001). Social play behaviour. Cooperation, fairness, trust, and the evolution of morality. *Journal of Consciousness Studies, 8*(2), 81–90.

Bekoff, M., Allen, C., & Burghardt, G. M. (2002). *The cognitive animal: Empirical and theoretical perspectives on animal cognition*. Cambridge, MA: MIT Press.

Bekoff, M., & Pierce, J. (2009). *Wild justice: The moral lives of animals*. Chicago, IL: University of Chicago Press.

Blazina, C. (2011). Life after loss: Psychodynamic perspectives on a continuing bonds approach with "pet companion". In C. Blazina, G. Boyraz, & D. Shen-Miller (Eds.), *The psychology of the human-animal bond* (pp. 203–224). New York, NY: Springer Publishing.

Blazina, C., & Bartone, A. (2015). Moving beyond essentialism in the psychoanalytic theories of masculinity: Implications for theory, practice, and research. In S. Wester & J. Wong (Eds.), *APA handbook of men and masculinity* (pp. 105–122). Washington, DC: APA Press.

Blazina, C., Boyraz, G., & Shen-Miller, D. S. (2011). *The psychology of the human-animal bond.* New York, NY: Springer.

Blazina, C., & Watkins, C. E, Jr. (2000). Separation/individuation, parental attachment, and male gender role conflict: Attitudes toward the feminine and the fragile masculine self. *Psychology of Men & Masculinity, 1*(2), 126–132. doi:10.1037/1524-9220.1.2.126

Bowlby, J. (1979). *The making and breaking of affectional bonds*. London: Brunner-Routledge.

Bowlby, J. (1999). *Attachment and loss: Vol I* (2nd ed., pp. 13–23). New York: Basic Books.

Brennan, K. A., Clark, C. L., & Shaver, P. R. (1998). Self-report measurement of adult attachment: An integrative overview. In J. A. Simpson & W. S. Rholes (Eds.), *Attachment theory and close relationships* (pp. 46–76). New York, NY: Guilford Press.

Brown, S. (2004). The human-animal bond and self-psychology: Toward a new understanding. *Society & Animals, 12*(1), 67–86.

Brown, S. E. (2007). Companion animals as self-objects. *Anthrozoos, 20*(4), 329–343.

Bustad, L. K. (1987). Investigators' interrelationship with laboratory animals. *Laboratory Animal Science, 37*, 167–170.

Butler, S. (1912). *The note-books of Samuel Butler*. London: A.C. Fifield.

Buttner, A. P., Thompson, B., & Strasser, R. (2015). Evidence for a synchronization of hormonal states between humans and dogs during competition. *Physiology & Behavior, 147*(2015), 54–62.

Cachia, P. (2001). *The interplay of gender role conflict and adult attachment*. Unpublished master's thesis, University of Malta.

Cain, A. O. (1983). A study of pets in the family system. In H. Katcher & A. M. Beck (Eds.), *New perspectives on our lives with companion animals* (pp. 72–81). Philadelphia, PA: University of Pennsylvania Press.

Cassidy, J. (1999). The nature of the child's ties. In J. Cassidy & P. R. Shaver (Eds.), *Handbook of attachment: Theory, research, and clinical applications* (pp. 3–20). New York, NY: Guilford Press.

Charnetski, C. J., Riggers, S., & Brennan, F. (2004). Effect of petting a dog on immune system functioning. *Psychological Reports, 3*(2), 1087–1091. doi:10.2466/pr0.95.3f.1087-1091

Cohen, S., & Janicki-Deverts, D. (2012). Who's stressed? Distributions of psychological stress in the United States in probability samples from 1983, 2006, and 2009. *Journal of Applied Social Psychology, 42*(6), 1320–1334. doi: 10.1111/j.1559-1816.2012.00900.x

Cohen, S., Kamarck, T., & Mermelstein, R. (1983). A global measure of perceived stress. *Journal of Health and Social Behavior, 24*(4), 385–396. doi:10.2307/2136404

Corson, S. A., Corson, E. O., Gwynne, P. H., & Arnold, L. E. (1977). Pet dogs as nonverbal communication links in hospital psychiatry. *Comprehensive Psychiatry, 18*(1), 61–72. doi:10.1016/S0010-440X(77),80008-4

DeFranc, W., & Mahalik, J. R. (2002). Masculine gender role conflict and stress in relation to parental attachment and separation. *Psychology of Men & Masculinity, 3*(1), 51–60. doi:10.1037/1524-9220.3.1.51

Del Giudice, M. (2011). Sex differences in romantic attachment: A meta-analysis. *Personality and Social Psychology Bulletin, 37*(2), 193–214. doi:10.1177/0146167210392789

DeMello, L. R. (1999). The effect of the presence of a companion-animal on physiological changes following the termination of cognitive stressors. *Psychology & Health, 14*(5), 859–868. doi:10.1080/08870449908407352

Dudukovic, N. M., Marsh, E. J., & Tversky, B. (2004). Telling a story or telling it straight: The effects of entertaining versus accurate retellings on memory. *Applied Cognitive Psychology, 18*(2), 125–143. doi: 10.1002/acp.953

Fischer, A. R. (2007). Parental relationship quality and masculine gender-role strain in young men mediating effects of personality. *The Counseling Psychologist, 35*(2), 328–358. doi:10.1177/0011000005283394
Fischer, A. R., & Good, G. E. (1998). Perceptions of parent–child relationships and masculine role conflicts of college men. *Journal of Counseling Psychology, 45*(3), 346–352. doi:10.1037/0022-0167.45.3.346
Fonagy, P. (2001). *Attachment theory and psychoanalysis*. New York, NY: Other Press.
Friedmann, E., Katcher, A. H., Lynch, J. J., & Thomas, S. A. (1980). Animal companions and one-year survival of patients after discharge from a coronary care unit. *Public Health Reports, 95*(4), 307–312. PMCID: PMC1422527.
Gentzler, A., & Kerns, K. (2006). Adult attachment and memory of emotional reactions to negative and positive events. *Cognition and Emotion, 20*(1), 20–42. doi:10.1080/02699930500200407
Gross, James J. (1999). The emerging field of emotion regulation: An integrative review. *Review of General Psychology, New directions in research on emotion, 2*(3), 271–299. doi: 10.1037/1089-2680.2.3.271
Guitard, P., Ferland, F., & Dutil, É. (2005). Toward a better understanding of playfulness in adults. *OTJR: Occupation, Participation and Health, 25*(1), 9–22. doi:10.1177/153944920502500103
Handlin, L., Hydbring-Sandberg, E., Nilsson, A., Ejdebäck, M., Jansson, A., & Uvnäs-Moberg, K. (2011). Short-term interaction between dogs and their owners: Effects on oxytocin, cortisol, insulin and heart rate—An exploratory study. *Anthrozoos: A Multidisciplinary Journal of the Interactions of People & Animals, 24*(3), 301–315. doi:10.2752/175303711X13045914865385
Hazan, C., & Shaver, P. R. (1987). Romantic love conceptualized as an attachment process. *Journal of Personality and Social Psychology, 52*(3), 511–524. doi:10.1037//0022-3514.52.3.511
He, J., Li, N., & Li, T. (2011). Adult attachment and incidental memory for emotional words. *Interpersonal: An International Journal on Personal Relationships, 5*(Suppl. 1), 1–20.
Henricks, T. (2008). The nature of play: An overview. *American Journal of Play, 1*(2), 157–180.
Hines, L. M. (2003). Historical perspectives on the human-animal bond. *American Behavioral Scientist, 47*(1), 7–15. doi:10.1177/0002764203255206
Horowitz, A. C., & Bekoff, M. (2007). Naturalizing anthropomorphism: Behavioral prompts to our humanizing of animals. *Anthrozoos: A Multidisciplinary Journal of the Interactions of People & Animals, 20*(1), 23–35. doi:10.2752/089279307780216650
Humane Society of the United States. (2013, September 27). *Pets by the numbers*. Retrieved from http://www.humanesociety.org/issues/pet_overpopulation/facts/pet_ownership_statistics.html
Johnson, T. P., Garrity, T. F., & Stallones, L. (1992). Psychometric evaluation of the Lexington Attachment to Pets Scale (LAPS). *Anthrozoos: A Multidisciplinary Journal of the Interactions of People & Animals, 5*(3), 160–175. doi:10.2752/089279392787011395
Jones, A. C., & Josephs, R. A. (2006). Interspecies hormonal interactions between man and the domestic dog (Canis familiaris), *50*(3), 393–400.
Knight, S., & Edwards, V. (2008). In the company of wolves. The physical, social, and psychological benefits of dog ownership. *Journal of Aging and Health, 20*(4), 437–455. doi:10.1177/0898264308315875
Kobak, R. (2009). Defining and measuring of attachment bonds: Comment on Kurdek. *Journal of Family Psychology, 23*(4), 447–449. doi:10.1037/a0015213
Kohut, H. (1984). *How does analysis cure?*. Chicago: University of Chicago Press.
Kurdek, L. A. (2008). Pet dogs as attachment figures. *Journal of Social and Personal Relationships, 25*(2), 247–266. doi:10.1177/0265407507087958
Kurdek, L. A. (2009). Pet dogs as attachment figures for adult owners. *Journal of Family Psychology, 23*(4), 439–446. doi:10.1037/a0014979
Lancy, D. F., & Grove, M. A. (2011). Marbles and Machiavelli: The role of game play in children's social development. *American Journal of Play, 3*(4), 489–499.
Land, L. N., Rochlen, A. B., & Vaugh, B. K. (2011). Correlates of adult attachment avoidance: Men's avoidance of intimacy in romantic relationships. *Psychology of Men and Masculinity, 12*, 64–74.

Levinson, B. M. (1978). Pets and personality development. *Psychological Reports, 42*(3c), 1031–1038. doi:10.2466/pr0.1978.42.3c.1031
Lyons, M. (1987). A taxonomy of playfulness for use in occupational therapy. *Australian Occupational Therapy Journal, 34*(4), 152–156. doi:10.1111/j.1440-1630.1987.tb01589.x
Main, M. (2000). The organized categories of infant, child, and adult attachment: Flexible vs. inflexible attention under attachment-related stress. *Journal of the American Psychoanalytic Association, 48*(4), 1055–1096. doi:10.1177/00030651000480041801
Main, M., & Solomon, J. (1986). Discovery of an insecure-disorganized/disoriented attachment pattern. In T. B. Brazelton & M. W. Yogman (Eds.), *Affective development in infancy* (pp. 95–124). Westport, CT: Ablex Publishing.
Margolies, L. (1999). The long goodbye: Women, companion animals, and maternal loss. *Clinical Social Work Journal, 27*(3), 289–304. doi:10.1023/A:1022894320225
Melson, G. F. (2002). Psychology and the study of human-animal relationships. *Society and Animals, 10*(4), 347–352. doi:10.1163/156853002320936791
Messner, M. (1995). *Power at play: Sports and the problem of masculinity*. Boston: Beacon Press.
Mikulincer, M., & Shaver, P. R. (2001). Attachment theory and intergroup bias: Evidence that priming the secure base schema attenuates negative reactions to out-groups. *Journal of Personality and Social Psychology, 81*(1), 97–115. doi:10.1037/0022-3514.81.1.97
Mikulincer, M., & Shaver, P. R. (2003). The attachment behavioral system in adulthood: Activation, psychodynamics, and interpersonal processes. *Advances in Experimental Social Psychology, 35*, 53–152. doi:10.1016/S0065-2601(03)01002-5
Miller, S. C., Kennedy, C., DeVoe, D., Hickey, M., Nelson, T., & Kogan, L. (2009). An examination of changes in oxytocin levels in men and women before and after interaction with a bonded dog. *Anthrozoos: A Multidisciplinary Journal of the Interactions of People & Animals, 22*(1), 31–42. doi:10.2752/175303708X390455
Mitchell, R. W., & Thompson, N. S. (1990). The effects of familiarity on dog-human play. *Anthrozoos: A Multidisciplinary Journal of the Interactions of People & Animals, 4*(1), 24–43. doi:10.2752/089279391787057314
Morrison, M. L. (2007). Health benefits of animal-assisted interventions. *Complementary Health Practice Review, 12*(1), 51–62. doi:10.1177/1533210107302397
Müller, C. A., Schmitt, K., Barber, A. L. A., & Huber, L. (2015). Dogs can discriminate emotional expressions of human faces. *Current Biology, 25*, 5, 2, 601–605.
Nagengast, S. L., Baun, M. M., Megel, M., & Leibowitz, M. J. (1997). The effects of the presence of a companion animal on physiological arousal and behavioral distress in children during a physical examination. *Journal of Pediatric Nursing, 12*(6), 323–330. doi:10.1016/S0882-5963(97)80058-9
O'Neil, J. M. (1982). Gender-role conflict and strain in men's lives. In K. Solomon & N. B. Levy (Eds.), *Men in transition: Theory and therapy* (pp. 5–44). New York, NY: Springer Publishing.
Odendaal, J. S. J., & Lehmann, S. M. C. (2000). The role of phenylethylamine during positive human-dog interaction. *Acta Veterinaria Brno, 69*(3), 183–188. doi:10.2754/avb200069030183
Odendaal, J. S., & Meintjes, R. A. (2003). Neurophysiological correlates of affiliative behaviour between humans and dogs. *The Veterinary Journal, 165*(3), 296–301. doi:10.1016/S1090-0233(02)00237-x
O'Neil, J. M. (2008). Summarizing 25 years of research on men's gender role conflict using the gender role conflict scale new research paradigms and clinical implications. *The Counseling Psychologist, 36*(3), 358–445. doi:10.1177/0011000008317057
O'Neil, J. M., Helms, B. J., Gable, R. K., David, L., & Wrightsman, L. S. (1986). Gender-role conflict scale: College men's fear of femininity. *Sex Roles, 14*(5–6), 335–350. doi:10.1007/BF00287583
Pasupathi, M. (2003). Emotion regulation during social remembering: Differences between emotions elicited during an event and emotions elicited when talking about it. *Memory, 11*(2), 151–163. doi:10.1080/741938212

Piaget, J. (1972). Intellectual evolution from adolescence to adulthood. *Human Development, 15*(1), 1–12. doi:10.1159/000271225

Pietromonaco, P. R., & Barrett, L. F. (1997). Working models of attachment and daily social interactions. *Journal of Personality and Social Psychology, 73*(6), 1409–1423. doi:10.1037/0022-3514.73.6.1409

Pollack, W. (1999). *Real boys: Rescuing our sons from the myths of boyhood.* New York, NY: Holt, Henry & Company Inc.

Proyer, R. T. (2012). Examining playfulness in adults: Testing its correlates with personality, positive psychological functioning, goal aspirations, and multi-methodically assessed ingenuity. *Psychological Test and Assessment Modeling, 54*(2), 103–127.

Roth, B. (2005). Pets and psychoanalysis: A clinical contribution. *Psychoanalytic Review, 92*, 453–457.

Rowe, A., & Carnelley, K. B. (2003). Attachment style differences in the processing of attachment–relevant information: Primed–style effects on recall, interpersonal expectations, and affect. *Personal Relationships, 10*(1), 59–75. doi: 10.1111/1475-6811.00036

Sadler, W. (1966). Play: A basic human structure involving love and freedom. *Review of Existential Psychology and Psychiatry, 6*(Fall), 237–245.

Samuelsson, I. P., & Carlsson, M. A. (2008). The playing learning child: Towards a pedagogy of early childhood. *Scandinavian Journal of Educational Research, 52*(6), 623–641. doi:10.1080/00313830802497265

Sanders, C. (1999). *Understanding dogs: Living and working with canine companions.* Philadelphia, PA: Temple University Press.

Sanders, C. R. (2003). Actions speak louder than words: Close relationships between humans and nonhuman animals. *Symbolic Interaction, 26*(3), 405–426. doi:10.1525/si.2003.26.3.405

Saunders, I., Sayer, M., & Goodale, A. (1999). The relationship between playfulness and coping in preschool children: A pilot study. *The American Journal of Occupational Therapy, 53*(2), 221–226. doi:10.5014/ajot.53.2.221

Schwartz, J. P., Waldo, M., & Higgins, A. J. (2004). Attachment styles: Relationship to masculine gender role conflict in college men. *Psychology of Men and Masculinity, 5*, 143–146.

Serpell, J. (1991). Beneficial effects of pet ownership on some aspects of human health and behaviour. *Journal of the Royal Society of Medicine, 84*(12), 717–720. doi:10.1177/014107689108401209

Serpell, J. A. (2010). Animal-assisted interventions in historical perspective. In A. H. Fine (Ed.), *Handbook on animal-assisted therapy: Theoretical foundations and guidelines for practice* (3rd ed., pp. 17–32). San Diego, CA: Academic Press.

Sharkin, B. S., & Bahrick, A. S. (1990). Pet loss: Implications for counselors. *Journal of Counseling & Development, 68*(3), 306–308. doi:10.1002/j.1556-6676.1990.tb01378.x

Sharkin, B. S., & Knox, D. (2003). Pet loss: Issues and implications for the psychologist. *Professional Psychology: Research and Practice, 34*(4), 414. doi:10.1037/0735-7028.34.4.414

Shaver, P. R., & Mikulincer, M. (2002). Attachment-related psychodynamics. *Attachment & Human Development, 4*(2), 133–161. doi:10.1080/14616730210154171

Shiverdecker, M. D., Schiml, P. A., & Hennessy, M. B. (2013). Human interaction moderates plasma cortisol and behavioral responses of dogs to shelter housing. *Physiology & Behavior, 109*, 75–79.

Siegel, J. M. (1990). Stressful life events and use of physician services among the elderly: The moderating role of pet ownership. *Journal of Personality and Social Psychology, 58*(6), 1081–1086. doi:10.1037/0022-3514.58.6.1081

Siegel, J. M. (1993). Companion animals: In sickness and in health. *Journal of Social Issues, 49*(1), 157–167. doi:10.1111/j.1540-4560.1993.tb00915.x

Stern, D. (2000). *The interpersonal world of the infant: A view from psychoanalysis and developmental psychology*. New York: Basic Books.

Sutton-Smith, B. (2008). Play theory: A personal journey and new thoughts. *American Journal of Play, 1*(1), 82–125.

Téglás, E., Gergely, A., Kupán, K., Miklósi, A., & Topál, J. (2012). Dogs' gaze following is tuned to human communicative signals. *Current Biology*, (22)3, 209–212. doi:10.1016/j.cub.2011.12.018

Voith, V. L. (1985). Attachment of people to companion animals. *The Veterinary Clinics of North America. Small Animal Practice, 15*(2), 289–295.

Vygotsky, L. S. (1978). The role of play in development. *Mind in society*, 92–104.

Walsh, F. (2009). Human-animal bonds I: The relational significance of companion animals. *Family Process, 48*(4), 462–480. doi:10.1111/j.1545-5300.2009.01296.x

Wells, D. L. (2009). The effects of animals on human health and well-being. *Journal of Social Issues, 65*(3), 523–543. doi:10.1111/j.1540-4560.2009.01612.x

Wester, S. R., Vogel, D. L., O'Neil, J. M., & Danforth, L. (2012). Development and evaluation of the gender role conflict scale short form (GRCS-SF). *Psychology of Men & Masculinity, 13*(2), 199–210. doi:10.1037/a0025550

Wexler, D. B. (2009). *Men in therapy: New approaches for effective treatment*. New York, NY: WW Norton & Company.

Winnicott, D. (1971). *Playing and reality*. New York: Brunner-Routledge.

Wood, L., Giles-Corti, B., & Bulsara, M. (2005). The pet connection: Pets as a conduit for social capital? *Social Science and Medicine, 61*(6), 1159–1173. doi:10.1016/j.socscimed.2005.01.017

Chapter 9
Pen Pals: An Examination of Human–Animal Interaction as an Outlet for Healthy Masculinity in Prison

Angela K. Fournier

This chapter discusses interactions between dogs and men who may be especially primed for the benefits of human–animal interaction (HAI) and at the same time a potentially risky group to entrust animals to—men in prison. After describing male imprisonment and the impact on expressed masculinity, prison-based animal programs are introduced and discussed. Following this review, an empirical study is described, which examined a dog training program in a men's prison. Researchers examined specific behaviors emitted by inmates when interacting with dogs, focusing on men in the general population. Findings are discussed in the context of prisonization and toxic masculinity. The chapter concludes with recommendations for future research.

Men in Prison

Beginning in the 1970s, the role of incarceration in the United States shifted from an effort to provide rehabilitation for inmates to an emphasis on "incapacitation" and "containment" (Ogloff 2002). As a result, psychological treatment for inmates was drastically reduced, despite an increase in the number of incarcerations (Haney 1997). The United States incarcerates a larger percentage of its population than any other country in the world. According to the Bureau of Justice Statistics (BJS) over 6.8 million men and women are under the supervision of adult correctional systems (BJS 2014a). That figure includes 1.5 million people incarcerated in prison, with men making up 93 % of the population.

A.K. Fournier (✉)
Department of Psychology, College of Health Sciences & Human Ecology,
Bemidji State University, 1500 Birchmont Dr. NE, Bemidji, MN, 56601, USA
e-mail: afournier@bemidjistate.edu

C. Blazina and L.R. Kogan (eds.), *Men and Their Dogs*,
DOI 10.1007/978-3-319-30097-9_9

Each year, a proportion of incarcerated men are released from prison and returned to society. Unfortunately, a large percentage of those released resume criminal behavior and are then sentenced to additional incarceration. In 2005, the U.S. Department of Justice tracked prisoners released in 30 states. Recidivism was extremely high; of the 286,829 prisoners released, 67.8 % were rearrested within three years and 76.6 % were rearrested within 5 years (BJS 2014b). Poor psychosocial functioning is just one of many variables that put men at risk for recidivism. Research suggests this poor functioning can be present prior to incarceration, but psychosocial abilities can also decline as a function of taking on the norms of the prison environment.

Prisonization

The Stanford Prison Experiment (Haney et al. 1973) is likely the most notable demonstration of the detrimental effects of incarceration. In this investigation into the power of the situation, psychologically healthy college students placed in a prison-like environment quickly took on the role of an inmate, becoming blindly obedient and suffering acute psychological trauma (Haney and Zimbardo 1998). Prisonization is a process in which inmates take on the customs, habits, and general culture of a correctional facility (Clemmer 1940). The prison culture includes adopting the inmate code, a code specifying an alliance *with* fellow inmates and *against* the facility administration and its policies (Clemmer 1940). In this process of socialization to the prison environment, inmates reject societal norms. The two primary theories used to explain prisonization postulate that (1) inmates take on the characteristics of prisonization as a way of coping with life in prison, called the deprivation model (Sykes 1958), or (2) prisonization is the result of maladaptive behaviors and values from the community entering the prison via those incarcerated, referred to as the importation model (Irwin and Cressey 1962). There is evidence for both models and many experts agree both sources contribute to the prisonization process (e.g., Rhodes 1979).

In a study of prisonization, Walters (2003) compared criminal thinking and criminal identity in novice inmates (i.e., never before incarcerated) and experienced inmates (i.e., having at least one prior incarceration) at the time of incarceration and after 6 months of their sentence. Both groups showed an increase in criminal thinking and identity after 6 months of incarceration, particularly the novice inmates. Although these changes related to prisonization may be adaptive for an inmate while incarcerated (e.g., reduces inmate-to-inmate violence), they are maladaptive for the man who is released back into the community, and may contribute to criminal behavior and subsequent return to prison. Haney (1997) suggests incarcerated men and women undergo a psychological "deep freeze" in prison and must recover from the negative effects of incarceration prior to reentering society. Men may be particularly at risk for the detrimental effects of incarceration, as they are forced to adapt their expression of masculinity to the confines of the prison environment.

Masculinity

Gender role conflict occurs when the gender roles ascribed someone by society have negative outcomes for them and others (O'Neil et al. 1995). For men, this can mean socialization of restricted emotionality, obsession with achievement and success, restrictive sexual and affectionate behavior, socialized control and power, extreme competitiveness, and homophobia (O'Neil 2008). The prison environment can magnify these characteristics. Research indicates gender role conflict is prevalent in incarcerated men and is a significant predictor of violence in prison samples (Amato 2012).

Phillips (2001) suggests that men in prison are deprived of all resources for enacting manhood, including women, money, clothing, weapons, and access to goods and services. Instead, inmates must demonstrate manhood through acts of bravery and physical power. This results in a constricted version of masculinity. Sabo et al. (2001) describe prison as an "ultramasculine world where nobody talks about masculinity" (p. 3). In their discussion of gender and punishment, they suggest prison facilitates and accentuates the relatively maladaptive behaviors of hegemonic masculinity, in which inmates, staff, and administration stress male dominance, violence, and competition. Kupers (2001a) refers to this constellation as *toxic masculinity*, a term that delineates socially destructive masculinity from prosocial expressions of masculinity (e.g., pride, achievement orientation). This is beyond the fear of the feminine (e.g., Blazina 1997, 2003; Neumann 1994) and normative male alexithymia (Levant 1998) that the average man in Western society is subject to. According to Sabo et al. (2001), prisons have four earmarks of a patriarchal institution. These earmarks are (1) homsociality—all inmates and most staff/administrators are men, (2) sex segregation—men only interact with women, including family, in infrequent and highly controlled visits, (3) hierarchy—status is carefully regulated, with violence-prone men at the top of the hierarchy and feminized men at the bottom, and (4) violence—relations between men, including inmate–inmate and staff–inmate, are negotiated and maintained through violence. These characteristics support a culture of violence in which many inmates are victims of physical and sexual assault (Kupers 2001b). In addition to being limited to expressing and falling prey to toxic masculinity, men in prison are unable to fulfill important roles in life that are meant to be continued once they are released, such as fatherhood.

Fatherhood

Approximately 51 % of men incarcerated in state prisons and 63 % in federal prisons are parents of at least one minor child (BJS 2010). Of those in prison, 78 % are in contact with their child(ren) via mail, telephone, or face-to-face visit. However, only 38.5 % are in contact weekly or more and all contact is under the close supervision of prison staff. Most incarcerated fathers will eventually be released, but many struggle to reestablish family connections. Dyer (2005) credits unsuccessful reunification to interrupted confirmation of the inmate's identity as a father. While incarcerated, the inmate is not able to behave in ways that are meaningful to his identity as a father. As such, he may abandon this aspect of his self to bring his perceived identity into congruence with his actual experience. Dyer suggests this father identity disruption can negatively influence reestablishment of family connections upon release. This is important because children with a parent in prison are at risk for problems such as depression and anxiety, behavior problems, and academic difficulties (Dawson et al. 2013). Moreover, successfully maintaining connection to family is associated with decreased problems for children (Pleck and Masciadrelli 2004) and reduced recidivism for inmates (Hughes 1998). It is possible the relatively new advent of working with animals in prison allows for inmates to enact some roles relevant to their identity as a father. In fact, inmates in a dog training program did report improved parenting skills as a result of working in the program (Turner 2007).

In summary, most U.S. prisons incarcerate men. Men's prisons are characterized as hypermasculine, where manhood is expressed through extreme competition, dominance, and violence. These norms may be adaptive while incarcerated but are maladaptive upon release into the community. Maintaining the toughness required to do "hard time" upon release can hinder reunification with family and reconnection with children for the large percentage of prisoners who are fathers. Given the increasing number of prison-based animal programs, one wonders whether interacting with animals can help to instill or extract the other side of masculinity, allowing men to express their full self.

Prison-Based Animal Programs

There is a significant history of prison inmates interacting with animals, whether adopting those that wandered onto the prison yard (e.g., Conover 2000; Paluch 2004) or working with livestock on a prison farm (Strimple 2003). However, many current interactions are the result of planned programming with HAI at the core. Furst (2006) refers to such programs as prison-based animal programs (PAPs). And although there is an underlying premise that programs will benefit the inmates, there is a clear distinction between PAPs and typical animal-assisted interventions. Prison programs are not primarily designed to be therapeutic for the inmates. They are generally designed as a type of work for the inmates, for the purpose of benefiting the animals and/or humans who will eventually keep the animals as pets or service providers (Furst 2011). Potentially improved functioning and reduced recidivism for the inmates are secondary objectives. Although inmates most often work with dogs, animals as diverse as birds, horses, and fish are involved in PAPs (Strimple 2003). Inmates' duties range from controlling the day-to-day operation of fisheries to training dogs for adoption or human service. The latter is the type of program evaluated in the present research.

Furst (2006) conducted a national survey of state department of corrections offices. Of the 46 states that completed the survey, 78 % ($n = 36$) reported having at least one PAP. Administrators reported a total of 159 sites across the country. The most common type of PAP reported was a community service model, in which animals are rehabilitated and adopted by someone in the community. For a discussion of the impact of acting as a teacher or mentor to animals, see Arluke (2007). Furst (2006) found that dogs were the most common animal reported in PAPs, making up 66 % of cases. Also quite common were service animal socialization programs and livestock care programs. The PAPs were implemented with men (56.7 %) more than women (22.4 %), and 20.9 % were implemented with *both* men and women. When asked their opinion of the program, administrators reported overwhelmingly that they would recommend the PAP to other prison administrators, with a lack of revenue being the only negative factor identified. Administrators reported the main benefit for the inmates was a sense of responsibility, instilled from having an animal depend on them. Other benefits reported included job skills, parenting skills, a sense of pride or accomplishment, and relationship skills. These reported benefits were anecdotal; empirical evidence of PAP outcomes is relatively sparse.

A review of the literature on PAPs shows there is a great deal yet to be understood about the impact of these programs. There are many descriptions of PAPs, reporting subjective evidence of program outcomes (e.g., Deaton 2005). Although empirical investigation of PAPs has increased in recent years, studies are limited by small sample sizes, selection bias, and nonexperimental research design. Evaluations of PAPs have considered a variety of dependent measures, including but not limited to: symptoms of psychological disorders (e.g., Suthers-McCabe et al. 2005), self-esteem (e.g., Walsh and Mertin 1994), self-confidence (Moneymaker and Strimple 1991), and vocational skills related to animal care (e.g., Bustad 1990). In addition to the methodological issues already listed, there is a significant shortcoming in the research. There are no studies investigating exactly *how* the inmates interact with the animals. Instead, HAI is treated as an independent variable—some inmates receive it and some do not—and psychosocial variables are the measured dependent variables.

For example, Turner (2007) reports on a qualitative study investigating the experiences of male prisoners who participated in a dog training program. Themes from interviews suggest inmates experienced increased patience and self-esteem; gained skills in parenting, helping others, and socializing; and experienced a greater sense of normalcy and calm. But their discussion of HAI is limited to describing the PAP as a community service program in which inmates train future service dogs in a wide variety of tasks.

Given the contrast between the toxic masculinity of men's prisons and positive psychosocial outcomes reported by investigators, it is important to understand the underlying processes governing PAPs. The specific ways in which inmates interact with the animals is one yet unexplored factor. A second gap in the research relates to the boundaries of HAI. Researchers describe the outcomes of PAPs for inmates directly involved in the program, whether training dogs (e.g., Turner

2007) or caring for livestock (e.g., Adams 2001; Blowen 2001). But there are no data regarding the degree to which nonparticipating inmates interact with the PAP animals. Since the average number of inmates involved in a PAP is around 20 (Furst 2006) and prisons hold hundreds or thousands of inmates (BJS 2008), it is important to know whether there are any spill over effects for inmates who are at a prison with a PAP but not actually involved in the program. The present study improves upon these shortcomings in the literature by (1) asking inmates to describe the actual behaviors they engage in with PAP animals and (2) studying HAI in inmates from the general population. In addition, data were analyzed in the context of men's issues, exploring the ways in which a PAP might impact men's expressions of masculinity. Regarding the latter, analysis of inmate reports was guided by the overall question—can PAPs provide an outlet for healthier gender expression and buffer men from the toxic masculinity of prison?

The Present Study

Pen Pals

Pen Pals is a dog training program in which dogs are selected from local shelters and trained by inmates in prison for 8 weeks (Virginia Department of Corrections 2015). During that time, dogs live with selected inmates who are educated in dog training skills from a certified animal trainer. Working as a team, four inmates are assigned to one dog, providing for the dogs' basic needs (i.e., food, shelter, grooming), and training them in obedience. After the training period, the dog is adopted by individuals in the community. Inmates become involved in the program by first applying for the position and then being selected by the coordinating correctional officer. Participation in the program is voluntary and is in addition to the inmate's regular responsibilities.

Pen Pals is located at a minimum-security men's prison in southwest Virginia. The prison has been in operation since 1960 and has a maximum capacity of 352 inmates. Men are housed in two buildings, where they live in a dormitory-style setting. Exclusion criteria for this facility include inmates serving sentences for kidnapping or abduction, violent sex offenders and those inmates determined to be escape risks. All inmates have fewer than 5 years of incarceration left to serve on their sentence. In addition to these criteria, the facility is limited to inmates with a history of substance abuse or legal charges related to alcohol or other drugs.

Participants

A total of 102 male inmates participated in the research. Fifty-four of those participants would go on to be studied in a quasi-experiment assessing the outcomes of the program. The detailed findings of the quasi-experiment are presented elsewhere, but in general, results suggested the program had a positive impact on social skills, reduction of institutional infractions, and enhanced progress in substance-related treatment (Fournier et al. 2007). This discussion describes the 102 inmates who initially signed up to participate in the research, prior to any formal participation in the PAP.

Participants ranged in age from 21 to 50 ($M_{age} = 32$) and had completed a mean of 11.9 years of education. All participants were able to read at an eighth grade reading level or higher, as indicated by intake assessment scores reported in their institutional file. With regard to race or ethnicity, 40.2 % of the participants identified as White or Caucasian, 17.6 % as Black or African American, 8.3 % identified as Hispanic, and 2.1 % identified as American Indian or Native American.

Materials

Materials included the Human Animal Interaction Scale, inmate applications to the PAP, and focus group transcripts.

Human Animal Interaction Scale (***HAIS***). In order to better understand the specific interactions that occurred between the inmates and the dogs, the research required a measure of HAI. While there were validated measures of constructs that may *predict* human behavior toward animals, such as attitudes toward animals (e.g., Herzog et al. 1991), empathy for animals (e.g., Paul 2000), and animal preference (e.g., Daly and Morton 2003), there were no measures to assess behavior emitted when a person interacts with an animal. Thus the Human–Animal Interaction Scale (HAIS) was created, consisting of an 11-item 4-point rating scale on which participants were asked to report their interactions with Pen Pals dogs over the past week.

To develop the scale, a pool of items was created by the authors based on a thorough review of the literature on HAI, observations during animal-assisted interventions, and informal interviews with animal-assisted therapy providers. Items were written to reflect the range of behaviors that may be emitted by a human while interacting with an animal. These initial items were then piloted in a laboratory. Volunteers interacted briefly with an animal and then responded to the items, providing feedback on content and clarity. Researchers also observed these interactions, adding or deleting items based on observations. The reliability and validity of the measure was tested with 161 adult volunteers who completed the HAIS in one of several different contexts.

A total of 41 undergraduate men and women completed the HAIS, reporting on any HAI experienced in the past six months; 57 undergraduate men and women completed the HAIS after a brief unstructured interaction with either a companion animal (e.g., dog or cat) or a small caged animal (i.e., rat, rabbit, hedgehog); and 63 men and women completed the HAIS following an equine-assisted growth and learning session. Participant ratings on the HAIS were compared with the Companion Animal Bonding Scale (Poresky et al. 1987) and the Companion Animal Semantic Differential (Poresky et al. 1988), providing convergent and divergent validity, respectively. Researchers observed interactions and also completed the HAIS, recording the interactions they observed between participants and the animals. Correlations between observers' and participants' ratings on the HAIS were above 0.70, providing initial evidence for concurrent validity. Analyses indicate good internal consistency, with a Cronbach's alpha of 0.822 overall and alpha's of 0.724 and higher across the different species and settings (Fournier et al. 2015).

Procedures[1]

The research was announced to all inmates through flyers placed in the dormitories, stating that research was being conducted on the prison dog program and that any inmate who had not already been a part of the program could participate in the research. As an incentive, inmates were informed that research participants would earn a Certificate of Participation to put in their institutional file. Those interested in participating attended a single mass testing session in which the principal investigator administered the HAIS to all volunteer participants at once. After data collection was complete, participants attended a 90 min focus group. Lastly, since each participant had applied to the PAP, program applications were reviewed, with participant consent, for qualitative data related to the research questions.

Results

A total of 102 men participated. Although each of them had applied to the PAP, only 35 of them met criteria for the program. At the time of data collection, all participants were in the general population (i.e., not working in the dog training program).

HAI

Table 9.1 provides descriptive data for the HAIS. For each item, the mean score is provided, as well as the percent of participants endorsing each response on that item. For example, when responding to the item, "How much did you *talk* to the dog(s) in the past week?" 42.3 % of the participants responded with a 4. Total HAI ranged from 0 to 44 ($M = 24.9$, $SD = 12.3$). Scores ranged from 0, indicating "*Not*

[1]All procedures were subject to full review and were approved by the Virginia Tech Institutional Review Board for Research with Human Subjects and the Human Subjects Review Board for the Virginia Department of Corrections.

Table 9.1 Reported human–animal interaction ($N = 102$)

Item	*M* (SD)	Percent rating				
		0	1	2	3	4
Watch	2.90 (1.20)	4.2	6.0	23.2	22.6	44.0
Hear	2.11 (1.34)	6.5	23.2	24.4	16.7	29.2
Talk	2.81 (1.21)	2.4	11.9	20.2	23.2	42.3
Pet	3.08 (1.12)	2.4	5.4	20.8	19.0	52.4
Play	2.62 (1.46)	6.6	13.9	15.1	16.9	47.6
Hold	1.79 (1.66)	24.4	11.9	17.3	11.9	34.5
Hug or kiss	1.79 (1.65)	26.2	9.5	13.1	17.3	33.9
Groom	0.87 (1.37)	47.0	12.5	16.7	6.0	17.9
Feed	1.49 (1.67)	31.7	15.0	16.2	10.2	26.9
Train	1.19 (1.56)	38.6	14.5	14.5	9.0	23.5
Walk	1.10 (1.62)	41.3	12.6	6.6	12.0	27.5
Total HAI	21.19 (12.21)	–	–	–	–	–

Table 9.2 Percent of participants rating the item 1 or higher

Item	Percent
Watch	94.1
Hear	90.1
Talk	96.0
Pet	97.0
Play	90.0
Hold	65.3
Hug or kiss	64.4
Groom	36.6
Feed	54.0
Train	45.0
Walk	39.0

at All" to 4, indicating "*A Great Deal*" on every item. As can be seen from the table, there was variability in ratings between the different items, with *Pet* rated the highest and *Groom* rated the lowest. Table 9.2 provides another view of the data, showing the percent of inmates who engaged in each behavior at all. The data were recoded from the 0 to 4 rating scale to a dichotomous yes/no variable. Responses of 1 or higher were coded as Yes, the behavior was reported. This illustrates the high rate of HAI, as several behaviors were reported by 90 % of the sample or more.

Figure 9.1 provides a comparison of reported HAI between inmates who had been approved for future entry into the PAP with those inmates who had applied but did not meet criteria, according to prison staff. Note that although some inmates had been approved for the PAP, none had begun the program at this point. Still, all inmates reported experiencing HAI, and there appear to be differences in HAI between these two groups of inmates. One-way ANOVAs were calculated,

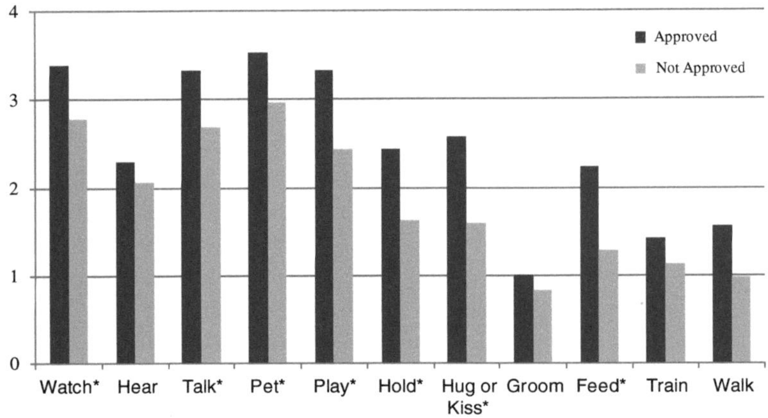

Fig. 9.1 Reported HAI by participants who were approved for the PAP ($n = 35$) and those who applied to the program but were not approved to join ($n = 67$). Groups were compared with one-way ANOVAs, $*p < 0.05$

comparing HAI between the two groups. There was an overall pattern of men who were approved for the PAP reporting more HAI than those who applied but were not approved, with those reports being significantly different for 7 of the 11 items.

The items on the HAIS included a variety of behaviors one could emit when interacting with an animal. Note that the list included behaviors that anyone in the general population who came across a Pen Pals dog might have been able to engage in, (e.g., *Watch*, *Hear*, *Pet*, *Talk*), while other items addressed more intimate behaviors, perhaps reserved for inmates who were dog trainers or otherwise more familiar with a particular dog (e.g., *Hold*, *Hug or Kiss*). Still other items addressed behaviors specific to caretaking, which would likely have been reserved for the dog trainers (e.g., *Train*, *Feed*, *Groom*). However, that was not the case, as *all* items were endorsed and *none* of the participants were working in the PAP. Even the more intimate items were endorsed by a large proportion of men, with over 64 % of them reporting they had hugged or kissed a dog in the past week. It is possible inmates approved for the program sought out interactions in preparation for their future role in the PAP. But looking again at Fig. 9.1, it is clear that there was no interaction between the different behaviors and the two groups of inmates. Inmates approved for the PAP rated all items higher than inmates not approved, regardless of how active, intimate, or relevant to dog training the behavior was.

Qualitative Data

Qualitative data were collected from two sources—Pen Pals applications and focus group responses. Applications had been completed prior to beginning the research; the focus group was held at the conclusion of the study.

Pen Pals applications. Each participant in this research had applied to work in the Pen Pals program and consented to researchers reviewing their program applications. The application form was written by staff at the facility and all selections for the PAP were made by the coordinating correctional officer. Researchers read and coded responses to the question, "Explain why you want to participate in the dog program, and how your participation will benefit the program." A content analysis of the participants' responses was performed in order to identify common themes, following the constant comparative method (Bruner 2004). The most prominent motivation reported for wanting to work in the program was love for animals in general or dogs specifically. For some men, this was the only response. For others, they expressed additional reasons. In these cases, five themes emerged as motivators for applying to the program. Inmates perceived the program as (1) a means of coping with incarceration, (2) an application of the inmate's talents, (3) a connection to family, (4) a way to contribute to society, and (5) identification with the dogs as unwanted or abused.

First, men indicated the program would help them cope, stating it would help them "*stay positive*," give them "*something to do that's positive while I'm here*," and decrease stress, "*I feel that being able to deal with the animals, that I won't sustain too much stress*."

In a second theme, the men described positive attributes they had that would help the program. Some of the attributes listed were related to dog training. Participants reported knowing about dogs, having experience with dogs as pets, and having experience training dogs. Another group of men discussed more interpersonal attributes, including patience, kindness, caring, and responsibility.

References to the dogs as family provided a third theme. Several inmates wrote about the dogs as "*kids*," "*children*," or "*family*." They compared their commitment to care for the dogs to a parents' commitment to a child, stating "*I will treat the dogs as if they were my kid*." They also referred to the significant commitment required, writing "*our pets depend on us 365 days a year*."

A fourth theme consisted of wanting to make a positive contribution. Men reported wanting to help the dogs, wanting to "*give back*," and wanting to help the families who will adopt them. For example, one man stated he wanted to help "*prepare the dog for some little boy or girl who needs a best friend*."

Finally, several applications indicated the men identified with the dogs specifically because they were shelter dogs and could relate to their situation:

> I care deeply for dogs, especially ones that no one else wants….I can relate to these animals because they have been left behind, abandoned, mistreated, etc. I know how it feels to be unwanted, but I also know how to love something that needs and wants love.

Overall, the program applications reflected an altruistic tone, with men reporting an interest in promoting the Pen Pals program, the dogs, and the community. Expected personal rewards were psychological in nature; inmates expected the program to be positive and to reduce stress. The applications suggested none of the toxic attributes of masculinity described in prison literature. Conversely, comments reflected a sense of nurturance, sacrifice, emotional sensitivity. This tone was presented even more strongly in the focus groups.

Focus groups. Fifteen of the 102 volunteers participated in a focus group, in which they were encouraged to discuss their impressions of the Pen Pals program. Focus group participants were recruited through announcements by prison staff. The focus group was scheduled by the prison staff according to inmate schedules and safety policies. Although there was substantial interest in attending the focus group, only 15 inmates were approved by staff and available at the scheduled time. Because the factor determining focus group attendance was practical rather than personal, there is no reason to suspect the other inmates would have responded differently to the researcher's questions.

Comments were reviewed and analyzed following the same methods described for reviewing applications, resulting in several distinct themes. First, participants reported that they were glad to be helping the dogs. It was a way they could give back to the community, to make up for what they took in committing their crime. A second theme centered around benefits to the inmates that made up for what prison takes away. Men reported having new feelings of accomplishment when helping to care for and train the dogs. The men also said that the dogs give them "*a sense of humanity*," describing how they felt like they mattered to the dog and to the other inmates on the [dog training] team. They also related interacting with the dogs to a sense of freedom:

> I always had dogs. I was surprised to see dogs in prison. I think the whole environment is different. It's like therapy – it's a little bit like home. It helps me feel less homesick. And it's like a little freedom. Just watching 'em play is like a little freedom.

Finally, the most prominent theme consisted of reported benefits to the inmates regarding mental health and well-being. The men described interacting with the dogs as helping them cope with and reduce stress, increasing self-esteem, helping them learn responsibility and patience, and facilitating emotion regulation:

> You learn how to deal with emotions, when you get frustrated or when you're sad about one of the dogs leaving.

The men were quite open, even in a large group of peers, discussing the sadness and grief they experienced when a dog would graduate from the program and leave prison to be adopted. They reported feeling sad and even talked about "*shedding tears*" over the loss. They also described feelings of joy and excitement at meeting a new dog entering the program. This open expression of emotions is counter to the stoicism expected in typical prison settings and is an example of the ways in which PAPs might be countering the toxic masculinity of prison.

Findings in the Context of Masculinity

Results from the HAIS, Pen Pals applications, and focus groups were analyzed in the context of masculinity. Specifically, data were reviewed using the positive psychology/positive masculinity framework (Kiselica and Englar-Carlson 2010),

Table 9.3 Findings in the context of healthy masculinity

Reported by inmates	Healthy masculinity[a]	May be experienced by	
		Pen Pals	General pop.
Playing, grooming, training behaviors	Action-oriented relating	x	x
Identify with dog as unwanted and care for them	Action empathy	x	x
Care for dogs as family, children	Generative fatherhood	x	
Interact with dogs to cope with incarceration	Self-reliance	x	x
Work with dogs in addition to regular job	Worker/provider	x	
Facing fears of dogs	Courage, risk-taking	x	x
Work in teams of 4 to care for/train dog	Group orientation	x	
Contribute to community, society	Humanitarian service	x	
Playing and laughing with dogs and teammates	Humor to attain intimacy	x	x
Train dog to save from euthanasia	Heroism	x	

[a]Positive aspects of traditional masculinity, from Kiselica and Englar-Carslson (2010)

a framework for studying men's issues that focuses on men's strengths rather than deficits. Table 9.3 lists each factor in the positive masculinity framework, alongside findings from the present study. The third and fourth columns indicate whether the factor could be expected to exist for inmates in the Pen Pals program, inmates from the general population, or both. For example, the positive masculinity framework suggests men relate with others through action (i.e., action-oriented relating) (Kiselica 2010). It is likely that both inmates in Pen Pals and in the general population could experience playing, grooming, and training behavior, suggesting the PAP could be an outlet for men to express this aspect of their masculinity. Note that while each of the healthy masculinity factors could apply to inmates in the Pen Pals program, inmates in the general population would likely be more limited. For example, inmates from the general population could use HAI to cope with incarceration (i.e., self-reliance), but because they are not responsible for the care and training of the dog, may not feel responsible for saving the dogs from euthanasia (i.e., heroism) or caring for them like their children (i.e., generative fatherhood). These findings suggest a prison environment quite different from the toxic masculinity (e.g., violence, dominance, competition) expressed in many men's prisons. Since factors of toxic and healthy masculinity were not measured, we cannot say whether a shift from toxic to healthy masculinity occurred as a result of HAI or the PAP. However, given that the major themes relate to these more prosocial aspects of masculinity, there is cause for study of these variables in future research.

Discussion

The purpose of this study was to determine the extent to which inmates in the general population interact with animals in a PAP program, gain insight into the actual behaviors inmates emit when interacting with PAP animals, and to examine inmate–animal interaction as it intersects with expressions of masculinity. Overall, the results indicate that inmates from the general population were experiencing a significant amount of HAI. A range of behaviors were endorsed, including passive behaviors like watching or hearing the dogs, as well as more intimate behaviors like holding, hugging or kissing the dogs. And even though none of the inmates were active participants in the PAP, many of them reported behaviors relevant to the dog training program, including grooming, feeding, and training the dogs. These data suggest that in addition to PAPs benefiting the select few who are chosen to participate in the programs, inmates in the general population can have substantial exposure to the animals and may also be benefitting. Considering prisons are in need of cost-effective rehabilitation programs, PAP programs are quite prevalent, and PAP programs tend to employ a small number of inmates, it is important that future evaluations of PAPs include an analysis of the program as it impacts inmates in the general population. Anecdotally, staff and administrators of the facility studied here reported significant improvements in the "culture" of the prison, stating there was a more positive atmosphere in general since the dogs had arrived. The findings of the present research warrant further study to determine whether HAI in the general population is specific to this particular facility or if it is common among PAPs.

Beyond the *quantity* of HAI occurring between the inmates and the dogs, the *kinds* of behaviors emitted by inmates are more consistent with healthy aspects of masculinity (Kiselica and Englar-Carlson 2010) than the toxic masculinity found in men's prisons (Kupers 2005). With 64.4 % of participants hugging or kissing dogs, 65.3 % holding dogs, and 90 % playing with dogs, one gets the image of inmates who are more nurturing than aggressive, more expressive than stoic, and more cooperative than competitive. Likewise, qualitative data from PAP applications indicate inmates saw the program as a way to give back to society and experience a family-like connection. Inmates also reported identifying with the dogs because they were shelter dogs who had been locked up, unwanted and in many cases abused. Themes from the focus groups reinforced statements made on applications regarding a desire to give back to society; they also suggested having the dogs at the prison returned a sense of humanity and helped them cope with the stresses of incarceration.

All of these data go against the prison code of acting tough, working against the law, and avoiding emotion at all costs (Sabo et al. 2001). It is important that research replicate the present findings and extend them by exploring *how* PAPs might be facilitating a different expression of masculinity by inmates. It is possible that the inmates feel freer to express healthy masculinity with animals present. Research indicates dogs can serve as a nonjudgmental other, more so than humans (e.g., Allen et al. 1991). Perhaps the animals are more salient than the unwritten rules of the prison, allowing inmates to respond innately to another living thing (Wilson 1984), rather than conforming to the constricted behavior typically allowed in prison.

Although toxic and healthy masculinity were not measured explicitly, the findings warrant their study in future work. Using an objective self-report measure, such as the Gender Role Conflict Scale (GRCS) (O'Neil et al. 1986), would be useful for comparing scores facility-wide before and after implementation of a PAP, as well as for individual inmates before and after participating in a PAP. These kinds of pre–post comparisons would shed light on the impact of PAPs on inmates. Studying GRCS and HAIS scores together would extend our understanding beyond PAP outcome, providing information on underlying processes as well as providing more information about HAI in general.

This research should also be followed up to determine the limits of these findings related to masculinity. Although the inmates were not yet involved in the PAP, they had all applied to work in the program. It is unknown how these men differ from men who chose not to apply. They could differ in ways unrelated to the question at hand (e.g., presence or absence of dog allergies) or in ways that are directly related (e.g., expressed masculinity). Even for the men in the study, who made reports consistent with healthy masculinity, it is unknown whether that gender expression was constricted to their interactions with the dogs and dog trainers, or whether it generalized to other aspects of their lives. While any movement in the direction of healthier gender expression is important, a global improvement in gender expression could have lasting implications for inmates. A global shift toward healthy masculinity might result in improved functioning during incarceration and increased success upon release. Anecdotally, reports from inmates, staff, and administration suggested a global improvement in inmate behavior—toward each other and toward staff. However, the data collected do not address this question and further research is required.

Participants reported engaging in significant caretaking behaviors, with 36.6 % grooming dogs, 45 % training dogs, and 54 % feeding dogs. Several of them were committed to caring for the dogs like they would a child, and compared the dogs to "kids" or "family." This is consistent with Turner's finding (2007) that male inmates credited a prison-based dog training program with improved parenting skills. Although this research did not study father identity, these data warrant further investigation into the ways in which PAPs might allow inmates to enact fatherly roles (e.g., provider, teacher, nurturer). Doing so might promote confirmation of the father identity, which is an important factor in reunification with children upon release from prison (Dyer 2005).

Finally, research is needed to explore the clinical utility of PAPs in facilitating physical and mental health. Comments from the focus groups suggest the inmates experience a full range of emotions with the dogs, which is quite different from the constricted emotional expression allowed by the prison code (Clemmer 1940) or even normative male alexithymia evidenced in many otherwise healthy men (Levant 1998). It is possible that emotions experienced with the dogs could be used as an avenue for exploring deeper issues. Currently, PAP work is reserved for the healthiest inmates and serves the animals and animal organizations, with inmates involved solely as workers. Staff and administrators report clinical implications for inmates; empirical evidence is limited by ceiling effects (i.e., trying to find healthy inmates getting even healthier). A more useful approach would be to determine the impact of PAP animals on the health of inmates with physical impairment (e.g., dog walking for inmates with cardiovascular disease) and mental health issues (e.g., animal-assisted therapy for inmates with anxiety or depression). Animals and our relationships with them can serve as metaphors for other aspects of life, a cornerstone of some animal-assisted interventions (EAGALA 2009). With some guidance, it's possible inmates could use PAP animals to conduct a transderivational search (Gordon 1978), learning about themselves through HAI. For the average inmate without physical or mental health problems, animal-assisted learning (Friesen and Delisle 2012) might be used to address everyday psychosocial functioning. In this way, relationships with animals are used to learn about interpersonal and intrapersonal functioning (e.g., social performance, self-disclosure, empathy) (e.g., Seiz and Koralewicz 2003).

Limitations

The findings and implications of the present research must be considered in light of several limitations. Perhaps the most important limitation is that the data rely on self-report. Inmates reported specific behaviors on the HAIS but those reports were not corroborated with observations. It is possible the inmates reported more interaction than had actually occurred, in order to please the researchers or to improve their chances of being selected for the PAP. Researchers tried to prevent this by stating clearly that selection and participation in the PAP was not at all related to their participation in the research. On the other hand, given the tenets of the prison code, it is surprising these participants rated the more intimate behaviors so highly. Playing, holding, hugging and kissing a dog are hardly consistent with doing "hard time." In that regard, it's possible the HAIS reports were actually conservative. Future research would be improved by asking staff to also complete the HAIS based on their observations of inmate–animal interactions.

The applications and focus groups are subject to the same limitation. Inmates applying for the program were likely motivated to write socially desirable statements that would promote their selection into the program. During the focus groups, the men may have wanted to give positive reports in order to please the researcher, please the staff, or ensure the program continues. This could explain the absence of any negative reports, but does not explain the particular content of their positive statements. Even if the inmates used a positive filter when making statements on their applications or in the focus groups, there are an infinite number of positive comments they could have made. Yet, there were focused themes to their reports that are relevant to men's issues. They paint a picture of a "softer" setting, of men expressing a form of masculinity more adaptive to life with family, friends, and the community outside prison walls.

It is important to note that this research investigated a specific PAP within a prison. The participants and the setting are unique, which make the generalizability of the findings questionable. This was a sample of convenience; inmates self-selected to apply to the PAP and to participate in the research. These inmates likely differ from inmates who did not apply or participate in the research. At the very least, it is probable the participants are interested in interacting with dogs and thus may seek out more HAI than other inmates. In that case, the reports on the HAIS may be overestimations of the HAI experienced by inmates in the general population. Generalizability may be limited to similar institutions. This prison was of minimum security and all inmates had less than 5 years to serve. It is likely the environment and the inmates differ in important ways from higher security prisons housing inmates with longer or even life sentences. Research suggests PAPs are being implemented in a range of different facilities (Furst 2006, 2011) and it's important to study their impacts.

All participants had at least an eighth grade reading ability and 72.2 % had reportedly completed high school, obtained a GED, or higher degree. According to the BJS (2003), approximately 49 % of inmates in state prisons have a high school diploma or GED. Thus, the present sample may not be representative of the typical prison inmate with regard to education. It is unknown how level of education might have impacted HAI, actual or reported. The nature of this research (i.e., self-report measures) required that inmates be able to read. Future research involving observations of inmate–animal interactions could reduce this limitation, allowing for a more representative sample. An observation study would also reduce selection bias.

Conclusion

PAPs are quite prevalent in the U.S. and around the world (Furst 2006). Although still in its infancy, research suggests the programs are effective in serving the animals and the community, and may have rehabilitative effects for the inmates involved (Furst 2011). PAPs tend to employ a small number of carefully selected inmates, making it difficult to determine whether positive outcomes are truly a result of the PAP or if they are just a reflection of the healthiest inmates rising to the top (Fournier et al. 2007). The data presented here suggest inmates from the general population may also be experiencing a significant amount of interaction with animals. The men reported substantial interactions with PAP dogs, acknowledging passive, active, and intimate behaviors, including caretaking and training.

Clearly, more research is needed to fully understand the processes and outcomes of PAPs for all inmates. Ideally, research should follow an experimental design, in which prisons are randomly assigned to have a PAP or serve as a control site. Within PAP prisons, a sample of appropriate inmates could be selected and then randomized to treatment or wait-list control conditions. Research investigating PAPs should continue to study the actual behaviors inmates engage in with the animals, including inmates from the general population as well as facility staff. Finally, since the majority of inmates are men, investigations should be sensitive to men's issues and the ways in which interacting with animals impacts healthy gender expression.

Researchers have long discussed the harsh conditions of prison and their failure to deter criminal behavior (e.g., Haney 1997). Adapting to prison often means accepting a code, aligning *with* fellow inmates and *against* the facility administration, and rejecting societal norms (Clemmer 1940). For men in particular, the prison experience means proving one's manhood through violence, dominance, and competition, as other expressions of masculinity are unacceptable (e.g., expression of a range of emotions) or unattainable (e.g., sense of accomplishment through work, sense of pride in protecting and providing for family) (Phillips 2001). Assimilating to these norms can interrupt connections to family and hinder reentry to the community when released from prison. The men in the present study reported behaviors and feelings of healthier, more complete masculinity. Although more research is needed to be certain, it seems the presence of animals in prison, whether the inmate is directly involved in a PAP or not, could serve as a buffer to taking on or perpetuating the "hardness" of prison. If so, this could be a less threatening way for men to do "softer" time, and facilitate a more adaptive transition to the community upon release.

References

Adams, K. (2001, March/April). 2nd chances. *Backstretch*, 32–37.

Allen, K. M., Blascovich, J., Tomaka, J., & Kelsey, R. M. (1991). Presence of human friends and pet dogs as moderators of autonomic responses to stress in women. *Journal of Personality and Social Psychology, 61*(4), 582–589.

Amato, F. J. (2012). The relationship of violence to gender role conflict and conformity to masculine norms in a forensic sample. *The Journal of Men's Studies, 20*(3), 187–208.

Arluke, A. (2007). *Animal assisted activates for at-risk and incarcerated children and young adults: An introductory ethnography of five programs*. Paper presented at the National Technology Assessment Workshop on Animal Assisted Programs for Youth at Risk, Baltimore.

Blazina, C. (1997). The fear of the feminine in the Western psyche and the masculine task of disidentification. *The Journal of Men's Studies, 6*, 55–68.

Blazina, C. (2003). *The cultural myth of masculinity*. Westport: Praeger Publishers.

Blowen, M. (2001, January 16). In prison, a happier trail. *Boston Globe*, A1.

Bruner, J. (2004). Life as narrative. *Social Research, 71*, 691–711.

Bureau of Justice Statistics. (2003). *Education and correctional populations*. Special Report NCJ 195670. U.S. Department of Justice.

Bureau of Justice Statistics. (2008). *Census of state and federal correctional facilities, 2005*. Special Report NCJ 222182. U.S. Department of Justice.

Bureau of Justice Statistics. (2010). *Parents in prison and their minor children*. Special Report NCJ 222984. U.S. Department of Justice.

Bureau of Justice Statistics. (2014a). *Correctional populations in the United States, 2013*. Special Report NCJ 248479. U.S. Department of Justice.

Bureau of Justice Statistics. (2014b). *Recidivism of prisoners release in 30 states in 2005: Patterns from 2005 to 2010*. Special Report NCJ 244205. U.S. Department of Justice.

Bustad, L. K. (1990). Prison programs involving animals. In L. K. Bustad (Ed.), *Compassion, our last great hope* (pp. 72–73). Renton, WA: Delta Society.

Clemmer, D. (1940). *The prison community*. New York: Prentice Hall.

Conover, T. (2000). *Newjack: Guarding sing-sing*. New York: Random House.

Daly, B., & Morton, L. L. (2003). Children with pets do not show higher empathy: A challenge to current views. *Anthrozoös, 16*(4), 298–314.

Dawson, A., Brookes, L., Carter, B., Larman, G., & Jackson, D. (2013). Stigma, health and incarceration: Turning the tide for children with a parent in prison. *Journal of Child Health Care, 17*(1), 3–5.

Deaton, C. (2005). Humanizing prisons with animals: A closer look at "Cell Dogs" and horse programs in correctional institutions. *The Journal of Correctional Education, 56*(1), 46–62.

Dyer, W. J. (2005). Prison, fathers, and identity: A theory of how incarceration affects men's paternal identity. *Fathering: A Journal of Theory, Research, and Practice About Men as Fathers, 3*(3), 201–219.

Fournier, A. K., Geller, E. S., & Fortney, E. (2007). Human-animal interaction in a prison setting: Impact on criminal behavior, treatment progress, and social skills. *Behavior and Social Issues, 16*(1), 89–105.

Fournier, A. K., Letson, E., & Krog, L. (2015). *Development of the human-animal interaction scale: An instrument to quantify human-animal interaction*. Poster presented to the International Society on Anthrozoology, Saratoga Springs, NY.

Friesen, L., & Delisle, E. (2012). Animal-assisted literacy: A supportive environment for constrained and unconstrained learning. *Childhood Education, 88*(2), 102–107.

Furst, G. (2006). Prison-based animal programs: A national survey. *The Prison Journal, 86*(4), 407–430.

Furst, G. (2011). *Animal programs in prison: A comprehensive assessment*. Boulder, CO: First Forum Press.

Gordon, D. C. (1978). *Therapeutic metaphors: Helping others through the looking glass*. USA: Meta Publications.

Haney, C. (1997). Psychology and the limits to prison pain: Confronting the coming crisis in eighth amendment law. *Psychology, Public Policy, and Law, 3*(4), 499–588.

Haney, C., Banks, W., & Zimbardo, P. (1973). Interpersonal dynamics in a simulated prison. *International Journal of Criminology and Penology, 1*, 69–97.

Haney, C., & Zimbardo, P. (1998). The past and future of U.S. prison policy: Twenty-five years after the Stanford Prison Experiment. *American Psychologist, 53*(7), 709–727.

Herzog, H., Betchart, N., & Pittman, R. (1991). Gender, sex role orientation, and attitudes towards animals. *Anthrozoös, 4*(3), 184–192.

Hughes, M. (1998). Turing points in the lives of young, inner-city men forgoing destructive criminal behaviors: A qualitative study. *Social Work Research, 22*, 143–151.

Irwin, J., & Cressey, D. R. (1962). Thieves, convicts, and the inmate culture. *Social Problems, 10*, 142–155.

Kiselica, M. S., & Englar-Carlson, M. (2010). Identifying, affirming, and building upon male strengths: The positive psychology/positive masculinity model of psychotherapy with boys and men. *Psychotherapy Theory, Research, Practice, & Training, 47*(3), 276–287.

Kupers, T. (2001a). Psychotherapy with men in prison. In G. Brooks & G. Good (Eds.), *A new handbook of counseling and psychotherapy approaches for men: A comprehensive guide to setting, problems, and treatment approaches* (pp. 170–184). San Francisco: Jossey-Bass.

Kupers, T. A. (2001b). Rape and the prison code. In D. Sabo, T. A. Kupers, & W. London (Eds.), *Prison masculinities* (pp. 111–117). Philadelphia, PA: Temple Universities Press.

Kupers, T. A. (2005). Toxic masculinity as a barrier to mental health treatment in prison. *Journal of Clinical Psychology, 61*(6), 713–724.

Levant, R. F. (1998). *Desperately seeking language: Understanding, assessing, and treating normative male alexithymia*. John Wiley & Sons Inc.

Moneymaker, J. M., & Strimple, E. O. (1991). Animals and inmates: A sharing companionship behind bars. *Journal of Offender Rehabilitation, 16*(3–4), 133–152.
Neumann, E. (1994). *The fear of the feminine and other essays on feminine psychology*. Princeton, NJ: Princeton University Press.
Ogloff, J. R. (2002). Offender rehabilitation: From "nothing works" to what next? *Australian Psychologist, 37*(3), 245–252.
O'Neil, J. M. (2008). Summarizing 25 years of men's gender role conflict using the gender role conflict scale: New research paradigms and clinical implications. *The Counseling Psychologist, 36*(3), 358–445.
O'Neil, J. M., Good, G. E., & Holmes, S. (1995). Fifteen years of theory and research on men's gender role conflict: New paradigms for empirical research. *A new psychology of men*, 164–206.
O'Neil, J. M., Helms, B. J., Gable, R. K., David, L., & Wrightsman, L. S. (1986). Gender-role conflict scale: College men's fear of femininity. *Sex roles, 14*(5–6), 335–350.
Paluch, J. J. (2004). *A life for a life: Life imprisonment: America's other death penalty*. Los Angeles, CA: Roxbury.
Paul, E. S. (2000). Empathy with animals and with humans: Are they linked? *Anthrozoös, 13*(4), 194–202.
Phillips, J. (2001). Cultural construction of manhood in prison. *Psychology of Men & Masculinity, 2*(1), 13–23.
Pleck, J. H., & Masciadrelli, B. P. (2004). Paternal involvement by US residential fathers: Levels, sources, and consequences. In M. Lamb (Ed.), *The role of the father in child development* (4th ed., pp. 222–271). Hoboken, NJ: Wiley.
Poresky, R. H., Hendrix, C., Mosier, J. E., & Samuelson, M. L. (1987). The companion animal bonding scale: Internal reliability and construct validity. *Psychological Reports, 60*, 743–746.
Poresky, R. H., Hendrix, C., Mosier, J. E., & Samuelson, M. L. (1988). The companion animal semantic differential: Long and short form reliability and validity. *Educational and Psychological Measurement, 48*(1), 255–260.
Rhodes, M. L. (1979). The impact of social anchorage on prisonization. *Dissertation Abstracts International, 40*, 1694A. (UMI No. 79–19, 101).
Sabo, D., Kupers, T. A., & London, W. (2001). Gender and the politics of punishment. In D. Sabo, T. A. Kupers, & W. London (Eds.), *Prison Masculinities* (pp. 3–18). Philadelphia, PA: Temple Universities Press.
Seiz, R., & Koralewicz, L. (2003). *Evaluation research project on New Leash on Life program: Final report*. CBR Youth Connect/Colorado Boys Ranch.
Strimple, E. O. (2003). A history of prison inmate-animal interaction programs. *American Behavioral Scientist, 47*(1), 70–78.
Suthers-McCabe, H. M., Van Voorhees, E., & Fournier, A. K. (2005). *Prison PUP: An examination of the human-animal bond in an American prison*. Unpublished manuscript.
Sykes, G. M. (1958). *The society of captives: A study of a maximum security prison*. Princeton, NJ: Princeton University Press.
Turner, W. G. (2007). The experiences of offenders in a prison canine program. *Federal Probation, 71*(1), 38–43.
Virginia Department of Corrections. (2015). *Pen Pals*. Retrieved August 13, 2015, from https://vadoc.virginia.gov/offenders/institutions/programs/penpals.shtm
Walsh, P. G., & Mertin, P. G. (1994). The training of pets as therapy dogs in a women's prison: A pilot study. *Anthrozoös, 7*(2), 124–128.
Walters, G. D. (2003). Changes in criminal thinking and identity in novice and experienced inmates prisonization revisited. *Criminal Justice and Behavior, 30*(4), 399–421.
Wilson, E. O. (1984). *Biophilia*. Cambridge: Harvard University Press.

Chapter 10
Animal Companions and Military Veterans: How Dogs Can Help America's Heroes

Teri L. Carper, Anne S. Bartone and Frederick C. Petty

The effects of Western socialization on gender role norms and men's psychological development, self-concept, and behaviors have been well documented (e.g., O'Neil 2008). Specifically, traits such as dominance, stoicism, independence, physical prowess, and emotional restriction are heavily emphasized in the United States, and become internalized and valued among men. As strongly ingrained as these expectations are for American men in general, their importance is even more profoundly indoctrinated within our military culture (Brooks 2005; Eisenhart 1975).

In their classic paper, Arkin and Dobrofsky (1978) refer to "secondary socialization," wherein both male and female service personnel become immersed in a culture that reinforces traditional masculine ideology. This is particularly true among men in combat roles, as "the training program for the masculine sex role is operationalized via skills and techniques deemed necessary for a man's survival in combat; combat training and masculine sex-role socialization are never separated from one another" (p. 159). The authors also suggest that men who already place a strong value on stereotypical gender roles may be attracted to the military to aid them in "becoming a man." As such, the relationship between hypermasculinity

T.L. Carper (✉) · A.S. Bartone · F.C. Petty
Orlando VA Medical Center, 13800 Veterans Way, Orlando, FL 32827, USA
e-mail: Teresa.Carper@va.gov

A.S. Bartone
e-mail: bartonea@hotmail.com

F.C. Petty
e-mail: Frederick.Petty2@va.gov

T.L. Carper
University of Central Florida College of Medicine, 6850 Lake Nona Blvd, Orlando, FL 32827, USA

C. Blazina and L.R. Kogan (eds.), *Men and Their Dogs*,
DOI 10.1007/978-3-319-30097-9_10

and military service is likely bidirectional; men who endorse traditional gender roles gravitate toward the military and the military training reinforces societal views of masculinity. Indeed, male military personnel tend to report high levels of conformity to these norms (Jakupcak et al. 2006; Kurpius and Lucart 2000). Moreover, troops involved in Operation Enduring Freedom or Operation Iraqi Freedom (OEF/OIF) may be particularly susceptible to these socialization processes, given that their relative youth makes them more vulnerable to this type of indoctrination (Levant and Richmond 2007).

Military Veterans and Attachment

Attachment theory assumes a universal need to form a bond to a specific attachment figure deemed stronger and wiser who can protect and increase one's chances of survival in infancy (Bowlby 1969, 1982). One's attachment orientation or style can be understood as a complex network of cognitive and affective processes and mental representations, including episodic, context-related, relationship-specific, and general attachment representations (Mikulincer and Shaver 2003). Attachment orientations are initially formed in interactions with primary caregivers during childhood. Although there is evidence to suggest that one's orientation can change subtly or dramatically depending on context and recent experiences (e.g., Mikulincer and Shaver 2001), there is ongoing support for the idea that a caregiver's response to the infant's needs shapes the internal working model and ultimately guides the emotional development and choices and behaviors in adult life (e.g., Hazan and Shaver 1987).

Several theorists have postulated that early attachment bonds are affected by gender socialization (e.g., Pollack 1995). Norms and expectations of gendered behavior, characterized as masculine for boys and feminine for girls in Western culture, are learned and reinforced via direct and indirect messages from parents and through observation and imitation of parents (MacNaughton 2006). As such, beginning in infancy, a child is exposed to myriad expectations and attitudes, generally determined by anatomical identification of the infant as a male or a female (Elise 1997). Though no specific research has directly examined attachment styles within military personnel, studies on gender differences within adult attachment styles can provide a useful framework for understanding how emotional attachment may impact men who strongly espouse masculine ideals, such as military personnel.

Hazan and Shaver (1987) were the first to extend attachment theory to the study of adult relationships, finding that individual differences in adult attachment styles mimic Ainworth's observations in infant–caregiver relationships. Contemporary work on adult attachment has altered initially proposed attachment styles into two dimensions: (1) anxious–ambivalence and (2) avoidance (Fraley et al. 2000). Generally, highly anxious–ambivalent people desire closeness and intimacy yet are unable to achieve a stable sense of either. Highly avoidant individuals on the other hand, have difficulty relying on others and prefer to limit intimacy and interdependence. With respect to gender differences, a recent meta-analysis found that women scored higher than men on anxiety and men scored higher than women on avoidance, particularly within community samples (Del Giudice 2011). Furthermore, gender differences in anxiety were largest in early adulthood, while gender differences in avoidance were relatively small in early adulthood. In another study using a large Internet sample, Chopik et al. (2013) found that women scored slightly higher on attachment anxiety, particularly in early adulthood. These findings suggest that women use anxiety as a secondary coping style when a secure attachment is not available.

Men comprise 84 % of the United States military and modal enlistment age is in early adulthood (Department of Defense 2012). As such, recruits tend to be relatively disinvested in cultivating a sense of closeness and intimacy with others. Superimposed on top of this is military training, which reinforces this predisposition via the promotion of hypermasculine values. The instilment of such values is intentional due to their importance on the battlefield. For example, emotional stoicism promotes survival, hardiness, and mission completion, a sense of dominance over trainees extends to the enemy as well as personal fears and weaknesses, and the embodiment of the "rugged warrior" helps acculturate the individual to violence and risk-taking (Alfred et al. 2014; Arkin and Dobrofsky 1978).

However, this embracement of hypermasculinity is not to say that military personnel do not form relationships with each other during deployment. In fact, loyalties between servicemen, referred to as unit cohesion, are also purposefully instilled during training. King et al. (2003) define unit cohesion as the perception of support and encouragement from leaders and peers. This is thought to be fairly easy to facilitate among service personnel, given that military units share characteristics of primary groups such as personal and affective bonding, reunification or separation by members from other commitments and relationships, formal membership requirements and/or initiation rites, and ideological commitments. It is thought that cohesive bonds begin forming during basic training and grow to be most intense during combat assignments (Morris 1996).

Numerous studies have examined the impact of unit cohesion on the functioning and adjustment of military personnel both during and post deployment (e.g., Brailey et al. 2007; Iversen et al. 2008; McTeague et al. 2004; Whitesell and Owens 2012). In one of the first longitudinal examinations of unit cohesion, Elder and Clipp (1988) found that veterans of the World War II and Korea eras who served in combat were more likely than their noncombat counterparts to maintain enduring interpersonal ties with their fellow servicemen. The authors posited that this relationship was mediated by war trauma, particularly related to the loss of comrades and friends in theater. Oliver et al. (1999) conducted a meta-analysis of military cohesion research and found that group cohesion was positively related to multiple desirable outcomes, including group performance, individual performance, job/military, satisfaction, retention, well-being, readiness, and indiscipline.

Although masculinized traits and relatively low attachment may be beneficial on the battlefield, individuals often have difficulty contextualizing these values to the war environment, and thus remain indoctrinated even after the transition back to civilian life. Unfortunately, this lack of connectedness often leads to impairments in emotional awareness and expression, including affective flattening (the inability to experience a full range of emotions), interpersonal detachment (feeling distant or cut off from others), and anhedonia (a significant reduction in the enjoyment of activities)—all of which are all symptoms of PTSD and depression. With respect to the aforementioned sense of group solidarity, a war veteran's ability to form bonds and develop trust with nonveteran civilians can be particularly problematic.

Traditional Masculine Ideology as a Barrier to Care

Within the general population, myriad psychological barriers to mental health care exist, such as perceived stigma, distrust of others, and cynicism regarding the efficacy of treatment approaches. These barriers are amplified among men, with research consistently demonstrating that masculinity conflicts and attitudes serve to impede the likelihood of seeking or adhering to mental health treatment. While the ideal therapy client has been described as "emotionally expressive, comfortable with ambiguity and vulnerability, and able to ask for help (p. 628)," the stereotypical male is known to have difficulty admitting a problem exists, asking for help, identifying emotional states, and a fear of intimacy (e.g., Rochlen 2005). Cultural values promoting stoicism, constricted emotionality, and self-reliance among men are incompatible with all stages of seeking help. Furthermore, because men are socialized to ignore and/or minimize their pain (Lisak 2001), they tend to underreport their emotions (Jansz 2000; Pollack 1999). However strong the desire to uphold traditional male ideology, it is clear that sheer denial of problems does not eliminate them as hoped. Rather, men tend to express their inner turmoil via methods that are more consistent with stereotypical male behavior, including anger outbursts, drug or alcohol use, and social isolation. Such methods serve to exacerbate the existing problems, potentially increasing social stressors (e.g., legal problems, marital discord), and can result in a more urgent need for mental health intervention. Therefore, men's socialized adversity toward help-seeking behavior for mental health problems results in a snowball effect, wherein the negative coping behaviors create additional complications that underscore the need for professional intervention.

Given the hypermasculine culture of the military, it is unsurprising that service personnel and veterans are at an even greater risk of not seeking out needed psychological services. Even when veterans do seek clinical care, it may be difficult for them to fully engage in therapy, as their masculine gender roles "create avoidance, rigid emotional control, and can make veterans reluctant or unwilling to experience the emotions they learned to 'turn off'" (Lorber and Garcia 2010, p. 297). Furthermore, the unspoken collusion to conceal any psychological or adjustment difficulties may lead veterans to inaccurately believe that such experiences are abnormal and that they are alone in their suffering, perpetuating feelings of shame and the pressure to "keep holding it together" (Lorber and Garcia 2010).

OEF/OIF Veterans in particular may be especially reticent to seek treatment due to perceived social stigma, self-stigma, and feelings of shame (Blais and Renshaw 2013; Hoge et al. 2004; Kehle et al. 2010; Seal et al. 2010). Among OEF/OIF Veterans seeking treatment at a VA facility, 21 % are estimated to have a major depressive disorder and 29 % are believed to have PTSD (Vaughan et al. 2014). Unfortunately, treatment utilization rates are staggeringly low; approximately 31–47 % of those with suspected PTSD or depression do not receive psychiatric intervention (Elbogen et al. 2013; Schell and Marshall 2008). Additionally, evidence suggests that OEF/OIF Veterans are more likely than their older counterparts to terminate treatment prematurely and/or miss mental health appointments (Erbes et al. 2009; Schell and Marshall 2008). As such, although individual differences exist that impact incidence and treatment rates of military-related mental health issues (Meredith et al. 2011), many veterans in need of psychological care are not receiving the treatment that they need. Although highly structured and evidence-based treatments exist for a multitude of mental health problems, a treatment is only as good as the extent to which it is deemed acceptable to the individual.

Human–Animal Interaction (HAI) for Military Personnel and Veterans

The symbiotic relationship between humans and animals has endured globally and throughout history (Yeager and Irwin 2012). Throughout modern warfare, animals have played a vital role as both battle comrades and supportive companions. From the essential role of horses in World War I, to the homing pigeons used in World War II, to the utilization of dolphins to detect mines during the Vietnam War, to the many stories of United States grounds troops bonding with (and in some cases, taking home) stray Iraqi dogs, animals have had a stable presence in American military operations. The use of animals as a therapeutic tool for service personnel dates back to 1919, when the US military first endorsed the use of dogs as a therapeutic intervention for psychiatric patients at Saint Elizabeth's Hospital in Washington, DC. The Department of Defense then began facilitating a human–animal bond program in the 1940s at Pawling Army Air Force Convalescent Center in Pawling, New York which integrated farm animals into the treatment milieu for emotionally traumatized veterans (Chumley 2012). Although interest in the use of animals in therapy has increased throughout the past century, empirical evidence supporting its use is still in its infancy.

The many benefits of HAI in diverse patient populations have been well documented. Specifically, interactions with animals, particularly dogs, lowers blood pressure and heart rate below even baseline (resting) levels (Friedmann et al. 1983), and regular human–canine interactions are associated with a 50 % or greater decrease in physiological response to stress as measured by blood pressure in hypertensive individuals (Allen et al. 2001). With respect to psychological functioning, HAI is related to increased self-reliance, motivation (Cusack 1988), and social interaction (Corson et al. 1977; Messent 1983), and decreased aggressive behavior (Cusack 1988). HAI is also associated with improved overall physical and psychological health (Allen et al. 2001; Sachs-Ericsson et al. 2002), and functions as a buffer against the adverse effects of chronic health and disease (Serpell 2003). Although the evidence unequivocally suggests that animals are beneficial for mental health patients in general, dogs may prove particularly therapeutic for active duty service personnel and veterans of war.

As previously discussed, military service personnel are at risk for developing emotional stoicism and affective constriction even above and beyond that which civilian men have been socialized to embody. As such, displaying empathy, compassion, patience, and affection toward others are socially undesirable in the military and can even result in ridicule or the accusation that one has gone "soft." Interestingly, these expectations do not translate to relationship with dogs. The presence of the eight canines deployed to Afghanistan and Iraq by Combat and Operational Stress Control teams (COSC) reduced negative attitudes associated with participating in stress-relieving activities and enhanced the facilitation of mental health care services (Gregg 2012; Krol 2012). For military personnel, knowing that they could interact with animals during sponsored activities increased the number of people who participated as well as enhanced rapport with COSC teams (Chumley 2012; Gregg 2012).

The fact that dogs are one of the few socially acceptable venues for displaying emotional connections in the military makes HAI a compelling option for ameliorating emotional numbing in veterans and facilitating therapeutic processes reliant on emotional identification and disclosure. Simply stated, dogs can be a nonthreatening, indirect way of loosening some of the constriction around affective experience and expression that has been so deeply ingrained into military culture.

The introduction of animals to individuals with varying needs can occur in multiple modalities. Table 10.1 provides an overview of some of the most relevant terms. It is important to note that these terms are often inconsistently defined in the literature (even within the same field). Therefore, the theoretical definitions are generally at the author's discretion. *Animal Assisted Activities* (AAA) provide opportunities for motivational, educational, recreational, and/or therapeutic benefits to enhance quality of life. AAA are delivered in a variety of environments including nursing homes and hospice care centers, wherein dogs or cats are taken to visit or interact with patients (Mills and Yeager 2012).

Resident/Facility Animals (RA) can be used in a form of AAA or Animal-Assisted Therapy (AAT, described below), wherein the animal may reside in the patient facility. These animals may be part of formal therapeutic activities or present to spontaneously interact with the patients and visit intermittently (Mills and Yeager 2012). In VAs across the country, it is growing increasingly commonplace to have RA. For example, the Orlando Veterans Affairs Medical Center in Orlando, Florida has an aviary in its Community Living Center (CLC), a facility for senior

Table 10.1 Animals used in various settings and situations

Term	Definition
Service (assistance) animals (e.g., guide dogs, hearing dogs, service dogs)	Dogs that are individually trained to do work or perform tasks for people with disabilities. Examples of such work or tasks include guiding people who are blind, alerting people who are deaf, pulling a wheelchair, alerting and protecting a person who is having a seizure, reminding a person with mental illness to take prescribed medications, calming a person with posttraumatic stress disorder (PTSD) during an anxiety attack, or performing other duties. In addition, the Department's revised ADA regulations have a new, separate provision about miniature horses that have been individually trained to do work or perform tasks for people with disabilities (Department of Justice 2011)
Animal-Assisted Activities (AAA)	Provide opportunities for motivational, educational, recreational, and/or therapeutic benefits to enhance quality of life. AAA are delivered in a variety of environments by specially trained professionals, paraprofessionals, and/or volunteers, in association with animals that meet specific criteria (Delta Society n.d.a)
Animal-Assisted Therapy (AAT)	A goal-directed intervention in which an animal that meets specific criteria is an integral part of the treatment process. AAT is directed and/or delivered by a health/human service professional with specialized expertize, and within the scope of practice of his/her profession (Delta Society n.d.b)
Resident/Facility Animals (RA)	Animals are trained to participate in a facility's planned and spontaneous activities and therapies with patients or residents. Resident/Facility Animals can be AAT or AAA animals and are comparable because each works with a volunteer or professional who has been trained by a formal program. Although RA are often personal pets of the handlers and accompany their handlers to the sites they visit, they may also reside at a facility (Mills and Yeager 2012)
Emotional Support Animals (ESA)	A type of companion animal/pet that provides comfort to a person with a psychiatric disability, but does not perform trained tasks to assist their owners. ESA are only legally defined in some states (Mills and Yeager 2012)

citizens in need of residential care. In addition, a golden retriever affectionately named Pal used to live at the CLC and visit with the veterans throughout the day. The residents would feed, groom, and walk Pal and frequently commented how much they enjoyed his presence.

In *Animal-Assisted Therapy* (AAT), the animal is used as a component of a specifically designed treatment intervention. Unlike in AAA, the interaction is formalized and goal-driven, and results are documented. The role of the animal in AAT is typically to aid in traditional therapy by facilitating a sense of comfort, security, and healthy distraction during a psychotherapy session. For instance, a patient might be asked to stroke a dog or a cat to ease his or her distress while talking about emotionally difficult content. The presence of animals in this manner has been demonstrated to positively impact treatment engagement and completion rates. For example, Beck et al. (1986) reported that inclusion of a canine in the therapy process was associated with improved compliance with psychotherapy, such that group members attend more consistently and participate more actively when group treatment involves HAI. More recently, Fournier et al. (2007) reported similar results, such that HAI was associated with greater engagement in existing psychological treatment. Several examples exist demonstrating that the presence of an animal enhances client–clinician rapport and trust building in a number of populations (e.g., Barker et al. 2010; Ritchie and Amaker 2012; Yeager and Irwin 2012). Cole et al. (2007) also argue that dedicated interaction with canines promotes sociability and cushions the negative physiological effects of anxiety. In some forms of AAT, the interaction with the animal constitutes the majority of the therapy, as it is considered to be beneficial in and of itself. As such, AAT may serve a dual purpose, direct improvement of specific mental health symptoms through mere time spent interacting with an animal, and indirect improvement through increased treatment initiation, engagement, and completion.

Unlike AAA, AAT, *Emotional Support Animals* (ESA), *Service (Assistance) Animals* (SA) are owned by and live with the patient. ESA are a type of Companion Animal/Pet that do not require any specialized training because they do not perform trained tasks to assist the patient. Generally, ESA help the individual cope with his or her mental health symptoms by providing companionship, comfort, and affection. In most jurisdictions, ESA do not have special permission to accompany owners into restaurants, hospitals, and other public places that typically do not allow animals (Mills and Yeager 2012). SA, on the other hand, are individually trained to do work or perform tasks for people with disabilities (Department of Justice 2011). As discussed later in this chapter, much debate surrounds the extent to which mental illness is a permanent disability as opposed to an episodic and modifiable impairment.

One specific type of HAI with dogs that has not been defined into one of the above categories involves patient participation in *Animal Training* or working with the animal to learn simple commands and decrease undesirable behaviors. These types of training-based therapies have been hypothesized to ultimately improve the patient's mental health, either via the interaction with the animal itself, or via improvement on several key features that impact the outcomes of psychotherapy. Specifically, research has found that when individuals learn to train and care for difficult-to-adopt shelter dogs, they demonstrate increased interest and participation in meaningful activities, decreased feelings of detachment/estrangement from others, expanded range of affect, and an increased future-oriented outlook

(Britton and Button 2006; Harkrader et al. 2004; Messent 1983). For example, programs in which individuals experiencing emotional numbing are taught to train difficult-to-adopt shelter dogs (i.e., dogs with behavioral/psychological challenges including anxiety, fear, and hyperactivity) have found positive results for the human participants with respect to increases in social skills (Davis and Bunnell 2007; Fournier et al. 2007; Turner 2007), patience (Britton and Button 2006; Furst 2006), empathy (Strimple 2003), compassion (Harbolt and Ward 2001), and parenting skills (Britton and Button 2006; Turner 2007). Human participants in these studies have also demonstrated decreased social isolation, increased social contact, and increased corrective social interactions (Fournier et al. 2007; Messent 1983; Sachs-Ericsson et al. 2002; Serpell 2003; Strimple 2003). In addition, these programs are associated with decreased anger, violence, and need for medication (Harkrader et al. 2004). Studies are currently underway with combat veterans with PTSD to determine if participation in a shelter dog-training program will improve compliance, engagement, and retention in evidence-based therapies for PTSD.

Current Programs Pairing Dogs and Veterans

Although a wide variety of species of animals have been used in conjunction with therapy (AAT) including cats, birds, and rabbits (Sockalingam et al. 2008), the most common are dogs and horses. After conducting a comprehensive review, there are several types of programs throughout the country that recognize the importance of the human–animal bond for active military personnel and veterans in the United States (see Table 10.2). Specific purposes vary greatly by organization but generally seek to provide, assist, train, and match animals with active duty service members and veterans for one or more of the following purposes: (1) physical support; (2) psychological support; (3) physical disabilities; (4) psychological disabilities; (5) companionship; (6) therapy services at military and VA hospitals; (7) combat stress relief for in-theater deployment; and (8) resources and information for military personnel, veterans and their guide, service, assistance, or therapy dogs (e.g., contact information for individuals throughout the United States willing to board animals while owners attend to service commitments). Some of the more typical accrediting bodies include Assistance Dogs International (ADI) and the International Guide Dog Federation (IGDF).

Several of the above organizations have related affiliations and partnerships. For example, America's VetDogs®, which trains and provides dogs to veterans with disabilities, combat stress relief dogs for in-theater deployment, and therapy dogs to provide physical and emotional therapy services at select military and VA hospitals, maintains cooperative relationships with the military and the Department of Veterans Affairs (VA), sets the standards for measuring Assistance Dog schools, and is involved in reviewing provisional guidelines for the placement of dogs with veterans with PTSD. America's VetDogs® is also currently participating in a study with Western Kentucky University to determine the

Table 10.2 Animal organizations

Organization	Website	Location(s)
Paws for Purple Hearts	http://www.pawsforpurplehearts.org	Headquartered in Rohnert Park, CA, but has programs in Bethesda, MD (2 locations), Menlo Park, CA, and Fort Belvoir, VA
Canine Companions for Independence®	www.cci.org	Operates six regional training centers and four development offices in Santa Rosa, Oceanside, and Los Angeles, CA, Colorado Springs and Denver, CO, Chicago, IL, Irving, TX, Delaware, OH, Medford, NY, and Orlando, FL
Warrior Canine Connection	http://warriorcanineconnection.org	Headquartered in Brookeville, MD with programs in Bethesda, MD (2 locations), Menlo Park, CA, Germantown, MD, and Fort Belvoir, VA as well
America's VetDogs®	www.vetdogs.org	Smithtown, NY
Patriot PAWS	http://www.patriotpaws.org	Rockwall, TX
4 Paws 4 Patriots	http://4paws4patriots.org	Temecula, CA
Patriots and Paws	http://www.patriotsandpaws.org	Huntington Beach, CA
Companions for Heroes	http://companionsforheroes.org	Fairfax Station, VA
Paws for Veterans	www.pawsforveterans.com	Melbourne, FL
New Horizons Service Dogs, Inc.	www.newhorizonsservicedogs.org	Orange City, FL
Operation Freedom Paws	http://operationfreedompaws.org	San Martin, CA
Tower of Hope	www.thetowerofhope.org	New York, NY
Service Dog Project, Inc.	http://www.servicedogproject.org	Ipswich, MA
Freedom Service Dogs, Inc.	http://freedomservicedogs.org	Englewood, CO
Patriot PAWS	http://www.patriotpaws.org	Rockwall, TX
Southeastern Guide Dogs, Inc.-Paws for Patriots™	http://www.guidedogs.org	Palmetto and St. Petersburg, FL
NEADS, Dogs for Deaf and Disabled Americans	www.neads.org	Princeton, MA
Pets for Patriots®	http://petsforpatriots.org	Headquartered in Long Beach, NY but partners with approved shelters and rescues throughout the U.S.
Freedom Paws Assistance Dogs	http://www.freedompaws.org	Marysville, OH
Puppies Behind Bars®	http://www.puppiesbehindbars.com	New York metropolitan area
PACT for Animals	https://pactforanimals.org	Delaware Valley region (eastern PA, southern NJ, and DE)
Prison Pups and Pals, Inc.-Paws of Freedom	http://www.prisonpupsandpals.org	Daytona Beach, FL
Canines for Service, Inc.	http://www.caninesforservice.org	Wilmington, NC
The Sam Simon Foundation-Service Dogs for Veterans	http://www.samsimonfoundation.com	Malibu, CA

(continued)

Table 10.2 (continued)

Organization	Website	Location(s)
K9s for Warriors	http://www.k9sforwarriors.org	Ponte Vedra Beach, FL
Freedom Dogs	http://www.freedomdogs.org	San Diego, CA
Hawaii Fi-Do Service Dogs	http://www.hawaiifido.org	Oahu, HI
Paws and Stripes	http://www.pawsandstripes.org	Rio Rancho/Albuquerque, NM
Sherri's Project: Wounded Warrior Pack	http://www.woundedwarriorpack.org	North County San Diego and surrounding areas
Soldier's Best Friend	http://soldiersbestfriend.org	Headquartered in Peoria, AZ, but has programs in Phoenix, Tucson, Prescott, Flagstaff, and Sierra Vista, AZ
Paws4People®-Paws4Vets Assistance Dog Placement Program	http://paws4people.org	Headquartered in Wilmington, NC with multiple programs throughout the mid-Atlantic and southeast region
Dogs on Deployment	http://dogsondeployment.org	Headquartered in Santee, CA but is an online network that can be used throughout the U.S.
Vets Adopt Pets™	http://www.vetsadoptpets.org	Headquartered in San Francisco, CA, but works with many pet shelters and rescues across the country
Pets for Vets, Inc.	http://pets-for-vets.com	Operates several chapters throughout the U.S.
Dunes Dog-Training Club-Pets N Vets	http://dunesdogtrainingclub.tripod.com	Hebron, IN
Specialty Dog-Training-Shelter to Solider™	http://specialtydogtraining.com	San Diego, CA
The Battle Buddy Program-Service Dog Program	http://tbbf.org	West Chester, OH
Animal Service Animal Society	https://www.dogs4vets.org/index2.php	Chandler, AZ
Guardian Angels for Soldier's Pet©-Warriors' Angels Program	http://guardianangelsforsoldierspet.org	Headquartered in Gatesville, TX, but operates several other programs throughout the state

efficacy of placing service dogs with veterans with PTSD in symptom reduction. Another organization, NEADS, Dogs for Deaf and Disabled Americans, trains dogs for people with physical disabilities. Clients come for two weeks of training before receiving a dog. NEADS' Canine for Combat Veterans program provides dogs at no cost to Veterans whose war injuries resulted in physical disabilities. Interestingly, NEADS was the first Assistance Dog organization invited to Walter Reed Hospital to give an in-service about how Assistance Dogs can help wounded veterans and was the first Assistance Dog organization to develop a program specifically geared to Iraq and Afghanistan war Veterans. Among other organizations, NEADS is partnered with Disabled American Veterans (DAV), the Military Order of the Purple Heart, and the Tower of Hope.

Despite promising potential and growing acceptance, the number of empirical studies on the human–animal bond in therapeutic settings remains low (Walsh 2009). As such, the extent to which HAI may help combat veterans with PTSD or other mental health maladies remains uncertain. However, national funding agencies, such as the Department of Defense and the National Institute of Mental Health, have begun to earmark dollars specifically for HAI studies, and several empirical investigations on the use of HAI with veterans are underway. For example, the authors of this chapter are currently investigating the extent to which an adjunctive, HAI-based intervention improves adherence to current evidence-based treatments for PTSD. The Research Center for Human–Animal Interaction (ReCHAI) at the University of Missouri has been conducting ongoing research examining the impact of shelter dogs living in the homes of combat veterans. Given the momentum of HAI and the emphasis on treating returning war veterans, there should be much data emerging over the next decade.

Considerations in Designing HAI Programs for Veterans

Clearly, the conjectural and antidotal evidence regarding the use of dogs to help veterans with mental health concerns is promising. The literature consistently suggests that veterans (as well as any individual) experiencing transition issues, loneliness, or general life stressors may reap psychological benefits from having a companion animal. However, when psychopathology or a more serious, diagnosable mental health disorder is present, specific considerations must be attended to prior to uniformly suggesting an animal to help with treatment. More broadly, our enthusiasm as a field must be tempered until the scientific evidence: (1) supports the use of canines in mental health treatments as being equal or superior to the well-established evidence-based therapies; and (2) elucidates the specific role and context of the animal in the patient's overall treatment plan.

Regarding the first concern, there have been no randomized controlled trials comparing animal interaction (whether it be AAA, AAT, animal training, or the possession of a SA) with current treatments. These types of direct comparisons are the "gold star" litmus test in the field of psychology. In assessing the value of an intervention, it is necessary to determine if it is as good or better than our current best practices. It may be the case that although an animal makes people feel good, the degree of change or progress in recovering from their disorder is much less than that of existing efficacious treatments. It also may be that current treatments are superior for most, but a subset of the population with particular features may benefit more from an animal-based or adjunctive intervention. Finally, animal interventions may be equally as effective as our current best practices; in this case, questions of parsimony and complexity must be considered.

While most recognize the value in the human–animal bond, an argument the potential for overdependent relationships between humans and companion animals is not without merit. For instance, Stallones et al. (1990) found that individuals between the ages of 21 and 34 who were strongly attached to their pets were at risk of having fewer human social supports. In the same study, it was found that when strong attachments to pets existed in the absence of human supports for individuals between 35 and 44, the attachment was associated with emotional distress. More recently, the strength of the attachment bond has been recognized as a significant predictor of psychological distress experienced after the animal companion dies (Field et al. 2009). Psychological difficulties following the death of a companion animal include loss of motivation and increased stress levels (Brown 1996), social impairment (Walsh 2009), and depression (Sharkin and Knox 2003). Finally, Peacock et al. (2012) also highlight the psychological vulnerability of individuals reporting a strong bond with their animal companion. Interestingly, unlike the studies described above, strength of attachment to the animal companion did not mediate the impact of social isolation on psychological distress, suggesting that animal companionship may not compensate for a person's limited human social supports.

In addition to establish that incorporating animals into a therapy adds significant value to current gold-standard treatments, a second, related, need is to determine exactly how to integrate dogs into the treatment paradigm. As described throughout this chapter, the pairing of animals with veterans for the purposes of enhancing psychological functioning can take many different forms, from merely visiting with an animal (as in AAT), to dependency on the animal to leave one's house (as with a service dog). Historically, approaches have been somewhat atheoretical in that a particular mechanism of action to justify the introduction of a dog has not been considered. Ensuring that the HAI is aligned with the current knowledge base and scientific underpinnings for a particular problem is paramount. Otherwise, we run the risk of well-intentioned interventions having iatrogenic effects.

Contraindications of Service Animals for Veterans

As it relates to PTSD, experts in the field have raised concerns that AAT, ESA, and SA may do more harm than good. According to the National Center for PTSD,

> Although people with PTSD who have a service dog for a physical disability or emotional support dog may feel comforted by the animal, there is some chance they may continue to believe that they cannot do certain things on their own. For example, if the dog keeps strangers from coming too close, the owner will not have a chance to learn that they can handle this situation without the dog. Becoming dependent on a dog can get in the way of the recovery process for PTSD. Based on what we know from research, evidence-based treatment provides the best chance of recovery from PTSD. (U.S. Department of Veterans Affairs 2014)

Specifically, the treatment for PTSD—a disorder characterized by pathological avoidance—centers on exposure therapy. Although this may come in different forms (e.g., Prolonged Exposure, Trauma Management Therapy, Cognitive Processing Therapy, Eye Movement Desensitization and Reprocessing), the core component of all effective PTSD treatments is exposure. Exposure involves the individual confronting feared stimuli, either in a graduated approach (systematic desensitization) or all at once (flooding), and is highly effective for any disorder that involves avoidance, including social phobia or panic disorder. Any type of device that allows the individual to engage in avoidance, whether it be watching a TV show to take one's mind off of distressing thoughts (avoidance of internal emotions), an enabling wife that does all the grocery shopping (avoidance of crowds) or drinking a six pack of beer (avoidance of physiological arousal) is referred to as a "safety signal" and is contraindicated for the treatment of PTSD, no matter how well-intentioned it may be. For this reason, the National Center for PTSD treatment guidelines now strongly caution against the use of benzodiazepines for the treatment of PTSD. While it may make it so that a person feels able to go to a restaurant, it is actually prolonging the illness in the long run, as the person is not learning how to go to a restaurant without the medication.

An analogous principle applies to canine companions. For example, programs that train dogs to "clear" a room for a veteran so that he or she feels comfortable to enter are actually covering up a problem, instead of working with the veteran on his or her distorted views on safety and the ability to cope with being in an area which he or she has not "secured." Similarly, a veteran who engages in AAT within a PTSD treatment paradigm will likely experience decreased tension, blood pressure, and pulse rate based on previous literature (Allen et al. 2001; Friedmann et al. 1983). Though on the surface this may seem desirable, the goal of combat trauma treatment is to encourage the veteran to fully confront and subsequently master his or her emotional demons. Anything that artificially promotes a sense of relaxation, whether it a medication, a dog, or a diversion, serves to prolong the problem from being addressed at its root. With depressive and mood disorders, there has been research into the role of experiential avoidance and how this serves to strengthen and prolong depressive episodes (Hayes et al. 2004). Mindfulness and acceptance-based approaches, often termed the "third wave" of psychotherapy, have been garnering strong empirical support in the contemporary literature. These approaches emphasize being able to "sit with," or tolerate, one's emotional experiences without attempting to distract, avoid, or mitigate. The use of "Service Animals" to aid with mental health problems has been an area of much debate in recent policy creation, national listservs, and position statements. Typically, a Service Dog is supplied to an individual with a disability that the dog either compensates for (e.g., a seeing eye dog helping a blind person cross the street) or assists with (e.g., a dog giving a warning that a seizure is imminent). In these cases, the dog is vital to the person improving his or her quality of life due to a permanent disability. However, where mental health problems are concerned, there exists a fine line between validation of a struggle and disempowerment; that is, problems such as PTSD, depression, substance abuse, and other common psychological sequelae of war are not permanent disabilities akin to blindness. This is a notion that the VA and other treatment facilities have worked hard to dispel, and a preponderance of the evidence supports the idea that these problems are highly treatable and, thus, temporary. As such, there is concern that, in addition to the aforementioned role as a safety signal, giving a veteran a PTSD support dog (or permitting their ESA to accompany them at all times) sends a strong message that they are disabled and, due to their trauma, are incapable of navigating potential triggers without the protection or comfort of the animal. The VA does not currently provide veterinary care for SA secured through other avenues. However, research is currently underway within the VA to determine the extent to which a specially trained SA provides psychological benefit for PTSD above and beyond the general benefits of animal ownership.

Integrating Dogs into PTSD Treatment

This is not to say that there is no place for HAI in PTSD treatment; on the contrary, given that treatment acceptance rates are so low and attrition is so high, there is a vital need to develop palatable alternatives or adjunctive interventions to traditional therapy. Given the aforementioned heightened affective symptoms in male military veterans (e.g., affective flattening, interpersonal detachment), it appears that HAI is a viable option for such modifications, but it must be purposefully planned in a manner that augments, and not detracts from, existing best practices. Dogs may play a vital role in being a conduit for therapeutic rapport and trust, and can be an integral component to exposure therapy. For example, a veteran may first go outside only with his dog, then go outside with his dog for half the time and then alone half the time, eventually graduating going outside alone. Training dogs at a shelter typically relies on the same principles found in exposure therapy, particularly when using behavioral paradigms to decrease fear and increase sociability. For instance, teaching a dog that humans are nothing to be afraid of by coaxing the animal out of his kennel little by little approximates how a veteran might work with a therapist learn that the grocery store is nothing to be afraid of. This parallel process could be very valuable in increasing the veteran's "buy in" for engaging in exposure therapy.

Dogs may also help with mindfulness-based approaches that emphasize being "present" in the here and now. To accomplish this, a variety of grounding techniques are used to focus the senses on the current moment. AAT may be a compelling option for this, allowing the veteran to practice mindfulness by focusing on the feel of the dog's fur, the sounds he makes when happy, or the visual contrast between the colorings on his coat. With respect to depressive and mood disorders, behavioral activation or getting out and doing activities is a vital component of almost all evidence-informed treatment approaches. Volunteering at a shelter to train dogs, taking a dog on a walk, or simply running errands associated with caring for a dog are all great ways to impel a person to leave the house. Additionally, the removal of a disorder is not the sole goal of psychotherapy; an increased quality of life and enhanced level of functioning must also be attended to (Seligman and Csikszentmihalyi 2000). Canine interaction has a documented positive effect in these areas (Nordgren and Engstrom 2014).

Collectively, many opportunities exist to use dogs in psychotherapy with veterans while maintaining fidelity to the current knowledge base. Though this body of literature is in its infancy, it is encouraging that no risks to the animals have been systemically identified thus far in AAT programs. In fact, the evidence seems to support the opposite notion, suggesting that such programs are beneficial to the animals, and thus engendering a symbiotic relationship. For example, Odendaal and Lehmann (2000) found that the neurotransmitter phenyl ethylamine is secreted when humans and animals intermingle. The amphetamine-like chemical is mutually produced in the pleasure center of the brain in both species during interactions.

Future Directions

Currently, there appears to be a continuum within the field of psychology anchored by two end camps: those who adhere strictly to empiricism and data-driven tools and interventions, and those who take a holistic approach, highlighting the differences between efficacy and effectiveness that invoke the use of complementary and alternative medicines. In our efforts to expand the use of HAI, we must help to integrate it from its current categorization in the VA as a complementary and alternative medicine toward the direction of empiricism (i.e., medicine) before it can be widely appreciated, implemented, or reimbursed by insurance agencies. As Kruger and Serpell (2006) note, the acceptance of HAI for the treatment of mental health problems has been hampered by a lack of a "unified, widely accepted, or empirically supported theoretical framework for explaining how and why the relationship between humans and animals are potentially therapeutic" (pp. 25–26). As such, it is imperative that future work focuses on the design and evaluation of randomized controlled trials to determine, and subsequently dismantle, the impact of HAI on the mental health of military personnel and veterans.

References

Alfred, G. C., Hammer, J. H., & Good, G. (2014). Traditional masculinity, hardiness, and psychological well-being in male student veterans. *Psychology of Men & Masculinity, 15*, 95–99.

Allen, K., Shykoff, B. E., & Izzo, J. L. (2001). Pet ownership, but not ACE inhibitor therapy, blunts home blood pressure responses to mental stress. *Hypertension, 38*(4), 815–820.

Arkin, W., & Dobrofsky, L. R. (1978). Military socialization and masculinity. *Journal of Social Issues, 34*, 151–168.

Barker, S., Knisely, J., McCain, N., Schubert, C., & Pandurangi, A. (2010). Buffering response patterns from interaction with a therapy dog. *Anthrozoos, 23*(1), 79–91.

Beck, A. S., Seradarian, L. L., & Hunter, G. F. (1986). Use of animals in the rehabilitation of psychiatric inpatients. *Psychological Reports, 58*, 63–66.

Blais, R. K., & Renshaw, K. D. (2013). Perceptions of partners' attributions for depression in relation to perceptions of support and conflict in romantic relationships. *Journal of Marital and Family Therapy, 40*(4), 498–508.

Brown, B. H. (1996). Pet bonding and pet bereavement among adolescents. *Journal of Counseling & Development, 74*, 505–509.

Bowlby, J. (1969). *Attachment and loss: Attachment* (Vol. 1). New York, NY: Basic Books.
Bowlby, J. (1982). Attachment and loss: Retrospect and prospect. *American Journal of Orthopsychiatry, 52*(4), 664–678.
Brailey, K., Vasterling, J. J., Proctor, S. P., Constans, J. I., & Friedman, M. J. (2007). PTSD symptoms, life events, and unit cohesion in U.S. soldiers: Baseline findings from the neurocognition deployment health study. *Journal of Traumatic Stress, 20*(4), 495–503.
Britton, D. M., & Button, A. (2006). Prison pups: Assessing the effects of dog training programs in correctional facilities. *Journal of Family Social Work, 9*(4), 79–95.
Brooks, G. R. (2005). Counseling and psychotherapy for male military veterans. In G. E. Good & G. R. Brooks (Eds.), *A new handbook of counseling and psychotherapy with men* (pp. 206–228). San Francisco, CA: Jossey Bass.
Chopik, W. J., Edelstein, R. S., & Fraley, R. C. (2013). From the cradle to the grave: Age differences in attachment from early adulthood to old age. *Journal of Personality, 81*(2), 171–183.
Chumley, P. R. (2012). Historical perspectives of the human–animal bond within the Department of Defense. *U.S. Army Medical Department Journal, 2*, 18–20.
Cole, K., Gawlinski, A., Steers, N., & Kotlerman, J. (2007). Animal assisted therapy in patients hospitalized with heart failure. *American Journal of Critical Care, 16*(6), 575–585.
Corson, S. A., Arnold, L. E., Gwynne, P. H., & Corson, E. O. L. (1977). Pet dogs as nonverbal communication links in hospital psychiatry. *Comprehensive Psychiatry, 18*, 61–72.
Cusack, O. (1988). *Pets and mental health*. New York: Haworth Press.
Davis, M., & Bunnell, M. (2007). *Working like dogs: The service dog guidebook*. Crawford, CO: Alpine Publications.
Del Giudice, M. (2011). Sex differences in romantic attachment: A meta-analysis. *Personality and Social Psychology Bulletin, 37*(2), 193–214.
Delta Society. (n.d.a). Animal-Assisted Activities (AAA). Retrieved from http://www.petpartners.org/page.aspx?pid=319
Delta Society. (n.d.b). Animal-Assisted Therapy (AAT). Retrieved from http://www.petpartners.org/page.aspx?pid=320
Department of Defense. (2012). Demographics: Profile of the Military Community. Retrieved from http://www.militaryonesource.mil/12038/MOS/Reports/2012_Demographics_Report.pdf
Department of Justice. (2011). Service animals. Retrieved from http://www.ada.gov/service_animals_2010.htm
Eisenhart, R. W. (1975). You can't hack it little girl: A discussion of the covert psychological agenda of modern combat training. *Journal of Social Issues, 31*(4), 13–23.
Elbogen, E. B., Wagner, H. R., Johnson, S. C., Kinneer, P., Kang, H., Vasterling, J. J., et al. (2013). Are Iraq and Afghanistan veterans using mental health services? New data from a national random-sample survey. *Psychiatric Services, 64*(2), 134–141.
Elder, G. H., & Clipp, E. C. (1988). Wartime losses and social bonding: Influences across 40 years in men's lives. *Psychiatry, 51*, 177–198.
Elise, D. (1997). Primary femininity, bisexuality and the female ego ideal: A reexamination of female developmental theory. *Psychoanalytic Quarterly, 66*(3), 489–517.
Erbes, C. R., Curry, K. T., & Leskela, J. (2009). Treatment presentation and adherence of Iraq/Afghanistan era veterans in outpatient care for posttraumatic stress disorder. *Psychological Services, 6*(3), 175–183.
Field, N. P., Orsini, L., Gavish, R., & Packman, W. (2009). Role of attachment in response to pet loss. *Death Studies, 33*(4), 334–355.
Fournier, A. K., Geller, E. S., & Fortney, E. E. (2007). Human-animal interaction in a prison setting: Impact on criminal behavior, treatment progress, and social skills. *Behavior and Social Issues, 16*(1), 89–105.
Fraley, R. C., Waller, N. G., & Brennan, K. A. (2000). An item response theory analysis of self-report measures of adult attachment. *Journal of Personality and Social Psychology, 78*(2), 350–365.
Friedmann, E., Katcher, A. H., Thomas, S. A., Lynch, J. J., & Messent, P. R. (1983). Social interaction and blood pressure: Influence of animal companions. *The Journal of Nervous and Mental Disease, 171*(8), 461–465.

Furst, G. (2006). Prison-based animal programs: A national survey. *The Prison Journal, 86*(4), 407–430.
Gregg, B. T. (2012). Crossing the berm: An occupational therapist's perspective on animal-assisted therapy in a deployed environment. *U.S. Army Medical Department Journal, 2*, 55–56.
Harbolt, T., & Ward, T. H. (2001). Teaming incarcerated youth with shelter dogs for a second chance. *Society and Animals, 9*(2), 177–182.
Harkrader, T., Burke, T. W., & Owen, S. S. (2004). Pound puppies: The rehabilitative uses of dogs in correctional facilities. *Corrections Today, 66*(2), 74–79.
Hayes, S. C., Strosahl, K., Wilson, K. G., Bissett, R. T., Pistorello, J., Taormino, D., et al. (2004). Measuring experiential avoidance: A preliminary test of a working model. *The Psychological Record, 54*, 553–578.
Hazan, C., & Shaver, P. R. (1987). Romantic love conceptualized as an attachment process. *Journal of Personality and Social Psychology, 52*(3), 511–524.
Hoge, C. W., Castro, C. A., Messer, S. C., McGurk, D., Cotting, D. I., & Koffman, R. L. (2004). Combat duty in Iraq and Afghanistan, mental health problems, and barriers to care. *New England Journal of Medicine, 351*(1), 13–22.
Iversen, A. C., Fear, N. T., Ehlers, A., Hacker Hughes, J. G., Hull, L., Earnshaw, N. M., et al. (2008). Risk factors for posttraumatic stress disorder among UK Armed Forces personnel. *Psychological Medicine, 38*(4), 511–522.
Jakupcak, M., Osborne, T. L., Michael, S., Cook, J. W., & McFall, M. (2006). Implications of masculine gender role stress in male veterans with posttraumatic stress disorder. *Psychology of Men and Masculinity, 7*(4), 203–211.
Jansz, J. (2000). Masculine identity and restrictive emotionality. In A. H. Fischer (Ed.), *Gender and emotional: Social psychological perspectives* (pp. 166–186). New York, NY: Cambridge University Press.
Kehle, S. M., Polusny, M. A., Murdoch, M., Erbes, C. R., Arbisi, P. A., Thuras, P., et al. (2010). Early mental health treatment-seeking among U.S. National Guard soldiers deployed to Iraq. *Journal of Traumatic Stress, 23*(1), 33–40.
King, D. W., Vogt, D. S., & King, L. A. (2003). Risk and resilience factors in the etiology of chronic PTSD. In B. T. Litz (Ed.), *Early interventions for trauma and traumatic loss in children and adults: Evidence-based directions* (pp. 34–64). New York: Guilford Press.
Krol, W. (2012). Training the combat and operational stress control dog: A innovative modality for behavioral health. *U.S. Army Medical Department Journal, 2*, 46–50.
Kruger, K. A., & Serpell, J. A. (2006). Animal assisted interventions in mental health. In A. Fine (Ed.), *Handbook on animal-assisted therapy: Theoretical foundations and guidelines for practice* (pp. 21–38). London: Academic Press.
Kurpius, S. E. R., & Lucart, A. L. (2000). Military and civilian undergraduates: Attitudes toward women, masculinity, and authoritarianism. *Sex Roles, 43*(3–4), 255–265.
Levant, R. F., & Richmond, K. (2007). A review of research on masculinity ideologies using the Male Role Norms Inventory. *Journal of Men's Studies, 15*, 130–146.
Lisak, D. (2001). Homicide, violence and male aggression. In G. Brooks & G. Good (Eds.), *A new handbook of counseling and psychotherapy approaches for men* (pp. 278–292). San Francisco, CA: Jossey-Bass.
Lorber, W., & Garcia, H. A. (2010). Not supposed to feel this: Traditional masculinity in psychotherapy with male veterans returning from Afghanistan and Iraq. *Psychotherapy: Theory, Research, Practice Training, 47*(3), 296–305.
MacNaughton, G. (2006). Constructing gender in early-years education. In C. Skelton, B. Francis, & L. Smulyan (Eds.), *The SAGE handbook of gender and education* (pp. 127–138). Thousand Oaks, CA: Sage.
McTeague, L. M., McNally, R. J., & Litz, B. T. (2004). Prewar, warzone, and postwar predictors of posttraumatic stress in female Vietnam veteran health care providers. *Military Psychology, 16*(2), 99–114.

Meredith, L. S., Sherbourne, C. D., Gaillot, S., Hansell, L., Ritschard, H. V., Parker, A. M., et al. (2011). *Promoting psychological resilience in the U.S. Military*. Santa Monica, CA: RAND Corporation.

Messent, P. (1983). Social facilitation of contact with other people by pet dogs. In A. Katcher & A. M. Beck (Eds.), *New perspectives on our lives with companion animals*. Philadelphia: University of Pennsylvania Press.

Mikulincer, M., & Shaver, P. R. (2001). Attachment theory and intergroup bias: Evidence that priming the secure base schema attenuates negative reactions to out-groups. *Journal of Personality and Social Psychology, 81*, 97–115.

Mikulincer, M., & Shaver, P. R. (2003). The attachment behavioral system in adulthood: Activation, psychodynamics, and interpersonal processes. *Advances in Experimental Social Psychology, 35*, 53–152.

Mills, J. T., & Yeager, A. F. (2012). Definitions of animals used in healthcare settings. *U.S. Army Medical Department Journal, 2*, 12–17.

Morris, M. (1996). By force of arms: Rape, war, and military culture. *Duke Law Journal, 45*(4), 651–781.

Nordgren, L., & Engstrom, G. (2014). Animal-assisted intervention in dementia: Effects on quality of life. *Clinical Nursing Research, 23*, 7–19.

O'Neil, J. (2008). Summarizing 25 years of research on men's gender role conflict using the gender role conflict scale: New research paradigms and clinical implications. *The Counseling Psychologist, 36*(3), 358–445.

Odendaal, J., & Lehmann, S. (2000). The role of phenylethylamine during positive human-dog interaction. *ACTA Veterinaria, 69*(3), 183–188.

Oliver, L. W., Harman, J., Hoover, E., Hayes, S. M., & Pandhi, N. A. (1999). A quantitative integration of the military cohesion literature. *Military Psychology, 11*, 57–83.

Peacock, J., Chur-Hansen, A., & Winefield, H. (2012). Mental health implications of human attachment to companion animals. *Journal of Clinical Psychology, 68*, 292–303.

Pollack, W. (1995). No man is an island: Toward a new psychoanalytic psychology of men. In R. F. Levant & W. S. Pollack (Eds.), *A new psychology of men* (pp. 33–67). New York, NY: Basic Books.

Pollack, W. S. (1999). *Real boys: Rescuing our sons from the myths of boyhood* (18th ed.). New York, NY: Henry Holt & Company.

Ritchie, E. C., & Amaker, R. J. (2012). Canine-assisted therapy in military medicine. The early years. *U.S. Army Medical Department Journal, 2*, 5–7.

Rochlen, A. B. (2005). Men in (and out) of therapy: Central concepts, emerging directions, and remaining challenges. *Journal of Clinical Psychology, 61*(6), 627–631.

Sachs-Ericsson, N., Hansen, N. K., & Fitzgerald, S. (2002). Benefits of assistance dogs: A review. *Rehabilitation Psychology, 47*, 251–277.

Schell, T. L., & Marshall, G. N. (2008). Survey of individuals previously deployed for OEF/OIF. In T. Tanielian & L. H. Jaycox (Eds.), *Invisible wounds of war: Psychological and cognitive injuries, their consequences, and services to assist recovery* (pp. 87–115). Santa Monica, CA: RAND Corporation.

Seal, K. H., Maguen, S., Cohen, B., Gima, K. S., Metzler, T. J., Ren, L., et al. (2010). VA mental health services utilization in Iraq and Afghanistan veterans in the first year of receiving new mental health diagnoses. *Journal of Traumatic Stress, 23*, 5–16.

Seligman, M. E. P., & Csikszentmihalyi, M. (2000). Positive psychology: An introduction. *American Psychologist, 55*, 5–14.

Serpell, J. A. (2003). Anthropomorphism and anthropomorphic selection-beyond the "cute response". *Society and Animals, 11*, 83–100.

Sharkin, B. S., & Knox, D. (2003). Pet loss: Issues and implications for the psychologist. *Professional Psychology: Research and Practice, 34*(4), 414–421.

Sockalingam, S., Li, M., Krishnadev, U., Hanson, K., Balaban, K., Pacione, L., et al. (2008). Use of animal-assisted therapy in the rehabilitation of an assault victim with a concurrent mood disorder. *Journal of Mental Health Nursing, 29*, 73–84.

Stallones, L., Marx, M. B., Garrity, T. F., & Johnson, T. P. (1990). Pet ownership and attachment in relation to the health of U.S. adults, 21 to 64 years of age. *Anthrozoös, 4*(2), 100–112.

Strimple, E. O. (2003). A history of prison inmate-animal interaction programs. *American Behavioral Scientist, 47*, 70–78.

Turner, W. (2007). The experience of offenders in a prison canine program. *Federal Probation, 71*, 38–43.

U.S. Department of Veterans Affairs. (2014, April 29). Dogs and PTSD. Retrieved from http://www.ptsd.va.gov/PTSD/public/treatment/cope/dogs_and_ptsd.asp

Vaughan, C. A., Schell, T. L., Tanielian, T., Jaycox, L. H., & Marshall, G. N. (2014). Prevalence of mental health problems among Iraq and Afghanistan veterans who have and have not received VA services. *Psychiatric Services, 65*(6), 833–835.

Walsh, F. (2009). Human–animal bonds I: The relational significance of companion animals. *Family Process, 48*(4), 462–480.

Whitesell, A. A., & Owens, G. (2012). The impact of patriotism, morale, and unit cohesion on mental health in Veterans of Iraq and Afghanistan. *Traumatology, 18*, 1–7.

Yeager, A. F., & Irwin, J. (2012). Rehabilitative canine interactions at the Walter Reed National Military Medical Center. *U.S. Army Medical Department Journal, 2*, 57–60.

Chapter 11
The Roles Animal Companions Play in Middle-Aged Males' Lives: Examining the Psychometric Properties of a Measure Assessing Males' Human–Animal Interactions

Chris Blazina and Anne S. Bartone

If one traces the historical origins of the popular phrase, "man's best friend," there are several sources to consider. Derr (2011) is among those who argue that dogs evolved from wolves becoming a sort of domesticated ally aiding primitive man in hunting big game. Over the centuries, the canine shifted from the outer periphery of the fire circle into the backyards of the twentieth century man. Between those points in time, the special relationship between man and dog is referenced in some important literary pieces, including Homer's epic the *Odyssey,* which among the oldest.

As the story goes, when the Greek hero Odysseus returns to Ithaca after being away for twenty years, his dog Argos immediately recognizes him. In a moving piece of literature, Argos strains with his last bit of strength to draw closer to his master before dying.

> So they spoke. And a dog, lying there, lifted its head and pricked up its ears. Argus was the hound of noble Odysseus, who had bred him himself, though he sailed to sacred Ilium before he could enjoy his company. Once the young men used to take the dog out after wild goat, deer and hare, but with his master gone he lay neglected by the gate, among the heaps of mule and cattle dung that Odysseus' men would later use to manure the fields. There, plagued by ticks, lay Argus the hound. But suddenly aware of Odysseus' presence, he wagged his tail and flattened his ears, though no longer strong enough to crawl to his master. Odysseus turned his face aside and hiding it from Eumaeus wiped away a tear… (Homer: The Odyssey, Bk XVII: 290-322).

C. Blazina (✉)
Department of Counseling and Educational Psychology, New Mexico State University, College of Education, MSC 3CEP, PO Box 30001, Las Cruces, NM 88003, USA
e-mail: cblazina@nmsu.edu

A.S. Bartone
1821 5th Ave. Apt.7, Troy, NY 12180, USA
e-mail: bartonea@hotmail.com

C. Blazina and L.R. Kogan (eds.), *Men and Their Dogs*,
DOI 10.1007/978-3-319-30097-9_11

French philosopher, Voltaire, offers this definition for a dog in his *Dictionnaire philosophique* (1764). Translated it reads as follows:

> DOG—It seems that nature has given the dog to man for his defense and for his pleasure. Of all the animals it is the most faithful: it is the best friend man can have.

In 1789, Frederick, King of Prussia, wrote a poem about the merits of dogs that would later be printed in *The New-York Literary Journal*, (Volume 4, 1821: [5])

> The faithful dog—why should I strive to speak his merits, while they live: In every breast, and man's best friend. Does often at his heels attend (p. 6).

In his journal, Napoleon Bonaparte also comments about the aftermath of a battle where he encounters a dead soldier accompanied by his dog. The dog lay beside the soldier's body, licking his face and howling.

> It was a beautiful, calm, moonlight night. Suddenly a dog, which had been hiding under the clothes of a dead man, came up to us with a mournful howl, and then disappeared again immediately into his hiding place. He would lick his master's face, then run up to us again, only to return once more to his master. Whether it was the mood of the moment, whether it was the place, the time, the weather, or the action itself, or whatever it was, it is certainly true that nothing on any battlefield ever made such an impression on me. I involuntarily remained still, to observe the spectacle. This dead man, I said to myself, has perhaps friends, and he is lying there abandoned by all but his dog! What a lesson nature teaches us by means of an animal.' … I looked on, unmoved, at battles which decided the future of nations. Tearless, I had given orders which brought death to thousands. Yet here I was stirred, profoundly stirred, stirred to tears. And by what? By the grief of one dog (Tsouras 1992; Wines 2014).

Another source comes directly from a trial at the Johnson City Courthouse in Tennessee in which an attorney, who would later become a senator (Senator George Graham Vest), sought damages on behalf of his client whose dog, Old Drum, was shot by a neighbor. The following is an excerpt from the speech given on October 18, 1869 at the trial:

> Gentlemen of the jury:… The one absolutely unselfish friend that a man can have in this selfish world, the one that never deserts him and the one that never proves ungrateful or treacherous is his dog….A man's dog stands by him in prosperity and in poverty, in health and in sickness….If fortune drives the master forth an outcast in the world, friendless and homeless, the faithful dog asks no higher privilege than that of accompanying him to guard against danger, to fight against his enemies, and when the last scene of all comes, and death takes the master in its embrace and his body is laid away in the cold ground, no matter if all other friends pursue their way, there by his graveside will the noble dog be found, his head between his paws, his eyes sad but open in alert watchfulness, faithful and true even to death (Morrow 2012, p. 290).

Among the citations mentioned above, various qualities of how men perceive the bond are identified including: loyalty, steadfastness, protection, and a single-minded devotion. Each alone potentially sets the stage for a unique type of bond between man and dog. When these qualities are combined, a more complex understanding of the relationship between man and dog emerges.

More contemporary perspectives in the field of human–animal interactions also offer various underlying meanings of the bond. For example, Freud mentions the unambivalent nature of dogs—"They love their friends and bite their enemies" (Molnar 1996). Freud also suggests that many humans develop a sense of "pure love" for their dogs (Bossard 1944; Roth 2005). Others have built on his original suggestions, offering that the human–animal bond provides an experience of unconditional love or acceptance. Recent research has examined how psychoanalyst Bowlby's (1969) attachment figures' characteristics originally devised to describe the caregiver and child relationship (e.g., safe base, safe haven, proximity seeking, and distress at being apart) is applicable to the human–animal bond (Kobak 2009; Kurdek 2008, 2009; Sharkin and Knox 2003).

In this chapter, we consider the male context in discussing the bond. Our primary assumption is that the human–animal bond plays various roles in men's lives and that the resulting meaning(s) is partly responsible for the strong emotional tie. For instance, dogs become a safe connection that offers soothing when under distress. Brown (2004, 2007) suggested that part of the significance of the human–animal bond rests on dog's single-minded devotion to human counterparts, mirroring a sense of specialness. There are also roles that dogs play that may on the surface seem only utilitarian in nature. With closer examination, however, these roles also potentially deepen the bond. When men play and exercise with their dogs, or experience them as steadfast guardians of their home, the nature of the connection can change. Derr (2011) stated that evolution and selective breeding has played a key role in turning the wolf into a canine companion, offering assistance to mankind in various ways. It could also be argued that the role(s) of the dog have evolved over time aligned with the modern man's needs. The emphasis on being a "working dog" in the traditional sense of herding and hunting has become a secondary function for most. Today, many "working dogs" fill more exclusive psychological roles; ones that are of particular value to men given the sometime conflicting nature of traditional male gender roles.

We argue that men may perceive their canine companion as assuming more than one significant role, sometimes several at once. Ultimately, we suggest that the convergence of multiple roles results in the deepening of the bond. In essence, a canine companion earns the title "man's best friend" because he/she helps supply certain essential emotional/relational qualities, some of which, due to traditional male socialization, may be limited in various other contexts. It is important to consider the multifaceted nature of what will be perceived by some men as a welcomed amicable if not familial bond.

To fully appreciate the value of human–animal interactions in the lives of men, a contextual understanding is needed (see Blazina et al. 2011). A contextual analysis allows masculinity to be paired with other key variables such as age, prior relationship success, perceived social support, current life stress, and attachment history. These lines of inquiry further clarify the meaning of the human–animal bond for men. It is essential that we do not assume that all men are not part of a singular homogenous sample in terms of the meanings of the bond. This is a limitation of previous research, in conjunction with not adequately accounting for male socialization as a viable contextual variable. Herzog (2007) suggested that it is the within-group differences among men (and women) that account for some of the gender confusion about attitudes toward the human–animal bond. Therefore, variations even exist among men and dogs with the most solid bonds. For example, some males may discover the bond during early phases of development as boys to offset insecure attachments in the family; others may deepen their ties in adulthood, or old age amid life transitions and stressors. Others may have fulfilling lives in terms of work and love but find their relationship with their canine companions to be unique. One way to operationalize the nature of the meaning of the bond is through the essential psychological or functional roles that the dog is perceived to play. This chapter attempts to explore some of these roles and their potential impact on adult men's level of attachment to their dogs. These goals are accomplished in part by developing a new measure that assesses the various types of roles men perceive their dogs to be fulfilling.

Method

Participants

A convenience sample ($n = 211$) was solicited through social networking sites (Facebook, Twitter, and Craigslist Pet Forums). Eligible participants were adult-aged men, who currently had at least one canine companion. The mean age of the participants was 41.8 (SD = 13.6); the mean age of their dogs was 4.13 (SD = 3.48), having been together with their dogs for an average of 3.51 years (SD = 2.11). In terms of romantic relationship status, 47.3 % reported they were married, 29.3 % single, 14.0 % in a committed relationship, 6.3 % divorced, and 2.3 % separated. In terms of education obtained, 19.4 % reported high school diploma, 5.0 % GED, 11.3 % associates degree or technical certificate, 29.7 % some college, and 34.7 % college degree or higher.

Instruments

Companions Animal Role Scale (CARS)

The Companion Animal Roles Scale (CARS) was developed for this study by the researchers.

The CARS initial construct validity was established through use of trained raters, graduate psychology students familiar with the literature of the human–animal bond. Items were generated and retained based on a measure assessing how well the descriptor(s) fit with the belief that an animal companion is like a friend or family member. Items that reached the $p > 0.001$ level of significance were retained for use on the pre-factor analysis instrument. The preliminary version of the CARS had 18 items.

Comfort from Companion Animals Scale (CCAS)

The Comfort from Companion Animals Scale (CCAS) is a measure designed to gauge the level of pet attachment participants have toward their animal. The CCAS is an 11-item self-report instrument rated on a 4-point Likert-type scale, ranging from 1 (*Strongly Disagree*) to 4 (*Strongly Agree*) with a higher score indicating greater perceived comfort from the pet. Sample items include "Having a pet gives me something to care about," "My pet is a source of constancy in my life," and "My pet makes me feel needed." The alpha for this scale was 0.94 (Zasloff 1996).

Lexington Attachment Scale (LAPS)

The Lexington Attachment Scale (LAPS) is a measure designed to assess the emotional attachment of individuals to their pets. The LAPS is a 23-item self-report instrument rated on a 4-point Likert-type scale, ranging from 1 (*Strongly Disagree*) to 3 (*Strongly Agree*). Negatively worded items are reverse coded prior to scoring and missing items or *Do not Know or Refuse* responses are recoded as 0 before calculating the total score. The coding provides a range of values from 0 to 69, with higher scores indicating higher degrees of dog attachment. Sample items include "Quite often I confide in my pet," "I believe my pet is my best friend," and "I enjoy showing other people pictures of my pet." The psychometric properties of this instrument were investigated and the authors reported scores with a high degree of internal consistency, with an alpha coefficient of 0.93. Construct validity was also assessed by examining how responses to the LAPS were related to interviewer assessments of 412 respondents' attachment to their pets. A one-way ANOVA was used to examine the relationships between the LAPS and respondent characteristics as evidence (Johnson et al. 1992).

Normative Male Alexithymia Scale (NMAS)

The Normative Male Alexithymia Scale (NMAS) is a measure designed to assess normative male alexithymia. The NMAS is a 20-item self-report instrument rated on a 6-point Likert-type scale, ranging from (1) *Strongly Disagree* to (7) *Strongly Agree*, with higher scores indicating higher levels of alexithymia. Sample items include "I don't like to talk with others about my feelings," "I find it is very hard to cry," and "It does not usually occur to me to deal with my stress by talking about what is bothering me." Exploratory and confirmatory factor analyses indicated that the NMAS consisted of a single 20-item factor. Scores on the NMAS displayed evidence of internal consistency (coefficient $\alpha = 0.92$) and test-retest reliability ($r = 0.91$) over a 1–2 month period (Levant et al. 2006).

Procedures

Due to the involvement of human participants, this research study received a formal review by the Division of Research and Sponsored Program's Institutional Review Board/Human Subjects Committee. Permission was obtained. The demographic questions, as well as the four measures discussed above were made available via SurveyMonkey, a secure web-based program designed to assist researchers in survey construction, dissemination, and data collection. SurveyMonkey is Health Insurance Portability and Accountability Act (HIPAA) compliant. All information was collected through SurveyMonkey.

Data Analysis

An essential component in the process of validating *The Companions Animal Role Scale* was to examine the measure's reliability, as it is an essential prerequisite for validity. The reliability of a measurement instrument is the extent to which it yields consistent reproducible estimates of an underlying true score and some have argued that it is the foundation on which other psychometric properties rest (Hinkin 1995). Heppner et al. (2008) affirmed that reliability is the variance of scores that is a result of true difference among participants.

Results

Factor Analysis

Internal consistency reliability refers to the homogeneity of the items in the measure (Hinkin 1995). Based on the guidelines for scale development, it is important to establish an internal consistency estimate of a least 0.70. In this case, the internal consistency coefficient (Cronbach's alpha) for the total scale, based on the entire sample ($N = 211$) was 0.880. To assess construct validity, exploratory factor analysis was used. For the present study, factor analysis was used to measure construct validity with the hopes of understanding the degree to which the hypothetical constructs measured share information with one another. This allowed for an unbiased evaluation of the factor structure because factors emerge devoid of theoretical explanation (Devellis 1991). To enhance construct validity, researchers are advised to conduct content analyses and consult with domain experts as well as to pilot items to identify potential problems with their wording (Heppner et al. 2008).

Table 11.1 provides descriptive information showing the means, and standard deviations for each of the 17 variables included in this analysis. The Kaiser–Meyer–Olking (KMO) statistic is 0.906 and the Bartlett's test is significant. Three extracted factors account for 56.971 of the variance in the items' variance–covariance matrix. The fact that the reproduced matrix is not significantly different from

Table 11.1 Descriptive Statistics

	Mean	Standard Deviation
1	4.38	0.861
2	3.46	1.360
3	3.69	1.206
4	4.58	0.838
5	2.82	1.310
6	3.20	1.480
7	2.46	1.284
8	3.44	1.280
9	2.70	1.314
10	3.83	1.217
11	4.00	1.117
12	4.13	0.957
13	4.62	0.878
14	1.43	0.955
15	1.90	1.309
16	2.52	1.613
17	3.27	1.444

the observed matrix suggests goodness-of-fit. None of the three factors correlated, so we proceeded with an orthogonal rotation rather than an oblique rotation strategy. Table 11.2 displays the rotated factor matrix.

Using 0.30 as a cutoff for interpretation, the loadings suggested three distinct factors. Factor 1 was labeled as representing the *Emotional Bond* men have with their dogs and consisted of the following descriptors: *Friend, Confidant, Emotional Support, Family Member, Helpful Throughout Life Tough Times, Share Good Times with, Unconditional Love,* and *Watch TV/Movies With.* Factor 2 was labeled as *Personal Growth* for characteristics that men perceive about the bond with their dogs and included the following descriptors: *Helps Meet and Socialize, Instill Hope,* and *Teacher of Life Lessons.* Factor 3 was designated as the *Life Style* aspects of men's relationships with their dogs. We believe the Life Style factor or subscale represents the practical roles dogs can play in men's lives and included these descriptors: *Exercise Partner, Home Security Protector, Medical Assistance,* and *Playmate for Children.* One item was not retained on the final CARS Total score (*Companion for Another Pet*) because it did not meet the .30 cutoff on any of the three factors. This resulted in 16 items.

Convergent validity was established by correlating both the CARS total and subscale scores with the Lexington Attachment to Pets Scale (LAPS), a well-established measure of HAI emphasizing strength of attachment bond. The results showed that total scores combined from the three factors were significantly related to increased scores of the LAPS (i.e., greater perception of an attachment bond with a companion animal). The LAPS total score was also significantly correlated

Table 11.2 Rotated Factor Matrix

Factor	1	2	3	
1	0.807	0.156	0.160	Friend
2	0.637	0.465	0.052	Confident
3	0.637	0.480	0.040	Emotional Support
4	0.762	0.056	0.150	Family Member
5	0.226	0.117	0.543	Exercise Partner
6	0.272	0.113	0.714	Home Security/Protector
7	0.122	0.687	0.227	Helps Meet and Socialize with others
8	0.501	0.741	-0.006	Instills Hope
9	0.271	0.721	0.285	Teacher of Life's Lessons
10	0.630	0.513	-0.042	Helps Me Through Tough Times
11	0.726	0.447	0.170	Share Good Times with
12	0.727	0.290	0.251	Enjoy Playful Times with
13	0.793	-0.010	0.122	Unconditional Love
14	-0.142	0.482	0.532	Medical Assistance
15	-0.106	-0.049	0.447	Playmate for Children
16	0.217	0.195	-0.078	Companion for Another Pet
17	0.476	0.334	0.004	Watch Tv/Movies with

Note.
Factor 1: Friend, Confidant, Emotional Support, Family Member, Helps Me Through Tough Times, Share Good Times With, Enjoy Playful Times With, Unconditional Love, Watch Tv/ Movies With
Factor 2: Helps Meet And Socialize With Others, Instill Hope, Teacher of Life's Lessons
Factor 3: Exercise Partner, Home Security/Protector, Medical Assistance, Playmate for Children

with all three subscales: Emotional Bond ($r = 0.512$, $p < 0.000$), Personal Growth ($r = 0.367$, $p < 0.000$), and Life Style ($r = 0.238$, $p < 0.001$).

In terms of internal reliability, the Cronbach alpha is (0.880) for the entire sample ($N = 213$). The two-week test–retest measure yielded a significant correlation for the total CARS score (0.974, $p < 0.000$) and also for each of the subsequent factors: Emotional Bond (0.941, $p < 0.000$), Personal Growth (0.963, $p < 0.000$).

Multiple Regressions

A series of regression analyses were conducted utilizing the three subscales of the CARS (Emotional Bond, Personal Growth, and Life Style) separately and then as a total score with other main variables of interest that included NMAS, LAPS total score, and the CCAS total score.

The Personal Growth subscale of the CARS was significantly inversely related to scores on the NMAS $b = -.189$, $t = -2.231$, $p < 0.05$. Personal Growth also explained a significant proportion of variance in NMAS, $R^2 = .036$, $F(1, 134)$

$= 4.97$, $p < 0.05$. Males that reported higher scores on the CARS reported lower scores on NMAS (total score).

The total CARS score was also significantly related to the LAPS scores for males, $b = .482$, $t = 6.836$, $p < 0.000$ and also explained a significant proportion of variance in LAPS, $R^2 = .233$, $F(1, 154) = 46.726$, $p < 0.000$. Males who reported increased scores on the three CARS subscales were associated with stronger bonds with their dogs.

The total CARS score was also significantly related to the CCAS scores for males, $b = .788$, $t = 16.426$, $p < 0.000$. The total CARS also explained a significant proportion of variance in CCAS, $R^2 = 0.621$, $F(1, 165) = 269.798$, $p < 0.000$. Males who reported increased scores on the three subscales of the CARS was associated with a greater sense of receiving comfort from their dogs.

Discussion

Today, animal companions are visible in many facets of life. In some studies, upwards of 85 % of persons define their pets as having a status comparable to that of a close friend or family member (Cain 1983; Voith 1985). While the discovery of the human–animal bond may seem like a recent development, animals have long been a valued part of human life as evidenced by ancient cultures in their perceptions of animals as companions, spiritual guides, figures within folklore, and as symbols of luxury (Serpell 1991, 2010; Walsh 2009). All of these examples may be construed as animals playing various roles in our lives and sense of wellness.

In the current study, we explored the development of a new measure emphasizing animal companions' roles as a central part of an attachment bond in men's lives. The CARS has 3-subscales subsequently labeled, Emotional Bond, Personal Growth, and Lifestyle. In terms of scale development, the CARS' psychometric properties were promising. The total CARS scores was significantly related to the LAPS scores. The LAPS has been utilized extensively in HAI research. This result helps establishing convergent validity. We also found that the inter-item reliability was good and the two-week test-retest reliability was very high.

Perhaps the most significant finding in terms of clinical application was males that reported greater scores of Normative Male Alexithymia perceived their dogs as promoting various facets of Personal Growth including expanding social networks, learning various life lessons, and sustaining hope. All of these characteristics are of value in their own right but perhaps take on a unique contextual meaning in the lives of many men that struggle with the constricting aspects of male socialization. Various theorists and researchers have identified some of the limiting effects of constricted forms of traditional male gender roles (see Blazina 2001; Blazina and Shen-Miller 2010; Levant 2001; O'Neil 1982, 1986, 2008; 2015; Pleck 1981; Pollack 1998). Male roles can include overly restricted emotionality, fear of intimacy, striving for skewed versions of success and power, and unyielding attempts to balance work, and family demands. An abundance of research supports the link between gender role conflict in men and psychological distress such as increase in depression, anxiety, substance use, and interpersonal problems (O'Neil 2008). Men who feel constricted by traditional gender roles are also adversely impacted by limited opportunities for intimacy (O'Neil 1986, 1995, 2008). We suggest that the bond between man and dog has the potential to offset some of these challenges, in part through the various roles animal companions play. However, explaining the psychological significance of the human–animal bond is a complex endeavor.

The bond's importance is far more than just being utilitarian in nature and potentially takes on more than one psychological quality. This may include offsetting struggles with loneliness and having at least one meaningful relationship. While there seems to be at least a few of these generative/supportive roles for each of the men in the survey, statistics alone cannot determine their clinical importance. Is it the combination of roles that is emotionally significant leading to a tipping point for developing the strength of the attachment bond? Or, is there one type of role that is especially central for men to feel deeply attached to their dogs?

Men's ascribed meaning of the bond may also involve a form of what has been referred to as male 'covert intimacy' (Kiselica et al. 2008; Kiselica & Englar-Carlson; 2010). This involves how males show affection indirectly, or through action, like doing for others in caring ways. This approach is done in order to circumvent the gender role dictums about men not being overtly emotional or demonstrative. Covert intimacy potentially has application for the man–dog bond. Its occurrence may also confuse some researchers and clinicians, who are not aware of the dynamic when trying to understand the meaning of the bond in males' lives. We may not have full overt access to how males perceive their animal companions, leading some to suspect the bond is not quite as meaningful for men. Furthering the complicated relational dynamics is the point that it is not just what males receive from animal companions that potentially deepens the bond. For some males, it is equally if not more important when afforded the opportunity to give to their dogs. Within the human–animal bond this process involves how men look after their dogs, protect them, spend time together, and take care of their day-to-day needs. This type of relational exchange is in sync with how traditionally men are taught to enact masculinity within caring relationships. Not having those opportunities to reciprocate may leave some with a sense of having nothing of value to offer; a feeling that may be intensified amid other intense life frustrations and let downs. While we did not measure how men's perception of giving to their animal companions impacted the bond, but future research should consider those dynamics. Research with the CARS measure should consider the reciprocal nature of the man–dog dyad and psychological well-being. To explore this point, measures of well-being needs to be assessed along with the CARS in order to determine the significance of reciprocal roles impacting men's functioning. This should be investigated both with males that are currently attached with their dogs as well as among those who have lost them. Kohut (1984) pointed out that one best determines the essential place of a love object only after losing them.

That is, one's sense of being is greatly impacted when both the object and the roles they played in our lives are lost.

It also seems likely that the bond allows some men to circumvent psychological defensive styles that are customarily utilized in relational encounters and clinical settings (see Blazina and Bartone 2015; Del Giudice 2011; Wexler 2009). These strategies involve distancing from affect, denial of attachment needs, and circumventing emotional involvement and intimacy when under duress (see Cassidy and Kobak 1988). Male gender roles can include patterns of going-it-alone and solving one's own problems. It is argued that the HAI allows many men to move both beyond the usual perceptions and guarded expectations. When in the presence of an animal companion there may be a temporary gender renorming or neutralizing regarding affection felt and displayed. Therefore, future research should also include natural observation when accessing males true sentiments toward their dogs. As mentioned previously, Freud referred to the 'pure love' qualities that characterize our relationships with animal companions, involving the sense of unconditional love or acceptance, but also reliability and trust. Animal companions may witness males vulnerabilities, having access to parts others may not often see. What emerges is a unique type of encounter.

There is also a prevailing trend for males in North America to report very negative attitudes toward seeking psychological or medical support services (Addis and Cohane 2005). The culturally conditioned ways men are socialized to think, feel, and act (see Levant 2001; O'Neil 1986, 1995, 2008; Pleck 1981) seem to leave many men confused and in a double-bind (Good and Wood 1995). Males may often mistake self-reliance for total self-sufficiency and feel pressure to keep any forms of vulnerability firmly in check. While potentially benefiting from various forms of social support, they simultaneously feel blocked from accessing them. Needless to say, these acquired practices often have a negative impact with significant others, friends, and family (O'Neil 2008; Levant 2001; Pollack 1998). One of those frequently cited clinical scenarios involves the constriction of affect, not being able to label emotion, and recognize these qualities in others. Levant (2001) refers to this as normative male alexithymia. In this study, males that reported more levels of normative male alexithymia also relied on their dogs for what can be described as personal growth. Males felt their animal companions helped them realize more social possibilities, life complexities, and personal understanding. In some ways, the Personal Growth subscale of the CARS is similar to the safe base notion Bowl proposed for attachment figures (1969/1982). They encourage a person to stretch, reaching greater levels of personal development. When males are significantly bonded with their dogs, the nature of the bond may in some cases spur on this type of personal expansion.

Scholars in the psychology of men and masculinity argue that cultural competence and contextual understanding are essential for effective research and clinical practice with males (see Liu 2005; Vacha-Haase et al. 2011). This is where man's "best friend" may play a pivotal role. Future research involving animal assisted therapy may wish to understand more about men's emotional responsiveness when a dog is involved. Even more specifically is the need for research regarding designated emotional service dogs in offering males' psychological support. Scenarios include post-deployment soldiers, and those civilians experiencing depression, anxiety, and limited social networks. These circumstances will help address what psychological roles males' may deem more acceptable for their dog to fulfill versus a human friend, companion, or family member; or at least, how the presence of an animal companion may allow those that feel emotionally constricted to open up.

Future research also needs to consider adding additional roles to the CARS. Our sample was community based, largely middle-aged males (mean = 41 years of age) who were mostly in some form of a relationship. This speaks to a unique sample in some ways akin to the Kurdek (2009) study exploring the bond with noncollege, middle-aged males. In that study, males reported turning to their animal companions as safe haven, someone that augmented moments of distress. In the present study, the Emotional Bond factor may be interpreted in similar ways. Researchers should continue exploring if males' age is a contextual variable of interest that impacts levels of attachment to one's animal companion. It is likely that other significant CARS roles also exist for males in various other development points across the life span, that include being single or widowed, having experienced significant strain or trauma, and report limited social support networks. Therefore, the CARS should be viewed as a work in progress that holds some promise for understanding the unique contextual view of the HAI from the perspectives of males and its use should be continued with other diverse samples.

A limitation of the study in terms of generalization of findings is that the CARS was not normed using women. It remains to be seen if the same types of patterns found in this study emerge when the measure is utilized with women. More work is needed using both men and women as subjects, but not as means compare as much as to understand contextual similarities and differences. Also, we relied extensively on self-report measures and future directions should also consider observational data to corroborate that roles reported are actual roles that were performed by animal companions. Also, there still may be other roles to be reported that may be influenced by a recency effect on the part of the human companions recalling what the most common and frequently occurring roles are now. Given that the average age of the dogs was 4 years old, that is old enough to be different from puppy behavior, and far too young to be considered how roles may change when dogs are in the later years. Middle-aged men may shift their perception of how significant animal companions' roles are with their own aging process, but we also need to know more about how dog's roles actually change when they enter old age. As mentioned, part of the focus is not only understanding what men receive from their animal companions but how taking care of them when they are aged or infirmed actually allow males to give back, setting up another form of covert intimacy. In these scenarios, men care for their animal companions, and by doing so, receive a potential purpose, a meaning, or even confirming the care offered has value. All are important characteristics for men of any age but especially for aging males that may lack other tangle forms of bolstering their worth. In short, the roles of animal companions may vary across our life span and theirs.

The results from the CARS suggested that males perceive their dogs as performing several distinct roles. This perception was related to increased sense of emotional bonding with animal companions, receiving more emotional comfort from them, and decreased scores of Normative Male Alexithymia. The findings support the CARS being a measure of potential interest for research with males and having possibly clinical application. The results speak to a multidimensional and nuanced bond between men and their animal companions.

References

Addis, M. E., & Cohane, G. H. (2005). Social scientific paradigms of masculinity and their implications for research and practice in men's mental health. *Journal of Clinical Psychology, 61*, 633–647.

Blazina, C. (2001). Analytic psychology and gender role conflict: The fragile masculine self. *Psychotherapy: Theory, Research, Practice, Training, 38*, 50–59.

Blazina, C., & Bartone, A. (2015). Moving beyond essentialism in the psychoanalytic theories of masculinity: Implications for theory, practice, and research. In S. Wester & J. Wong (Eds.), *APA handbook of men and masculinity* (pp. 105–122). Washington, DC: APA Press.

Blazina, C., Boyraz, G., & Shen-Miller, D. S. (2011). *The psychology of the human-animal bond.* New York, NY: Springer Publishing.

Blazina, C., & Shen-Miller, D. (2010). *An international psychology of men: Theoretical advances, case studies, and clinical innovations*. New York: Routledge.

Bossard, J. H. S. (1944). Mental hygiene of owning a dog. *Mental Hygiene, 28*, 408–413. Retrieved from http://www.worldcat.org/title/mental–hygiene/oclc/1606164

Bowlby, J. (1969). *Attachment and loss: Attachment* (Vol. 1). New York, NY: Basic Books.

Brown, S. (2004). The human-animal bond and self-psychology: Toward a new understanding. *Society and Animals, 12*(1), 67–86.

Brown, S. E. (2007). Companion animals as self-objects. *Anthrozoos, 20*(4), 329–343.

Cain, A. (1983). A study of pets in the family system. In A. Katcher & A. Beck (Eds.), *New perspectives on our lives with companion animals* (pp. 72–81). Philadelphia, PA: University of Pennsylvania Press.

Cassidy, J., & Kobak, R. R. (1988). Avoidance and its relation to other defensive processes. In J. Belsky & T. Nezworski (Eds.), *Clinical implications of attachment* (pp. 300–323). Hillsdale, NJ: Erlbaum.

Del Giudice, M. (2011). Sex differences in romantic attachment: A meta-analysis. *Personality and Social Psychology Bulletin, 37*, 193–214.

Derr, M. (2011). *How dog's evolved into 'our best friend.'* (D. Davies, Interviewer). Retrieved from November 8, 2011 http://www.npr.org/2011/11/08/142100653/how-dogs-evolved-into-our-best-friends

Devellis, R. F. (1991). *Scale development.* Newbury Park, NJ: Sage.

Frederick, I. I. (1821). King of Prussia (1789). The faithful dog—Why should I strive to speak his merits, while they live: In every breast, and man's best friend. Does often at his heels attend. *The New-York Literary Journal, 4*, p. 6.

Good, G. E., & Wood, P. K. (1995). Male gender role conflict, depression, and help-seeking: Do college men face double jeopardy? *Journal of Counseling and Development, 74*, 70–75.

Herzog, H. A. (2007). Gender differences in human-animal interactions: A review. *Anthrozoös, 20*(1), 7–21. doi:10.2752/089279307780216687.

Heppner, P. P., Wampold, B., & Kivlighan, D. M, (2008). Research design in counseling (3rd Ed.) Chapters 17–21. Belmont, CA: Thomson Brooks/Cole.

Hinkin, T. R. (1995). A review of scale development practices in the study of organizations. *Journal of Management, 21*(5), 967–988.

Homer. The Odyssey. Bk XVII: 290-322. Translated by Robert Fagles.

Johnson, T. P., Garrity, T. F., & Stallones, L. (1992). Psychometric evaluation of the lexington attachment to pets scale. *Anthrozoös, 5*(3), 160–175. doi:10.2752/089279392787011395.

Kiselica, M. S., Englar-Carlson, M., Horne, A. M., & Fisher, M. (2008). A positive psychology perspective on helping boys. In M. S. Kiselica, M. Englar-Carlson, & A. Horne (Eds.), Counseling troubled boys (pp. 31– 48). New York: Routledge.

Kiselica, M. S., & Englar-Carlson, M. (2010). Identifying, affirming, and building upon male strengths: The positive psychology/positive masculinity model of psychotherapy with boys and men. *Psychotherapy Theory, Research, Practice and Training, 47*(3), 276–287.

Kobak, R. (2009). Defining and measuring of attachment bonds: Comment on Kurdek (2009). *Journal of Family Psychology, 23*(4), 447–449. doi:10.1037/a0015213.

Kohut, H. (1984). *How does analysis cure?*. Chicago: University of Chicago Press.

Kurdek, L. A. (2008). Pet dogs as attachment figures. *Journal of Social and Personal Relationships, 25*(2), 247–266. doi:10.1177/0265407507087958.

Kurdek, L. A. (2009). Pet dogs as attachment figures for adult owners. *Journal of Family Psychology, 23*(4), 439–446. doi:10.1037/a0014979.

Levant, R. F. (2001). Desperately seeking language: Understanding, assessing and treating normative male alexithymia. In G. R. Brooks & G. Good (Eds.), *The new handbook of counseling and psychotherapy for men* (Vol. 1, pp. 424–443). San Francisco: Jossey-Bass.

Levant, R. F., Good, G. E., Cook, S. W., O'Neil, J. M., Smalley, K., Owen, K., & Richmond, K. (2006). The normative Male Alexithymia Scale: Measurement of a gender-linked syndrome. *Psychology of Men & Masculinity, 7*(4), 212–224.

Liu, W. M. (2005). The study of men and masculinity as an important multicultural competency consideration. *Journal of Clinical Psychology, 61*(6), 685–697.

Molnar, M. (1996). Of dogs and doggerel. *American Imago, 53*(3), 269–280.

Morrow, L. B. (2012). *The giant book of dog names*. Gallery Books.

O'Neil, J. M. (1982). Gender-role conflict and strain in men's lives. In K. Solomon & N. B. Levy (Eds.), *Men in transition: Theory and therapy* (pp. 5–44). New York, NY: Springer Publishing.

O'Neil, J. M. (2008). Summarizing 25 years of research on men's gender role conflict using the gender role conflict scale new research paradigms and clinical implications. *The Counseling Psychologist, 36*(3), 358–445. doi:10.1177/0011000008317057.

O'Neil, J. M. (2015). *Men's gender role conflict: Psychological costs, consequences, and an agenda for change*. Washington, DC: APA Books.

O'Neil, J. M., Helms, B. J., Gable, R. K., David, L., & Wrightsman, L. S. (1986). Gender-role conflict scale: College men's fear of femininity. *Sex Roles, 14*(5–6), 335–350. doi:10.1007/BF00287583.

Pollack, W. S. (1998). *Real Boys: Rescuing our sons from the myth of boyhood.* New York: Random House.

Pleck, (1981). *The myth of masculinity*. Cambridge: The MIT Press.

Serpell, J. A. (1991). Beneficial effects of pet ownership on some aspects of human health and behaviour. *Journal of the Royal Society of Medicine*, *84*(12), 717–720. Retrieved from http://jrs.sagepub.com/

Roth, B. (2005). Pets and psychoanalysis: A clinical contribution. *Psychoanalytic Review, 92*, 453–457.

Serpell, J. A. (2010). Animal-assisted interventions in historical perspective. In A. H. Fine (Ed.), *Handbook on animal-assisted therapy: Theoretical foundations and guidelines for practice* (3rd ed., pp. 17–32). San Diego, CA: Academic Press.

Sharkin, B. S., & Knox, D. (2003). Pet loss: Issues and implications for the psychologist. *Professional Psychology: Research and Practice, 34*(4), 414. doi:10.1037/0735-7028.34.4.414.

Tsouras, P. G. (1992). *Warrior's words: A quotation book*. London, England: Arms and Armour Press.

Vacha-Haase, T., Wester, S. R., & Fowell-Christianson, H. (2011). *Psychotherapy with older men*. New York: Routledge Taylor and Francis Group.

Voith, V. L. (1985). Attachment of people to companion animals. *Veterinary Clinics of North America: Small Animal Practice, 15*, 289–295.

Voltaire. (1764/2008). *Philosophical dictionary* (*Dictionnaire philosophique*). Mobi Classics Series.

Walsh, F. (2009). Human-animal bonds I: The relational significance of companion animals. *Family Process, 48*(4), 462–480. doi:10.1111/j.1545-5300.2009.01296.x.

Wexler, D. (2009). *Men in Therapy: New Approaches for Effective Treatment*. New York: Norton.

Wines, J. A. (2014). *Dogs' miscellany: Everything you always wanted to know about man's best friend*. London: Michael O'Mara Books.

Zasloff, L. R. (1996). Measuring attachment to companion animals: a dog is not a cat is not a bird. *Animal Behaviour Science, 47*, 43–48.

Chapter 12
Exploring How the Human–Animal Bond Affects Men in a Relational Way: Attachment, Loss, and Gender Role Conflict in Middle-Aged and Young-Men

Anne Bartone and Chris Blazina

Within Western culture, masculine gender socialization emphasizes characteristics such as stoicism, independence, physical toughness, dominance, restrictive emotional expression, competition, and anti-femininity (Levant 2001; Mahalik et al. 2003). One implication of the traditional norms of the male role is the "loss of relational connection to the world" (Chodorow 1978, p. 110). Studies show a relationship between traditional masculine gender roles and struggles with psychological intimacy and interpersonal relationships among men (e.g., Mahalik et al. 2001; O'Neil et al. 1995). Tannen (1986) asserts that the traditional feminine gender role is a social orientation that emphasizes closeness and solidarity, while the traditional masculine gender role is a social orientation that emphasizes power and status. It is not that men are unconcerned about their degree of closeness or connection with others. Rather, the difference is one of emphasis and priority. While a masculine disposition is generally concerned about status and power in social exchange relations, the feminine disposition is usually concerned with solidarity and closeness (Ickes 1993). Women are, on average, more relationally oriented than men (e.g., Deaux and Major 1987). Researchers suggest that any behavioral differences that men and women may have, as a function of genes and hormones, are exaggerated and therefore more likely due to the impact of socialization and

A. Bartone (✉)
1821 5th Avenue, Apartment 7, Troy, NY 12180, USA
e-mail: bartonea@hotmail.com

C. Blazina
Department of Counseling and Educational Psychology, New Mexico State University,
College of Education, MSC 3CEP, PO Box 30001, Las cruces, NM, USA
e-mail: cblazina@nmsu.edu

C. Blazina and L.R. Kogan (eds.), *Men and Their Dogs*,
DOI 10.1007/978-3-319-30097-9_12

social norms. Therefore, despite an innate tendency to develop strong bonds, men are disadvantaged in this realm.

There is conflicting research concerning gender differences about companion animal attachment and grief reactions. While many suggest no differences (e.g., Gosse and Barnes 1994; Stallones et al. 1990; Williams et al. 2009), most studies have shown that females of various age groups exhibit stronger bonds and higher levels of grief symptoms/more intense grief reactions following a loss (e.g., Brown et al. 1996; Lue et al. 2008; Marks et al. 1994; Wrobel and Dye 2003). Furthermore, very few studies control for gender or explain gender differences as a function (at least partially) of cultural gender role stereotypes that influence men to be (or to report being) less emotional or more masculine in their behavioral roles (Mandell et al. 1980). Finally, conducting within-groups comparisons are a trend worth adopting. It appears that until very recently, there had only been one empirical study that strictly uses male dog owners in its sample (see Nagasawa and Ohta 2010). Because of the focus of this project, gender and type of pet were controlled for by recruiting current and/or past male dog owners and by selecting measures that attempted to counterbalance the likelihood that some instruments of affective expression are bias against men. With that said, canine companions may be particularly significant in men's lives, as the level of authenticity and depth inherent in this bond has the ability to surpass the constraints of gender socialization and is a powerful catalyst for relational benefits with other people.

A contextual exploration of attachment and loss within human–animal interactions is important work to the psychology of men and masculinity (Blazina et al. 2011). Although we emphasize the positive psychological impact animal companions (and in particular dogs) have in many male's lives in this chapter, it is obvious from the research on domestic abuse, neglect, animal fighting, and abandonment that not all men feel the same. Sometimes, those who identify as having meaningful and healthy bonds with animal companions struggle forming attachment bonds with human companions. In other cases, a relationship with an animal companion can be one important bond part of a larger social network consisting of various types of healthy attachments with human companions.

Purpose of the Study

The primary purpose of this chapter is to explore the bond between men and their canine companions through attachment behavior and gender socialization, and when applicable, the response to the loss of a canine companion. The investigation of the human–canine bond as it pertains to men is theoretically important for several reasons:

1. Because traditional male socialization can significantly impact a man's relational world, canine companions offer an opportunity to offset some of the issues often encountered in human relationships;
2. Animal companionship can be perceived as providing a source of support that could also help to facilitate the development of human-to-human relationships;
3. Expanding contextual knowledge of canine companionship among men will help add to the human–animal interaction literature on attachment and loss.

It is suggested that there would be a predictable pattern of grief based upon attachment and socialized gender role patterns. This includes differences found across cohorts of men (i.e., young, middle-aged, and older men). When one loses an animal companion that feels like a friend or family member, there will be a sense of grief. Therefore, we suggest that subjects will report more signs of mourning (i.e., intensity and duration), as the strength of attachment to their animal companion increases. However, cultural mechanisms such as stringent gender roles can derail outward expressions of grief and mourning for men, leading to disenfranchised grief, especially when those losses are not recognized by society as legitimate, such as the loss of an animal companion. Aspects of gender role conflict such as Restricted Emotionality (RE) can therefore impact the bereavement process.

Four hypotheses will be investigated in this study.

1. Gender role conflict (e.g., RE, Success, Power, Completion, Restricted Affectionate Behavior Between Men (RABBM), Conflict Between Work and Family) will be differ by age group (i.e., young, middle-aged, and older men).
2. The strength of the attachment bond and the level of perceived social support from the most significant canine companion will differ depending on age group (i.e., young, middle-aged, and older men).
3. A dissonant pattern of grief after the loss of the most significant canine companion will vary by age group (i.e., young, middle-aged, and older men).
4. A human avoidant attachment style will moderate the relationship between a human anxious attachment style and a dissonant pattern of grief after the loss of the most significant canine companion.

Method

Research Design

A cross-sectional survey design was used in the present study to test statistical differences between variables as well as statistical relationships between variables. Specifically, all four subscales of the Gender Role Conflict Scale-Short Form (GRCS-SF; Wester et al. 2012), the Pet Attachment Scale (PAS; Albert and Bulcroft 1988), one subscale of the Multidimensional Scale of Perceived

Social Support (MSPSS; Zimet et al. 1988), and one subscale of the Grief Pattern Inventory (GPI; Doka and Martin 2010) were examined for differences between the subgroups of male dog owners based on age. Moreover, an interaction effect between both subscales of the Experiences in Close Relationships Scale-Short Form (ECR-S; Wei et al. 2007) was assessed for its relationship with one subscale of the GPI (Doka and Martin 2010) among male dog owners.

Participants

A convenience sample was solicited through listservs, social networking sites, electronic classifieds, forums, dog parks, pet stores, animal hospitals, veterinary clinics, and personal referrals. Eligible participants were adult-aged men (aged ≥18 years) who have been/are currently in a romantic relationship and have/have had at least one special canine companion.

Instruments

Demographic Questionnaire (DQ)

In addition to a basic demographic questionnaire, the following measures were presented.

Gender Role Conflict Scale-Short Form (GRCS-SF)

Based on the Gender Role Conflict Scale (GRCS; O'Neil et al. 1986), the GRCS-SF was created to reflect greater conflict, increased situational focus, and better potential clinical use. The GRCS-SF is a 16-item self-report instrument measuring the four factors that gender role conflict affects. Items are rated on a 6-point Likert-type scale, ranging from (1) strongly disagree to (6) strongly agree. Subscale scores are obtained by summing the responses to the individual subscales, with higher scores indicating greater gender role conflict (O'Neil et al. 1986). Sample items include: "Winning is a measure of my value and personal worth," "I do not like to show my emotions to other people," "Affection with other men makes me tense," and "Finding time to relax is difficult for me" (Wester et al. 2012, p. 204).

Experiences in Close Relationships Scale-Short Form (ECR-S)

The ECR-S was devised as a shorter version of the Experiences in Close Relationships Scale (ECR; Brennan et al. 1998) to assess (human) adult (romantic) attachment (Wei et al. 2007). The ECR-S is a 12-item self-report measure with each item rated on a 7-point Likert-type scale, ranging from (1) strongly disagree to (7) strongly agree. Participants produce scores on each dimension. Those who score high on either or both of these dimensions are assumed to have an insecure adult attachment orientation. On the other hand, participants with lower scores are viewed as having a secure adult attachment orientation (Brennan et al. 1998). Sample items include: "I try to avoid getting too close to my partner" and "I turn to my partner for many things, including comfort and reassurance" (Wei et al. 2007, p. 194).

Multidimensional Scale of Perceived Social Support (MSPSS)

The MSPSS was created to assess perception of social support on various levels. A self-report measure, each of the 12-items are rated on a 7-point Likert-type scale, ranging from (1) very strongly disagree to (7) very strongly agree. Subscale scores are achieved by the summation of all four items and then dividing by 4. A total score can be obtained by the summation of all 12 items and then dividing by 12. The possible range for total score is (12) lowest to (84) highest. Higher scores indicate a greater degree of perceived social support. Sample items include: "My family is willing to help me make decisions" and "I can count on my friends when things go wrong" (Zimet et al. 1988, p. 35). The three subscales of support associated with the MSPSS are: (a) family (FA), (b) friends (FR), and (c) significant other (SO). Although SO is generally left to the participant to define for the purposes of this study, it was defined as "the most significant canine companion." During initial studies of the MSPSS, Zimet et al. (1988) encouraged the measurement of social support on a variety of populations, including pets.

Pet Attachment Scale (PAS)

The PAS was developed to measure feelings of intimacy, caring, and attachment to pets. The PAS is a 9-item self-report instrument based on a 5-point Likert-type scale, ranging from (1) strongly disagree to (5) strongly agree. Scores can range from (10) lowest to (44) highest, with higher scores indicating a higher level of pet attachment support. Sample items include: "I feel closer to (pet's name) than to many of my friends" and "There are times when (pet's name) is my closest companion" (Albert and Bulcroft 1988, p. 547).

Grief Pattern Inventory (GPI)

The GPI was designed to assess preferred pattern of grief. The GPI is a 30-item self-report measure based on a 5-point Likert-type rating scale from (+2) always to (−2) never. According to Doka and Martin (2010), there are two patterns of grief as end points on a continuum, Intuitive (IGP1) and Instrumental (IGP2).

However, some individuals exhibit more Blended (BGP) patterns, which draw from both intuitive and instrumental reactions and responses. Others show inconsistencies between the ways grief is experienced and expressed and are identified as Dissonant (DGP) patterns. Items on the GPI are generally summed, with higher scores on the IGP1 and IGP2 subscales indicating greater adherence to that particular grieving pattern. Blended grievers do not indicate a clear preference and employ a combination of both. While dissonant grievers can be either intuitive or instrumental, constraints hold them back from freely expressing their feelings. Such items should be evaluated separately and may be temporary in nature. Because the seven dissonant items correlated well in this study, they were evaluated together as its own subscale. Sample items include: "I appreciate when others encourage me to share my painful feelings with them," "I have been told that I am avoiding my grief even though I don't think that I am," "Since my loss, I feel like I'm just pretending to be strong in front of most people," and "I worry that I am not as upset by my loss as I should be and feel guilty that I don't have more intense feelings" (p. 207).

Procedures

Due to the involvement of human participants, this research study received a formal review by the Division of Research and Sponsored Program's Institutional Review Board/Human Subjects Committee at Tennessee State University. Permission was obtained. The demographic questions and measures discussed above were made available via SurveyMonkey, a secure web-based program designed to assist researchers in survey construction, dissemination, and data collection. SurveyMonkey is Health Insurance Portability and Accountability Act (HIPAA) compliant. All information was collected through SurveyMonkey.

At any time, participants were allowed to discontinue or refuse to answer any question with no penalty. No identifying information was obtained about the participant, as SurveyMonkey handles information concerning participation automatically without any processing from the researcher. Contact information for the primary researcher was provided in the event that the participant had any questions regarding the survey and/or the participant wanted to be included in the raffle of eight $25Amazon gift cards.

Once data were entered into the SurveyMonkey, the researcher extracted the data periodically and purged it from the system into SPSS 21.0 for Mac. No one but the researcher could access the data, as it was password protected. The researcher deactivated the study and purged it from the system at the conclusion of the project.

Results

Data Preparation

Due to the large sample size, a visual inspection approach was used in lieu of traditional statistical tests to evaluate the fulfillment of testing assumptions prior to analysis. Visual inspection was more appropriate because evaluating whether the data was normally distributed via tests such as the Kolmogorov–Smirnov test, as well as examining skewness and kurtosis, would all be prone to indicating violations of assumptions when in fact the data was appropriate for further analysis (Field 2009). All variables reasonably resembled a normal distribution with the exception of the Most Significant Canine Companion (SO) subscale of the MSPSS, which was distributed with a slight negative skew. The fact that scores generally fell toward the upper limit of the SO subscale is not completely unexpected given the recruitment strategies (e.g., dog parks). Given the fact that the use of transformations in general raise issues when interpreting data, the statistical tests used in this study were robust against violations of normality and because the sample was comprised of current and/or former dog owners (which are expected to have skewed responses and a distribution favoring high levels of SO), a data transformation was not used. A total of 944 male dog owners served as the sample. Forty-eight were not usable because the participant failed to answer *yes* for one or both of the validity checks in the survey. Another three surveys were removed for a straight-line response pattern. Outliers were detected by identifying values that exceeded ±2 standard deviations, which is theoretically expected to only account for about 4.6 % of normally distributed data (Moore 2009). SO was the only variable that exceeded this expectation, but the deviation was not noteworthy, as only 4.9 % of the respondents on this variable could be considered an outlier. As such, no other modifications to the dataset were made.

Demographic Information of the Sample

The sample was comprised of 911 predominately White (70.5 %), Christian (48.4 %), Married or In a Committed Relationship (52.1 %), male dog owners between the Ages of 25–34 (30.6 %). Table 12.1 includes the frequency distribution for all of the demographics collected.

Descriptive Statistics for the Study Instruments

The total number of participants included, mean scores, standard deviations, number of items, possible range (per item), and reliability coefficients are presented in

Table 12.1 Demographic information (N=911)

Variable		Frequency	Percent
Age	18–24	203	22.3
	25–34	279	30.6
	35–44	169	18.6
	45–54	128	14.1
	55–64	82	9.0
	65–74	23	2.5
	75 or older	6	0.7
	Missing	21	2.3
Religious affiliation	Christianity	441	48.4
	Buddhism	20	2.2
	Judaism	31	3.4
	Islam	11	1.2
	Hinduism	7	0.8
	Secular/Agnostic/Atheist	133	14.6
	Other	68	7.5
	None	177	19.4
	Missing	23	2.5
Race	White	642	70.5
	Black or African American	80	8.8
	Asian	38	4.2
	Native Hawaiian or other Pacific Islander	5	0.5
	American Indian	3	0.3
	Alaska native	0	0
	Mixed-race	70	7.7
	Other	47	5.2
	Missing	26	2.9
Highest level of school completed/highest degree received	Some high school	19	2.1
	High school degree or equivalent	115	12.6
	Some college (no degree)	279	30.6
	Skills training/apprenticeship	43	4.7
	Associate's degree	72	7.9
	Bachelor's degree	224	24.6
	Master's degree	91	10.0
	Doctoral degree	28	3.1
	Professional degree	15	1.6
	Missing	25	2.7
Approximate average household income	\$0–\$24,999	183	20.1
	\$25,000–\$49,999	257	28.2
	\$50,000–\$74,999	183	20.1
	\$75,000–\$99,999	118	13.0
	\$100,000 or More	129	14.2
	Missing	41	4.5

(continued)

Table 12.1 (continued)

Variable		Frequency	Percent
Marital status	Single (never married)	320	35.1
	Married	314	34.5
	In a committed relationship	160	17.6
	Widowed and not remarried	12	1.3
	Divorced and not remarried	69	7.6
	Married but separated	12	1.3
	Missing	24	2.6
Current living situation	Single person living alone	166	18.2
	Single person living with others	259	28.4
	Single parent (children at home)	17	1.9
	Living with spouse/partner (no children)	273	30.0
	Living with spouse/partner (children at home)	162	17.8
	Other	5	0.5
	Missing	29	3.2
Number of years owned	0–1	49	5.4
	1–3	102	11.2
	3–5	125	13.7
	5–7	97	10.6
	7–9	73	8.0
	9–11	57	6.3
	11–13	36	4.0
	13 or more	50	5.5
	Missing	322	35.3
Canine died/lost	Yes	194	21.3
	No	389	42.7
	Missing	328	36.0
Length of time since death/loss	1	14	1.5
	2	15	1.6
	3	52	5.7
	4	26	2.9
	5	54	5.9
	8	1	0.1
	Missing or declined to answer	32	3.4
	Missing or not applicable	717	78.9
Survey	Listservs	33	3.6
	Social networking sites	180	19.8
	Electronic classifieds and forums	253	27.8
	Dog parks, pet stores, animal hospitals, etc.	6	0.7
	Personal referrals	63	6.9
	Other	19	2.1
	Missing	357	39.2

Table 12.2 Descriptive statistics for study instruments

Scale/subscale	N	Mean (SD)	# of items	Possible range (per item)	α
Success, power, and competition (GRCS-SF/SPC)	673	14.14 (4.59)	4	1–6	0.76
Restricted emotionality (GRCSSF/RE)	669	13.04 (5.00)	4	1–6	0.82
Restricted affectionate behavior between men (GRCS-SF/RABBM)	672	12.06 (5.44)	4	1–6	0.86
Conflict between work and family relationships (GRCS-SF/CBWFR)	678	13.48 (4.90)	4	1–6	0.79
Human attachment anxiety (ECRSS/AA1)	593	22.46 (7.11)	6	1–6	0.72
Human attachment avoidance (ECRS-S/AA2)	601	17.01 (6.60)	6	1–7	0.77
Friends (MSPSS/FR)	577	19.78 (5.49)	4	1–7	0.91
Family (MSPSS/FA)	574	19.62 (5.80)	4	1–7	0.88
Significant other/canine companion (MSPSS/SO)	585	22.70 (5.38)	4	1–7	0.92
Pet attachment scale (PAS)	571	34.53 (7.76)	9	N/A	0.91
Intuitive grief pattern (GPI/IGP1)	169	36.18 (6.96)	11	+2 to 2	0.78
Instrumental grief pattern (GPI/IGP2)	168	35.60 (7.73)	12	+2 to 2	0.78
Dissonant grief pattern (GPI/DGP)	174	22.29 (5.31)	7	+2 to 2	0.72

Note. Scales/subscales: GRCS-SF = Gender Role Conflict Scale-Short Form; ECRS-S = Experiences in Close Relationship Scale-Short Form; MSPSS = Multidimensional Scale of Perceived Social Support; PAS = Pet Attachment Scale; GPI = Grief Pattern Inventory

Table 12.2. As shown, a Cronbach's alpha coefficient was calculated for each scale and subscale. All demonstrated reliability estimates above the acceptable standard of 0.70 (Nunnaly 1978).

Hypothesis Testing

As shown in Table 12.3, prior to conducting the main set of analyses, a Pearson Product Moment Correlation was computed on each variable. For the purposes of Hypotheses 1–3, three age groups [young (ages 18–34), middle-aged (ages 35–54), and older men (ages 55 and older)] were operationally defined based on the work of Rumbaut (2005).

Table 12.3 Pearson product-moment intercorrelations

V	1	2	3	4	5	6	7	8	9	10
1	1.00									
2	0.707**	1.00								
3	0.721**	0.318**	1.00							
4	0.698**	0.317**	0.398**	1.00						
5	0.646**	0.377**	0.271**	0.167**	1.00					
6	0.147**	0.145**	0.108**	0.028	0.142**	1.00				
7	0.476**	0.225**	0.394**	0.506**	0.182**	0.121**	1.00			
8	−0.249**	−0.120**	−0.208**	−0.225**	−0.121**	−0.133**	−0.265**	1.00		
9	−0.157**	−0.034	−0.184**	−0.034	−0.181**	−0.119**	−0.241**	0.469**	1.00	
10	−0.094*	−0.043	−0.074	−0.083*	−0.055	0.064	−0.174**	0.160**	0.137**	1.00
11	0.040	0.008	0.085*	0.035	−0.027	0.140**	0.044	−0.128**	−0.163**	0.357**
12	0.443**	0.271**	0.501**	0.250**	0.212**	0.112	0.372**	−0.145	−0.015	−0.108
13	0.076	0.052	0.028	0.009	0.135	0.286**	0.052	−0.069	−0.154*	0.100
14	0.476**	0.296**	0.580**	0.288**	0.146	0.259**	0.433**	−0.249**	−0.134	−0.075
15	0.428**	0.292**	0.528**	0.246**	0.122	0.284**	0.367**	−0.249**	−0.159*	−0.045
16	−0.123**	−0.239*	−0.086*	0.074	−0.111**	−0.082*	−0.002	−0.060	−0.035	0.031
17	−0.007	0.001	−0.045	−0.033	0.064	−0.034	−0.086*	0.108**	0.075	0.011
18	−0.099**	−0.067	−0.109**	−0.154**	0.060	−0.062	−0.136**	0.181**	0.133**	0.016
19	−0.043	−0.115**	−0.032	0.008	0.007	−0.047	−0.031	0.076	0.036	0.101*
20	−0.124	−0.019	−0.228**	−0.075	−0.020	−0.026	−0.144	0.007	0.053	−0.069

Note. Scales/Subscales: 1 = Gender Role Conflict Scale-Short Form/Total; 2 = Gender Role Conflict Scale-Short Form/Success, Power, and Competition; 3 = Gender Role Conflict Scale-Short Form/Restricted Emotionality; 4 = Gender Role Conflict Scale-Short Form/Restricted Affectionate Behavior Between Men; 5 = Gender Role Conflict Scale-Short Form/Conflict Between Work and Family Relationships; 6= Experiences in Close Relationship Scale-Short Form/Human Attachment Anxiety; 7 = Experiences in Close Relationship Scale-Short Form/Human Attachment Avoidance; 8 = Multidimensional Scale of Perceived Social Support/Friends; 9= Multidimensional Scale of Perceived Social Support/Family; 10 = Multidimensional Scale of Perceived Social Support/Significant Other/Canine Companion

* Statistically significant at the 0.05 level ** Statistically significant at the 0.01 level

Table 12.3 (continued)

V	11	12	13	14	15	16	17	18	19	20
1										
2										
3										
4										
5										
6										
7										
8										
9										
10										
11	1.00									
12	0.076	1.00								
13	0.130	0.118	1.00							
14	0.162*	0.576**	0.299**	1.00						
15	0.178*	0.503**	0.377**	0.955**	1.00					
16	0.116*	−0.118	0.140	−0.194**	−0.163*	1.00				
17	−0.054	−0.144	0.144	−0.126	−0.114	0.287**	1.00			
18	−0.130**	−0.142	−0.071	−0.292**	0.254**	0.125**	0.345**	1.00		
19	0.024	−0.041	−0.087	−0.190*	−0.197**	0.212**	0.196**	0.044	1.00	
20	−0.126	−0.136	−0.157*	−0.231**	−0.215**	0.234**	0.035	0.141	0.084	1.00

Note. Scales/Subscales: 11 = Pet Attachment Scale; 12 = Grief Pattern Inventory/Instrumental Grieving Pattern; 13 = Grief Pattern Inventory/Intuitive Grieving Pattern; 14 = Grief Pattern Inventory/Dissonant Grieving Pattern; 15 = Grief Pattern Inventory/Dissonant Grieving Pattern/Image Managers; 16 = Age; 17 = Approximate Average Household Income; 18 = Highest Level of School Completed/Highest Degree Received; 19 = Number of Years Owned; 20 = Length of Time Since Death/Loss

* Statistically significant at the 0.05 level ** Statistically significant at the 0.01 level

Hypothesis 1

Hypothesis 1 proposed that gender role conflict would vary depending on age. A MANOVA was conducted to test for significant mean differences on a combination of the four factors of gender role conflict between the subgroups of male dog owners based on age. The MANOVA results demonstrated a statistically significant main effect difference in pattern of gender role conflict based on age, $\Lambda = 0.898$, $F(8, 1372) = 9.489$, $p < 0.2001$, $\eta = 0.052$. Thus, Hypothesis 1 was confirmed.

Given the significance of the overall test, univariate follow-up tests for each dependent variable were conducted. These tests showed that a statistically significant difference between age groups pertained to the Success, Power, and Competition (SPC), $F(2, 696) = 19.58$, $p < 0.001$, the RABBM, $F(2, 693) = 6.22$, $p = 0.002$, and the Conflict Between Work and Family Relationships (CBWFR), $F(2, 697) = 4.65$, $p = 0.010$ subscales of the Gender Role Conflict Scale-Short Form (GRCS-SF).

Post hoc comparisons using the Tukey's HSD test indicated a number of group significant differences. First, regarding the SPC subscale, the mean score for young males ($M = 3.76$, SD = 1.11) was significantly greater than it was for middle-aged ($M = 3.40$, SD = 1.13, $p < 0.001$) and older males ($M = 3.00$, SD = 1.08, $p < 0.001$). Using Cohen's d (Cohen 1988), effect size differences were calculated. The effect size difference between young and middle-aged males was 0.29 (small), demonstrating that young males had higher levels of SPC. The difference between middle-aged and older males is 0.36 (small), indicating that middle-aged males had higher levels of SPC. The effect size difference between young and older males is 0.69 (medium), specifying that young males had higher levels of SPC. Second, in terms of the RABBM subscale, the mean score for middle-aged males ($M = 3.29$, SD = 1.44) was significantly greater than it was for young males ($M = 2.89$, SD = 1.28, $p = 0.001$). The effect size difference between young and middle-aged males was 0.29 (small), indicating that middle-aged males had higher levels of RABBM ($p = 0.001$). Finally, with respect to the CBWFR subscale, the mean score for young males ($M = 3.48$, SD = 1.18) was significantly greater than it was for older males ($M = 3.05$, SD = 1.32, $p = 0.007$). The effect size difference between young and older males was 0.35 (small), suggesting that young males had higher levels of CBWFR ($p = 0.007$). All other group differences were not significant at the 0.05 level.

Hypothesis 2

Hypothesis 2 stated that the strength of the attachment bond and level of perceived social support from the most significant canine companion would differ depending on age. A MANOVA was conducted to test for significant mean differences on a combination of the strength of the attachment bond and level of perceived social support between the subgroups of male dog owners based on age. The MANOVA results demonstrated a statistically significant main effect difference in strength of the attachment bond and level perceived social support from the most significant canine companion based on age, $\Lambda = 0.976$, $F(4, 1154) = 3.593$, $p = 0.2006$, $\eta = 0.012$. Thus, Hypothesis 2 was confirmed.

Given the significance of the overall test, univariate follow-up tests for each dependent variable were conducted. These tests showed that a statistically significant difference between age groups pertained to the PAS, $F(2, 579) = 5.19$, $p = 0.006$ and the Significant Canine Companion (SO) subscale, $F(2, 586) = 3.01$, $p = 0.050$ of the Multidimensional Scale of Perceived Social Support (MSPSS).

Post hoc comparisons using the Tukey's HSD test indicated two significant group differences. First, with regard to the PAS, the mean score for middle-aged males ($M = 3.97$, SD = 0.77) was significantly greater than it was for young males ($M = 3.73$, SD = 0.88, $p = 0.007$). The effect size difference between young and middle-aged males was 0.29 (small), indicating that middle-aged males had higher levels of PAS. Second, in terms of the SO subscale, the mean score for middle-aged males ($M = 5.88$, SD = 1.14) was significantly greater than it was for young males ($M = 5.57$, SD = 1.40, $p = 0.046$). The effect size difference between young and middle-aged males was 0.24 (small), demonstrating that middle-aged males had higher levels of SO. All other group differences were not significant at the 0.05 level.

Hypothesis 3

Hypothesis 3 predicted that a dissonant grief pattern (DGP) after the loss of the most significant canine companion would vary by age. An ANOVA was conducted to test for significant mean differences on a dissonant pattern of grief between the subgroups of male dog owners based on age. The ANOVA results demonstrated a statistically significant main effect difference in DGP based on age, $F(2, 178) = 4.74$, $p = 0.010$. Thus, Hypothesis 3 was confirmed.

Post hoc analyses using the Tukey's HSD test indicated one significant group difference. Regarding the DGP subscale, the mean score for young males ($M = -0.06$, SD = 0.77) was significantly greater than it was for middle-aged males ($M = -0.40$, SD = 0.67, $p = 0.015$). The effect size difference between young and middle-aged males was 0.47 (medium), indicating that young males had higher levels of DGP. The remaining group differences were not significant at the 0.05 level.

Hypothesis 4

Hypothesis 4 proposed that a human avoidant attachment style would moderate the relationship between a human anxious attachment style and a DGP after the loss of the most significant canine companion. A multiple linear regression (MLR) was calculated to test the moderating effect of attachment avoidance (AA2) on the relationship between attachment anxiety (AA1) and a DGP.

Prior to conducting this analysis, AA2 and AA1 were centered on their mean scores to prevent *multicollinearity* (as articulated by Aiken and West 1991). The interaction between AA2 and AA1 did not have a significant effect on DGP. Therefore, Hypothesis 4 was not supported. However, the overall model was significant, $F(3, 177) = 19.666$, $p < 0.01$ and accounted for 25 % of the variance. As such, AA2 ($B = 0.421$) and AA1 ($B = 0.246$) were both statistically significant ($p < 0.001$, $p < 0.001$) predictors of a DGP, but their interaction did not have a significant effect on DGP ($p = 0.644$, $B = -0.031$).

Discussion

The overarching goal of this study was to explore the bond between males and their canine companions across the developmental life span. To do so, differences in patterns of gender role conflict based on age were investigated. Although other studies have assessed age differences and patterns of gender role conflict using diverse samples of men, dog owners had not been one of them. Second, whether age affects the strength of the attachment bond, as well as the level of perceived social support was also tested. Numerous studies have analyzed the various roles and functions of human–animal companionship from childhood to old age with mixed results. Third, differences in a dissonant pattern of grief based on age had not been previously examined. Although there is some research on both the effects of human attachment style on the response/adjustment to the loss of an animal companion, and pet attachment orientation on the grief reactions to the loss of a companion animal, a DGP had not yet been evaluated.

Hypothesis 1
As predicted, a statistically significant main effect difference in gender role conflict (GRCS-SF; SPC, RE, RABBM, and CBWFR subscales) based on age group among male dog owners was found. This finding is bolstered by the results of several previous studies that have assessed age differences and patterns of gender role conflict. Although males are conflicted with their gender roles across the lifespan, the ways vary. For example, O'Neil (2008) reported that among adolescent boys, RE, RABBM, and CBWFR significantly predicted boys' family stress and problems with conduct, anger, and emotions. For retired men, as RE, RABBM, and CBWFR decreased, retirement satisfaction increased.

In the present study, separate univariate follow-up tests for each dependent variable revealed that a statistically significant difference between age groups pertained to the SPC, RABBM, and CBWFR subscales. Although there were no significant differences between age groups on the RE subscale, this finding is consistent with the existing literature. Over the course of 25 years (1982–2007) studying gender role conflict, O'Neil (2008) indicated "one of the most striking conclusions across all of the studies is that RE showed no significant age differences across the different age groupings" (p. 379). This finding may be especially important, as it implies that gender socialization continues to impact men and their relationships with human companions throughout the lifecycle. Any bond that transcends these barriers is significant. While additional research is needed, the bond between man and dog is poised to interest researchers from a variety of different fields.

Several significant group differences from the GRCS-SF subscales were also found. Young male dog owners had significantly greater SPC than both middle-aged and older males. This finding is substantiated by the results from two previous studies in which college-aged men reported significantly more SPC than middle-aged men (Cournoyer and Mahalik 1995; Theodore and Lloyd 2000). Furthermore, middle-aged males reported greater SPC than did older males.

According to O'Neil (2008), younger men report significantly more SPC than older men because as men age, they tend to resolve gender role conflict by recognizing the futility of such attitudes and behaviors or through reexamining their roles, which enables more freedom in defining themselves as men (O'Neil 1982). In the present study, young males also reported significantly more CBWFR than older males. These results are in-line with typical developmental aspirations and challenges (e.g., beginning careers and starting families) facing younger men in this society. Finally, middle-aged males had greater RABBM than young males. This finding may reflect a cohort effect, as there is evidence to suggest that younger men are less homophobic than older men (e.g., McCormack and Anderson 2010). Although sexual orientation was not asked about in this study, the finding may be explained by the results of another study. In examining gender role conflict in 20 homosexual men and 20 heterosexual men, McMahon (2009) found that although heterosexual men had higher scores of gender role conflict in all four subscales when means were tested, the only subscale in which heterosexual men scored significantly higher was the RABBM. This suggests that while some gay men react to societal expectations of the male gender role, their sexual orientation does not increase or cause higher gender role conflict.

Hypothesis 2

As hypothesized, a statistically significant main effect difference in the strength of the attachment bond (PAS total scale) and the level of perceived social support (Multidimensional Scale of Perceived Support (MSPSS); Most Significant Canine Companion (SO) subscale) derived from the most significant canine companion was based on age. Separate univariate follow-up tests for both dependent variables revealed that a statistically significant difference between age groups related to both PAS and SO. Two significant group differences were also found, suggesting that middle-aged males are more attached and feel more socially supported by their canine companions than do young males. These findings align with previous research in the areas of pet ownership and pet attachment. For example, in a sample of 592 men and women (totals by gender were not provided) using two measures of pet attachment, the 18–24-year old age group reported being the least attached to their dogs while the 35–49-year old age group reported being the most attached to their dogs. It was indicated that the 18–24-year olds did not have the time needed to establish the kinds of bonds that they wanted to with their dogs. On the other hand, the 35–49-year olds developed the attachments that they wanted to with their dogs because of the animal's importance in their lives (Reid and Anderson 2009).

In another study, Albert and Bulcroft (1988) reported that pet ownership was most prevalent in households where the oldest member was between 30 and 49 years old, reflecting the likelihood that families in the "middle" stages of the life cycle were pet owners. Unfortunately, household members' gender-related information was not provided. The fact that pets were found to be important sources of affection and attachment among divorced, never married, and widowed individuals as well as with childless couples, newlyweds, and empty nesters suggests that pets function as emotional substitutes for children and spouses. Middle-aged adults generally spend less time on child-rearing practices and animal companions may serve to fill this void. Baby talk is common and provides evidence that humans see animal companions as infants/children rather than adults (Hirsh-Pasek and Treiman 1982). Training and nurturing animal companions and feelings of pride and guilt associated with them (Sanders 1990) are other examples of the similarities between raising a human infant and an animal companion (Belk 1996). Based on Carstensen's socioemotional selectivity theory, Netting et al. (2013) proposed that social preferences shift throughout life. As people age, they tend to become more socially selective, thereby reducing their interaction with casual social partners in favor of close friends. This dynamic may be especially pronounced among aging males who report a shrinking network of intimate relationships and fewer opportunities to connect with others (Barbee et al. 1993). In such a scenario, familiar others, such as animal companions, may become a real source of comfort.

In a study conducted by Kurdek (2009), with a sample of male and female dog owners (mean age = 47.95), being male, widowed, highly involved in the care of the dog, and uncomfortable with self-disclosure, moderated the likelihood that the dog was viewed as an attachment figure. On average, participants were also more likely to turn to their dogs as a safe haven than they were to their mothers, fathers, brothers, sisters, best friends, and children in times of distress. The only bond that rivaled that of one's animal companion on the safe haven dimension was one's romantic partner. In examining the loss of either in a clinical context, we understand more fully how a man's life, his social network, and his sense of emotional soothing are derived from these few attachment bonds. As clinicians, being aware that a disproportionate amount of weight is carried by a small number of emotional supports is particularly relevant.

In the only other empirical study to include exclusively male dog owners in its sample, men who owned their first dog at an early age and more dogs later in life scored higher on scales of companionship and social support. The experience of dog ownership in childhood was related to the sociality of older men, indicating that the connection between humans and their animal companions helps to facilitate companionship with humans (Nagasawa and Ohta 2010). One explanation is that the bond between men and their dogs demonstrates the benefits of emotional support and meaningful connections. According to Wood et al. (2005), companion animals are important conduits of social capital, which has been conceptualized as "features of social life— networks, norms, and social trust—that enable participants to act together more effectively to pursue shared objectives, or to facilitate coordination and cooperation for mutual benefit" (p. 1159). Developmental psychologists have long argued in favor of children being raised with pets (e.g., Paul and Serpell 1993). Animal companions become unbiased providers of feedback and offer ways to learn about attachment and loss. Although animal companions may take on additional meanings in the lives of some, boys that experience rigid socialization and the accompanying expectations may turn to animal companions for respite. In fact, one might argue that this dyad enables the restrictions associated with being male to be temporarily relaxed, thereby allowing a more innate attachment tendency to emerge.

According to Bowlby (1980), the need for bonding and caretaking is present and active throughout life. While humans form bonds with animal companions at all ages, the relationship may be increasingly significant with age for men. Blazina (2016) suggested that as men get older, animal companionship becomes even more important amid health issues, fewer social supports, and the buildup associated with operating for years under the misconceptions of masculinity. The "pure love" of animal companions provides some respite for men trying to sort through the accumulation of frustrations that accompany challenges in work, love, and play. Maturational changes and losses are generally copious at this stage of development. In addition to the physiological and psychosocial ones, for middle-aged adults, mortality becomes an intimate personal issue. An awareness of one's own mortality can evoke existential angst. These feelings, which often result in a renewed search for meaning in life, require the individual to address questions related to freedom and responsibility, as well as a painful sense of isolation (Becker 2006). Middle-aged adults reportedly fear death more than both young and older adults (Santrock 2013) and yet, according to the Center for Disease Control and Prevention (CDC 2013), the suicide rate for middle-aged men (ages 35–64) increased more than 27 % from 1999 to 2010 (21.5 suicides per 100,000 people to 27.3). In fact, males are four times more likely to complete suicide and are responsible for 79 % of all U.S. suicides. Levinson and Mallon (1997) believe that humans attempt to recapture a sense of unity with nature because it provides a point of reference, support, and, for some, assuages existential anxiety. Animal companions may help provide this sense of unity.

Hypothesis 3

As postulated, differences in a DGP (GPI; DGP subscale) based on age group for male dog owners who lost their most significant canine companion existed. The dissonance or conflict associated with loss may be a function (at least in part) of family, cultural, and social traditions of masculinity. Because the importance and/or influence of masculinity ideology may change throughout the lifecycle, a DGP can also vary with age. According to Doka and Martin (2010), these maladaptive reactions *may* become a semi-permanent way of responding to loss and serve as the basis for complicated mourning or intense ambivalence that interfered with the detachment process (Bonanno and Kaltman 1999).

Stroebe et al. (2005) indicated that those who do not have a secure attachment are more prone to different forms of complicated grief. On the one hand, we socialize men to be strong, confident, and in control. On the other hand, if men do not show or express thoughts and feelings in the ways that women typically do, we assume that they are emotionally unavailable, avoidant, in denial, or not grieving at all. The fact that the loss of a companion animal is a disenfranchised loss in our society only complicates matters further. It would be reasonable to expect that men are hesitant to exhibit normative grief reactions with socially sanctioned losses. This is probably more pronounced with the loss of an animal companion.

Regarding specific significant group differences in this study, young males reported higher levels of DGP over the loss of their most significant canine companion than did middle-aged males. This finding may be explained by the theory that men and women become more androgynous as they age. That is, as people get older, they become less bound by rigid gender characteristics and sex roles. Interestingly, evidence suggests that androgyny is actually more characteristic of elderly men than it is of elderly women (Kausler et al. 2007). Furthermore, Doka and Martin (2010) point out that restrictive emotionality or "having difficulty and fears about expressing one's feelings and difficulty finding words to express basic emotions" (O'Neil et al. 1995, p. 176) is the concept most important to a discussion about DGP. Emotional restrictiveness is at the core of image managers (IM), the first of the two forms of dissonant grief. IM, especially male grievers, are generally toward the intuitive end of the continuum and often hide their feelings and thoughts from others and may avoid or withdraw from people because of it (Doka and Martin 2010). Wong et al. (2006) found that men with high emotional restriction are probably able to express their feelings but choose to inhibit instead. These explanations provide credence to this finding in the present study.

It should also be noted that while significant differences between age groups on the RE subscale of the GRCS-SF did not exist in Hypothesis 1, it can be argued that the emotional restrictiveness inherent in a DGP, as described by Doka and Martin (2010), provide a basis for further investigation of nuanced conceptual and measurement approaches to the RE concept. Future research that re-examines these constructs together with different samples is an important next step.

Hypothesis 4

Contrary to the hypothesis, human AA2 (Experiences in Close Relationships Scale-Short Form (ECR-S); AA2 subscale) did not moderate the relationship between human AA1 (Experiences in Close Relationships Scale-Short Form (ECR-S); AA1 subscale) and a DGP. Although previous studies have examined how a human attachment style affects the grief response to the death of an animal companion (e.g., Field et al. 2009), as well as how a pet attachment orientation affects the grief response to the death of an animal companion (e.g., Zilcha-Mano et al. 2011), no other empirical studies have looked specifically at DGP. The fact that a DGP may be a precursor to complicated mourning (Doka and Martin 2010), provided the basis for assessing this construct in the present study. Complicated grief is common in both anxious and avoidant individuals, as the insecurely attached often have a more difficult time adapting to loss than the securely attached (Shaver and Tancredy 2001; Wayment and Vierthaler 2002).

Although the interaction between AA1 and AA2 did not have a significant impact on DGP, AA1 and AA2 were both statistically significant predictors of a DGP in the loss of one's most significant canine companion. This hypothesis was developed based on a previous study that found high anxiety and high avoidance (categorized as fearful avoidance) to be predictive of more severe grief following the loss of a pet (Field et al. 2009). However, the Relationship Scales Questionnaire (RSQ; Griffin and Bartholomew 1994) used in that study distinguished between fearful avoidance (high anxiety and high avoidance described as a strong sense of distrust and expectation of rejection) and dismissive avoidance (low anxiety and high avoidance described as a reluctance to rely on others and a preference to maintain emotional distance). Conversely, the ECR-S used in the present study does not differentiate between the two types of avoidant attachment, which potentially influences results.

Nonetheless, both AA1 and AA2 were significant predictors of DGP. Assuming a relationship between DGP and complicated grief, the effect of AA1 and complicated grief replicates previous findings from studies of both human and pet loss (e.g., Field et al. 2009; Fraley and Bonanno 2004). Results are mixed in studies examining the effect of AA2 and complicated grief. As indicated previously, new research has suggested that individuals with an avoidant attachment style who fail to display grief symptoms may have some resilience and are able to adjust well to death in the long run.

Study Limitations

As with any study, there were limitations to this project. First, because this was a sample of convenience, participants who chose to participate may not accurately represent the larger population. With use of an online survey, certain populations are invariably less likely to have Internet access, to respond to such requests, or to have the skills necessary to complete online surveys. Furthermore, because the electronic and paper recruitment flyers were posted at sites where evaluations of pets would most likely be high, the sample was skewed toward owners with very positive perceptions of their dogs. Such findings may not generalize to samples of less dedicated owners. This potentially restricts the ability to fully investigate attachment and perceived social support. Moreover, due to minimal and conflicting research on demographic factors as they relate to attachment and perceived social support, a "profile" of male dog owners who are more/less attached and perceive more/less social support from their canine companions might enable professionals to better help their clients. Unfortunately, although the sample size was large, it consisted of predominately Caucasian Christians, limiting the ability to complete a cluster analysis as well as understand demographic differences across the main variables.

Second, this study relied on retrospective self-report data about grief experiences. Of those participants who responded to this portion of the survey, the mode for the length of time since the death or loss was 5 years. Great variability in the time elapsed since the death or loss as well. In this study, the range was from 1 to 8 years. Implicit and explicit memory for emotion bias is well established in the literature. Recent memories are generally better guides than distant memories for goal-directed behaviors because emotional memories fade over time (Hendersen 1985). Whether people generally overestimate or underestimate when recalling the intensity of past emotions is dependent on many factors.

Third, the GPI is a relatively new and understudied instrument. Moreover, a limited amount of information on the psychometric properties of the GPI is available. Although the dissonant grief-related items were supposed to be evaluated separately, they were combined for the purposes of this study. While the internal consistency of this set of items was high, this modification could have impacted the results.

Suggestions for Future Research

There are a number of areas where future research is merited. First, there are a lack of studies that have looked into how (and if) demographic differences impact companion animal attachment and adjustment to loss. Of the studies that do exist, the results vary tremendously (e.g., Archer and Ireland 2011; Bagley and Gonsman 2005; Brown 2002; Johnson et al. 1992). Recognizing that each contextual factor contributes to a better understanding of the individual differences in the degree to which someone bonds with and adapts to the loss of an animal companion, we attempted to run a cluster analysis. Unfortunately, the sample sizes in some of the categories were too small and a "profile" could not be developed. While the idea is not intended to stereotype pet owners, identifying demographic differences among male dog owners might help us to better serve our clients.

Second, additional moderator and mediator studies are also suggested. For example, exploring precisely how attachment style affects (both human and pet) grief response after the loss of an animal companion or by identifying the underlying mechanisms through which attachment style affects adaptation to loss (e.g., continuing bonds). In future studies, other measures of assessing attachment style should be used. Whether or not factors such as attachment and perceived social support moderate and/or mediate the relationship between gender role conflict in men and, for example, anxiety, depression, and loneliness during different developmental periods or ages is another area worthy of exploration.

Third, three other areas needing further exploration include the use of adult attachment instruments for measuring human attachment style to animal companions, the correlation between adult romantic attachment style and pet attachment style and the idea of displacement of attachment to an animal companion among those with insecure attachment styles.

Lastly, when assessing the male dog dyad, observer effects should be taken into consideration. While it is expected that attachment type behaviors are promoted in the dyad, (e.g., freer expression of tender feelings, play, etc.), when there is a concern that others may view this type of interaction as counter to rigid gendered expectations, the behavior is likely to change. In a human–animal interaction version of the well-known Hawthorne effect, men who want to appear more traditional in the presence of others may temporarily alter their attachment behavior or, minimally, feel conflicted about discussing it. This suggests a propensity for bias and underreporting when it comes to the significance of the bond both in terms of attachment and loss. That is, when queried by researchers, some males may actually think or feel more than they report. This includes emphasizing constricting affect or having little need for emotional closeness. Researchers have observed this in boys as young as 8 years old, when they were asked in a study to describe the special bond they shared with an animal companion (Kidd and Kidd 1987). Therefore in future research, it is important to move beyond the confines of self-report measures and also to control for the influence of observer effects.

Clinical Implications

The primary implication for the field of psychology is to increase our understanding of the importance of the human–animal bond throughout men's lives. Although a majority of the studies suggest that women form stronger attachments to their pets (e.g., Archer and Ireland 2011; Johnson et al., 1992; Poresky and Daniels, 1998) and grieve pet loss more intensely (e.g., Gage & Holcomb, 1991; Margolies, 1999), this study suggests that the human–canine bond is of profound relational significance for men and that previous researchers have not attended to the nuances of gender socialization in a way that would necessarily elicit this important information.

Although future research with male dog owners in the general population is warranted, the results of this study contribute to the current body of knowledge on the human–animal bond. Continued efforts to understand the many ways in which males respond to various aspects of gender socialization will help us to more comprehensively grasp the connection between man and dog. Based on the results of this study, mental health professionals might be more aware that some middle-aged men view the human–animal bond with distinct importance. This may include normalizing and encouraging male clients to discuss their bond with animal companions as significant objects in their lives. Moreover, in the therapeutic context, discussing the bond men have with their canine companions might provide a non-defensive way of garnering information.

Second, although much of the progress associated with the field of human–animal studies is attributed to veterinary medicine and today is considered interdisciplinary, this study attempted to further bridge the gap that exists between the field of psychology and veterinary medicine. While the role of the psychologist in educating and working with those practicing human medicine is well established, collaboration within veterinary medicine is not as typical. Psychologists could offer veterinary trainees and students, among other things, communication and self-care skills, training in ways to practically and emotionally support grieving animal owners, and valuable research skills and knowledge (Chur-Hansen and Winefield 2013).

The present study offers a new perspective regarding the significance of the human–animal bond in men's lives. While future research investigating the relationship between males and their canine companions is warranted, this study has provided some insight into the integral part that dogs can play in the lives of men. It is important for professionals to become sensitive to the potential cost associated with this type of loss. The development of services based on a more accepting, normalizing approach is also encouraged.

Finally, the bond between a male and his animal companion may offer a type of role renorming, albeit a momentary one. When in the company of an animal companion, whether it is going for a walk or just lying on the couch together, males at any age have more freedom to relax their psychological defenses and other aspects of traditional maleness. Future research will put these ideas to the test. In the meanwhile, many men who have a special relationship with a canine friend will quietly observe the meaning of their own bond, perhaps going unnoticed or not fully comprehended by others.

References

Aiken, L. S., & West, S. G. (1991). *Multiple regression: Testing and interpreting interactions*. London, England: Sage

Albert, A., & Bulcroft, K. (1988). Pets, families, and the life course. *Journal of Marriage and the Family, 50*(2), 543–552. doi:10.2307/352019

Archer, J., & Ireland, J. L. (2011). The development and factor structure of a questionnaire measure of the strength of attachment to pet dogs. *Anthrozoös, 24*(3), 249–261. doi:10.2752/175303711X13045914865060

Bagley, D. K., & Gonsman, V. L. (2005). Pet attachment and personality type. *Anthrozoös, 18*(1), 28–42. doi:10.2752/089279305785594333

Barbee, A. P., Cunningham, M. R., Winstead, B. A., Derlega, V. J., Gulley, M. R., Yankeelov, P. A., & Druen, P. B. (1993). Effects of gender role expectations on the social support process. *Journal of Social Issues, 49*(3), 175–190. doi:10.1111/j.1540-4560.1993.tb01175.x

Becker, D. (2006). Therapy for the middle-aged: The relevance of existential issues. *American Journal of Psychotherapy, 60*(1), 87–99. Retrieved from http://www.ajp.org/

Belk, R. W. (1996). Metaphoric relationships with pets. *Society and Animals, 3*(2), 121–145. doi: 10.1163/156853096X00115

Blazina, C. (2016). *Dog tracks: Understanding the last impressions of man's best friend* (Unpublished manuscript).

Blazina, C., Boyraz, G., & Shen-Miller, D. (2011). Preface. In C. Blazina, G. Boyraz, & D. Shen-Miller (Eds.), *The psychology of the human-animal bond: A resource for clinicians and researchers* (p. vii). New York: Springer.

Bonanno, G. A., & Kaltman, S. (1999). Toward an integrative perspective on bereavement. *Psychological Bulletin, 125*(6), 760–776. doi:10.1037/00332909.125.6.760

Bowlby, J. (1980). *Attachment and loss: Loss* (Vol. 3). New York, NY: Basic Books.

Brennan, K. A., Clark, C. L., & Shaver, P. R. (1998). Self-report measurement of adult attachment: An integrative overview. In J. A. Simpson & W. S. Rholes (Eds.), *Attachment theory and close relationships* (pp. 46–76). New York, NY: The Guilford Press.

Brown, S. E. (2002). Ethnic variations in pet attachment. *Society and Animals, 10*(3), 249–266. doi:10.1163/156853002320770065

Brown, B. H., Richards, H. C., & Wilson, C. A. (1996). Pet bonding and pet bereavement among adolescents. *Journal of Counseling & Development, 74*(5), 505–509. doi:10.1002/j.1556-6676.1996.tb01901.x

Center for Disease Control (CDC). (2013). Suicide among adults aged 35–64 years–United States, 1999–2010. *Morbidity and Mortality Weekly Report, 62*(72), 321–325. Retrieved from http://www.cdc.gov/mmwr/preview/mmwrhtml/mm6217a1.htm?s_cid=mm6217a1_w

Chodorow, N. (1978). *The reproduction of mothering: Psychoanalysis and the sociology of gender*. Berkeley, CA: University of California Press.
Chur-Hansen, A., & Winefield, H. R. (2013). Companion animals and physical health: The role of health psychology. In M. L. Caltabiano & L. A. Ricciardelli (Eds.), *Applied topics in health psychology* (pp. 134–142). Chichester, England: Wiley-Blackwell.
Cohen, J. (1988). *Statistical power analysis for the behavioral sciences* (2nd ed.). Hillsdale, NJ: Erlbaum
Cournoyer, R. J., & Mahalik, J. R. (1995). Cross-sectional study of gender role conflict examining college-aged and middle-aged men. *Journal of Counseling Psychology, 42*(1), 11–19. doi:10.1037/0022-0167.42.1.11
Deaux, K., & Major, B. (1987). Putting gender into context: An interactive model of gender related behavior. *Psychological Review, 94*(3), 369–389. doi:10.1037/0033-295X.94.3.369
Doka, K. J., & Martin, T. L. (2010). *Grieving beyond gender: Understanding the ways men and women mourn* (2nd ed.). New York, NY: Routledge.
Field, A. (2009). *Discovering statistics using IBM SPSS statistics* (3rd ed.). Thousand Oaks, CA: Sage Publications Ltd.
Field, N. P., Orsini, L., Gavish, R., & Packman, W. (2009). Role of attachment in response to pet loss. *Death Studies, 33*(4), 334–355. doi:10.1080/07481180802705783
Fraley, R. C., & Bonanno, G. A. (2004). Attachment and loss: A test of three competing models on the association between attachment-related avoidance and adaptation to bereavement. *Personality and Social Psychology Bulletin, 30*(7), 878–890. doi:10.1177/0146167204264289
Gage, M. G., & Holcomb, R. (1991). Couples' perception of stressfulness of death of the family pet. *Family Relations, 40*(1), 103–105. doi:10.2307/585666
Gosse, G. H., & Barnes, M. J. (1994). Human grief resulting from the death of a pet. *Anthrozoös, 7*(2), 103–112. doi:10.2752/089279394787001970
Griffin, D. W., & Bartholomew, K. (1994). Models of the self and other: Fundamental dimensions underlying measures of adult attachment. *Journal of Personality and Social Psychology, 67*(3), 430–445. doi:10.1037/0022-3514.67.3.430
Hendersen, R. W. (1985). Fearful memories: The motivational significance of forgetting. In F. R. Brush & J. B. Overmier (Eds.), *Affect, conditioning, and cognition: Essays on the determinants of behavior* (pp. 43–53). Hillsdale, NJ: Erlbaum.
Hirsh-Pasek, K., & Treiman, R. (1982). Doggerel: Motherese in a new context. *Journal of Child Language, 9*(1), 229–237. doi:10.1017/S0305000900003731
Ickes, W. (1993). Traditional gender roles: Do they make, and then break, our relationships? *Journal of Social Issues, 49*(3), 71–85. doi:10.1111/j.1540-4560.1993.tb01169.x
Johnson, T. P., Garrity, T. F., & Stallones, L. (1992). Psychometric evaluation of the Lexington Attachment to Pets Scale. *Anthrozoös, 5*(3), 160–175. doi:10.2752/089279392787011395
Kausler, D. H., Kausler, B. C., & Krupsaw, J. A. (2007). *The essential guide to aging in the twenty-first century: Mind, body, and behavior*. Columbia, MO: University of Missouri Press.
Kidd, A. H., & Kidd, R. M. (1987). Seeking a theory of the human/companion animal bond. *Anthrozoös, 1*(3), 140–145. doi:10.2752/089279388787058489
Kurdek, L. A. (2009). Pet dogs as attachment figures for adult owners. *Journal of Family Psychology, 23*(4), 439–446. doi:10.1037/a0014979
Levant, R. F. (2001). The crisis of boyhood. In G. R. Brooks & G. E. Good (Eds.), *The new handbook of psychotherapy and counseling with men: A comprehensive guide to settings, problems, and treatment approaches* (pp. 2355–2368). San Francisco, CA: Jossey-Bass.
Levinson, B. M., & Mallon, G. P. (1997). *Pet-oriented child psychotherapy* (2nd ed.). Springfield, IL: Charles C. Thomas Publishers.
Lue, T. W., Pantenburg, D. P., & Crawford, P. M. (2008). Impact of the owner-pet and client veterinarian bond on the care that pets receive. *Journal of the American Veterinary Medical Association, 232*(4), 531–540. doi:10.2460/javma.232.4.531
Mahalik, J. R., Locke, B. D., Ludlow, L. H., Diemer, M. A., Scott, R. P. J., Gottfried, M., et al. (2003). Development of the conformity to masculine norms inventory. *Psychology of Men & Masculinity, 4*(1), 3–25. doi:10.1037/1524-9220.4.1.3

Mahalik, J. R., Locke, B. D., Theodore, H., Cournoyer, R. J., & Lloyd, B. F. (2001). A cross national and cross-sectional comparison of men's gender role conflict and its relationship to social intimacy and self-esteem. *Sex Roles, 45*(1–2), 1–14. doi:10.1023/A:1013008800019

Mandell, F., McAnulty, E., & Reece, R. M. (1980). Observations of paternal response to sudden unanticipated infant death. *Pediatrics, 65*(2), 221–225. Retrieved from http://pediatrics.aappublications.org/

Margolies, L. (1999). The long goodbye: Women, companion animals, and maternal loss. *Clinical Social Work Journal, 27*(3), 289–304. Retrieved from http://link.springer.com/journal/10615

Marks, S. G., Koepke, J. E., & Bradley, C. L. (1994). Pet attachment and generativity among young adults. *The Journal of Psychology, 128*(6), 641–650. doi:10.1080/00223980.1994.9921292

McCormack, M., & Anderson, E. (2010). It's just not acceptable any more: The erosion of homophobia and the softening of masculinity at an English sixth form. *Sociology, 44*(5), 843–859. doi:10.1177/0038038510375734

McMahon, J. (2009). *Gender role conflict in gay men living in Ireland: A study to investigate gender role conflict in gay men living in Ireland and to compare these findings against their heterosexual peers* (Unpublished manuscript).

Moore, D. (2009). *The basic practice of statistics* (5th ed.). Gordansville, VA: W. H. Freeman.

Nagasawa, M., & Ohta, M. (2010). The influence of dog ownership in childhood on the sociality of elderly Japanese men: Influence of dog ownership in childhood. *Animal Science Journal, 81*(3), 377–383. doi:10.1111/j.1740-0929.2010.00741.x

Netting, F. E., Wilson, C. C., Goodie, J. L., Stephens, M. B., Byers, C. G., & Olsen, C. H. (2013). Attachment, social support, and perceived mental health of adult dog walkers: What does age have to do with it? *Journal of Sociology & Social Welfare, 40*(4), 261–284. Retrieved from http://wmich.edu/socialwork/journal/

Nunnally, J. C. (1978). *Psychometric theory* (2nd ed.). New York, NY: McGraw-Hill.

O' Neil, J. M., Helms, B., Gable, R., David, L., & Wrightsman, L. (1986). Gender role conflict scale (GRCS): College men's fear of femininity. *Sex Roles, 14*(5–6), 335–350. doi:10.1007/BF00287583

O'Neil, J. M. (1982). Gender-role conflict and strain in men's lives: Implications for psychiatrists, psychologists, and other human-service providers. In K. Solomon & N. B. Levy (Eds.), *Men in transition: Theory and therapy* (pp. 5–44). New York, NY: Plenum.

O'Neil, J. (2008). Summarizing 25 years of research on men's gender role conflict using the gender role conflict scale: New research paradigms and clinical implications. *The Counseling Psychologist, 36*(3), 358–445. doi:10.1177/0011000008317057

O'Neil, J. M., Good, G. E., & Holmes, S. (1995). Fifteen years of theory and research on men's gender role conflict. In R. F. Levant & W. S. Pollack (Eds.), *The new psychology of men* (pp. 164–206). New York, NY: Basic Books.

Paul, E. S., & Serpell, J. A. (1993). Childhood pet keeping and humane attitudes in young adulthood. *Animal Welfare, 2*, 321–338.

Poresky, R. H., & Daniels, A. M. (1998). Demographics of pet presence and attachment. *Anthrozoös, 11*(4), 236–241. doi:10.2752/089279398787000508

Reid, J. S., & Anderson, C. E. (2009). Identification of demographic groups with attachment to their pets. *Proceedings of the American Society of Business and Behavioral Sciences, 16*(1). Retrieved from http://asbbs.org/files/2009/PDF/A/AndersonC.pdf

Rumbaut, R. G. (2005). Immigration, incorporation, and generational cohorts in historical contexts. In K. W. Schaie & G. H. Elder (Eds.), *Historical influences on lives and aging* (pp. 43–88). New York, NY: Springer Publishing Co.

Sanders, C. R. (1990). The animal 'other': Self-definition, social identity and companion animals. In M. E. Goldberg, G. Gorn, & R. W. Pollay (Eds.), *Advances in consumer research* (pp. 662–668). Provo, UT: Association for Consumer Research.

Santrock, J. (2013). *Life-span development* (14th ed.). New York, NY: McGraw Hill.

Shaver, P., & Tancredy, C. (2001). Emotion, attachment, and bereavement: A conceptual commentary. In M. Stroebe, R. O. Hansson, W. Stroebe, & H. Schut (Eds.), *Handbook of bereavement research: Consequences, coping, and care* (pp. 63–88). Washington, DC: American Psychological Association.

Stallones, L., Marx, M. B., Garrity, T. F., & Johnson, T. P. (1990). Pet ownership and attachment in relation to the health of U.S. adults, 21 to 64 years of age. *Anthrozoös, 4*(2), 100–112. doi:10.2752/089279391787057206

Stroebe, M., Schut, H., & Stroebe, W. (2005). Attachment in coping with bereavement: Atheoretical integration. *Review of General Psychology, 9*(1), 48–66. doi:10.1037/1089-2680.9.1.48

Tannen, D. (1986). *That's not what I meant! How conversational style makes or breaks your relations with others*. New York, NY: Morrow.

Theodore, H., & Lloyd, B. F. (2000). Age and gender role conflict: A cross-sectional study of Australian men. *Sex Roles, 42*(11–12), 1027–1042. doi:10.1023/A:1007088617819

Wayment, H. A., & Vierthaler, J. (2002). Attachment style and bereavement reaction. *Journal of Loss and Trauma, 7*(2), 129–149. doi:10.1080/153250202753472291

Wei, M., Russell, D. W., Mallinckrodt, B., & Vogel, D. L. (2007). The experiences in close relationship scale (ECR)-short form: Reliability, validity, and factor structure. *Journal of Personality Assessment, 88*(2), 187–204. doi:10.1080/00223890701268041

Wester, S. R., Vogel, D. L., O'Neil, J. M., & Danforth, L. (2012). Development and evaluation of the gender role conflict scale short form (GRCS-SF). *Psychology of Men & Masculinity, 13*(2), 199–210. doi:10.1037/a0025550

Williams, J. M., Muldoon, J., & Lawrence, A. (2009). Children and their pets: Exploring the relationships between pet ownership, pet attitudes, attachment to pets and empathy. *Education and Health, 28*(1), 12–15. Retrieved from http://sheu.org.uk/content/page/education–and–health–journal

Wong, Y. J., Pituch, K., & Rochlen, A. B. (2006). Men's restrictive emotionality: An investigation of associations with other emotion-related constructs, underlying dimensions, and anxiety. *Psychology of Men and Masculinity, 7*(2), 113–126. doi:10.1037/1524-9220.7.2.113

Wood, L., Giles-Corti, B., & Bulsara, M. (2005). The pet connection: Pets as a conduit for social capital? *Social Science and Medicine, 61*(6), 1159–1173. doi:10.1016/j.socscimed.2005.01.017

Wrobel, T. A., & Dye, A. L. (2003). Grieving pet death: Normative, gender, and attachment issues. *OMEGA, 47*(4), 385–393. doi:10.2190/QYV5-LLJ1-T043-U0F9

Zilcha-Mano, S., Mikulincer, M., & Shaver, P. R. (2011). An attachment perspective on human-pet relationships: Conceptualization and assessment of pet attachment orientations. *Journal of Research in Personality, 45*(4), 345–357. doi:10.1016/j.jrp.2011.04.001

Zimet, G. D., Dahlem, N. W., Zimet, S. G., & Farley, G. K. (1988). The multidimensional scale of perceived social support. *Journal of Personality Assessment, 52*(1), 30–41. doi:10.1207/s15327752jpa5201_2

Chapter 13
Older Adults and Pets—Physical and Psychological Benefits

Lori Kogan

The next two chapters focus on the relationship older adults, and men in particular, have with their companion animals including the benefits, the challenges, and the programs designed to help preserve this bond.

This chapter provides background on older adults—who they are and the challenges they face. It then explores the psychological and physiological benefits of pet ownership for this population. The chapter ends with challenges of pet ownership for older adults; providing the background for the next chapter that describes intergenerational service learning and one example, Pets Forever, a course designed to support pet ownership for older adults.

Elderly—Demographics

Today in the US, approximately one in every seven people are 65 years and older; older adults now constitute 13.7 % of the U.S. population (43.1 million); an increase from 4.1 % since 1900 ("A Profile" 2013). The number of older Americans has increased by 21 % since 2002 compared to an increase of 7 % for people under 65. Average life expectancy for people in the US has also increased dramatically in recent years. Individuals approaching 65 years of age now have an average life expectancy of an additional 19.2 years (20.4 years for females and 17.8 years for males) ("A Profile" 2013).

L. Kogan (✉)
Clinical Sciences Department, College of Veterinary Medicine and Biomedical Sciences, Colorado State University, 1601 Campus Delivery, Fort Collins, CO 80523, USA
e-mail: Lori.kogan@colostate.edu

C. Blazina and L.R. Kogan (eds.), *Men and Their Dogs*,
DOI 10.1007/978-3-319-30097-9_13

Given the fact that the number of Americans aged 45–64 has also increased 24 % between 2002 and 2012, this trend is expected to continue. Between 2012 and 2050, the United States will experience considerable growth of the older generations. Largely due to the baby boomer generation, by 2030, more than 20 % of U.S. residents are projected to be 65 or older, and by 2050, this number is projected to be 83.7 million, almost double the population in 2012 (Ortman et al. 2014).

Furthermore, the older population itself is growing increasingly older. In 2012, the 65–74 age group was more than 10 times larger than in 1900; the 75–84 group was 17 times larger and the 85+ group was 48 times larger ("A Profile" 2013). The number of people aged 85 and over is projected to grow from 5.9 million in 2012 to 8.9 million in 2030. In 2050, those aged 85 and over are projected to account for 4.5 % of the U.S. population (Ortman et al. 2014).

Female life expectancy has long exceeded male life expectancy, resulting in women outnumbering men in all older age groups. While this trend is projected to continue within the foreseeable future, due to the more rapid increase in life expectancy for men projected over the next several decades, the gap between the number of older women and men is expected to narrow. Among those 65 years and over in 2050, 55.1 % are projected to be females, compared to 56.4 % in 2012. Among those 85 years and over, 61.9 % are projected to be females in 2050, down from 66.6 % in 2012 (Ortman et al. 2014).

The changing gender ratios, as well as where older populations choose to live, will likely have major impacts on communities. Currently, the percentage of older persons varies considerably by state, with some states experiencing much greater growth in their older populations. In 2012, the states with the highest percentages of people 65 and older included the following: Florida (18.2 %); Maine (17.0 %); West Virginia (16.8 %); Pennsylvania (16.0 %); Montana (15.7 %); Vermont (15.7 %); Delaware (15.3 %); Iowa (15.3 %); Hawaii (15.1 %); Rhode Island (15.1 %), and Arkansas (15.0 %) ("A Profile" 2013).

In addition to actual numbers, it is important to track which states are experiencing large increases in the 65+ population. There are 14 states in which the older population has increased 30 % or more between 2002 and 2012: Alaska (58.9 %), Nevada (49.3 %), Colorado (41.7 %), Georgia (40.1 %), Arizona (39.6 %); Idaho (39.1 %), South Carolina (39.1 %), Utah (36.6 %), North Carolina (34.6 %), Washington (33.9 %), New Mexico (33.6 %), Delaware (33.6 %), Texas (33.2 %), and Virginia (30.2 %).

Unfortunately, many older adults live below the poverty line. In 2013, the poverty rate for people aged 65 and older was 9.5 %, not statistically different from their 2012 estimates (United States Census Bureau 2014). Yet, the percentage of people 65 and older living below poverty varies a great deal state by state. In 2013, the District of Columbia (16 %), North Carolina (15 %), Louisiana (14 %), Arizona (13 %), and New Mexico (13 %) had the highest percentage of older persons at or below poverty. The states with the lowest poverty rates for older adults include Maine (5 %), Missouri (6 %), Wisconsin (6 %), Vermont (6 %), and Massachusetts (6 %).

These high poverty rates are especially concerning given that financial status impacts life expectancy. Reversing an earlier trend toward greater equality, there are significant differences in life expectancy between people with high and low socioeconomic status, and this difference has only widened over the past three decades (Burtless 2014). In fact, much of the recent increase in expected life spans is concentrated among those with above-average incomes, with life expectancy holding constant or declining for poorer Americans (Pear 2008).

Regardless of financial status, resources tailored for older adults will need to expand. These will include resources for both those who are able to remain living in their home (the majority of older adults) as well as those who move into some type of institution. Contrary to the popular conception, only a small percentage (3.5 %) of people 65 and older live in institutional settings (e.g., nursing homes). This percentage does increase with age, however, ranging from 1 % for persons 65–74 years to 3 % for persons 75–84 years and 10 % for persons 85 and older. In addition, approximately 2.7 % of elderly live in senior housing that offers at least one supportive service to their residents. Over half (57 %) of older noninstitutionalized people (71 % of men) live with their spouse yet this percentage decreases with age. About 28 % of all noninstitutionalized older persons live alone, representing about 19 % of all older men ("A Profile" 2013). The percentage of older adults living alone also increases with advanced age.

Although older adults are a heterogeneous group, there are many aspects related to aging that impact a large percentage of older adults, many of which can negatively affect their quality of life (Bourque et al. 2005; Paskulin and Molzahn 2007). As one ages, numerous physical and cognitive changes are common. In 2012, 58.7 % of adults 65 years and older had at least one basic action difficulty or complex activity limitation. Difficulties and limitations include challenges with movement, emotion, sensory ability (seeing or hearing), cognition, social or work limitations, or self-care; self-care defined as activities of daily living or instrumental activities of daily living (CDC 2015). Additional challenges include development of chronic conditions, loss of independence, and increased isolation (Bourque et al. 2005). The percentage of older adults needing assistance with everyday activities ranges from 9 % for those ages 65–69 to 50 % for those 85 years and older (APA 1998).

The most common physical changes include hearing and visual impairment. The number of older adults with vision loss is expected to double over the next 30 years (NYC Coalition 2015). Eighteen percent of the U.S. adults older than 70 have impaired vision. These impairments include problems with reading, difficulty seeing in dim light, and problems locating objects (APA 1998). These challenges can result in an increased risk of falling, overall poor health, and depression (NYC Coalition 2015). Although hearing impairment among older adults is often moderate or mild, it is widespread, experienced by 48 % of men over 75 years of age (APA 1998). Both visual and hearing impairments can significantly impact the ability to drive and other daily activities. Additionally, arthritis and chronic pain can both impact quality of life and the ability to care for oneself and others (Vacha-Haase et al. 2011).

Another serious health risk for older men is suicide. In the United States, men's suicides constitute 79 % of the total number of suicides each year. The risk for suicide among men is four times higher than among women, and this rate is highest for men 75 and older who live alone (APA 1998). According to the Centers for Disease Control and Prevention, about 51 of every 100,000 white men age 85 and older committed suicide in 2012, compared with the national average for all ages of 12.6. Additionally, White men 85 and older are more likely to commit suicide than Americans in any other age group, committing suicide at a rate of four times that of the general population (CDCP 2010).

Health and Loneliness

Depression and suicidal behaviors and can be the result of age-related physical changes and limitations, or the loss of social connections and resultant loneliness. The number of one's social relationships tends to decrease with age (Holwerda et al. 2012), most often due to the death of a spouse, parents, friends, colleagues, or neighbors (Krause-Parello and Gulick 2013). These often lead to situational factors (e.g., being single or living alone) that can increase an older adult's risk for social isolation (Coyle and Dugan 2012). According to the Administration on Aging, 29 % of noninstitutionalized older adults live alone, and as the number of elderly increase, so will the number of individuals living alone. Yet being socially connected is not only important for psychological and emotional well-being, but it also has a significant and positive influence on physical well-being and overall longevity (Uchino 2006; Holt-Lunstad et al. 2010; Shor et al. 2013).

Although loneliness is often associated with forms of emotional and social isolation, research suggests that social isolation and loneliness are not always correlated (Coyle and Dugan 2012; Perissinotto and Covinsky 2014). It has been postulated that even though there may be a great deal of overlap between social isolation and loneliness, these are not equivalent terms and should be assessed individually. For instance, some may be socially isolated but content with minimal social contact or actually prefer to be alone; others may have frequent social contact but still feel lonely. Living alone, having few social network ties, and having infrequent social contact are all indicators of social isolation (Holt-Lunstad et al. 2015). Loneliness, on the other hand, is the perception of social isolation and is therefore a more subjective measurement. For many, those who report a lack of human contact also report feeling lonely. Both loneliness and social isolation are associated with poor health behaviors including smoking, physical inactivity, and sleep problems (Theeke 2010), as well as negative physical aspects such as higher blood pressure, increased C-reactive protein, lipid profiles, and poorer immune functioning (Grant et al. 2009; Hawkley and Cacioppo 2010).

It is not surprising then, that social isolation and loneliness result in higher likelihood of mortality. One recent study found the increased likelihood of death of those reporting loneliness was 29 % for those reporting social isolation, and 32 % for those living alone (Holt-Lunstad et al. 2015). These findings are consistent with prior research suggesting that people who report being more socially connected have higher survival rates than those with fewer social connections (Holt-Lunstad et al. 2010; Cacioppo et al. 2015; Thoits 2011; Hawkley and Cacioppo 2010). The negative impact of loneliness cannot be overstated; it has been recognized as a clinically important frailty factor in older persons, and associated with psychosocial, psychological, and physical problems (Holwerda et al. 2012). In fact, the risks associated with social isolation and loneliness are comparable with well-established risk factors for mortality, including lack of physical activity, obesity, substance abuse, irresponsible sexual behavior, poor mental health, injury and violence, poor environmental quality, and lack of immunization and access to health care (Holt-Lunstad 2015).

Sadly, approximately 40 % of adults aged 65 years and older report feeling lonely at least part of the time, and 5–15 % report feeling frequently lonely; and given the numerous changes within society, these numbers appear to only be increasing (Pinquart and Sorensen 2001; Hawkley and Cacioppo 2010; Perissinotto et al. 2012; Victor and Yang 2012; Wilson and Moulton 2010). Considering that older adults are the fastest growing segment of the US population, the case can be made that loneliness is a significant public health risk (Cacioppo and Patrick 2008) and identifying ways to increase social connectedness should be a societal priority.

This need appears to perhaps be even more critical for men, given the fact that they are even more vulnerable to social isolation and loneliness, likely due to fewer close relationships outside marriage than women (Van Grootheest et al. 1999; Murray et al. 2006; Holwerda 2012; Dykstra and De Jong Gierveld 2004; Boomsma et al. 2005). For example, even after controlling for potentially confounding factors, Holwerda (2012) found that older men who reported feelings of loneliness were 30 % more likely to have died at a 10-year follow-up.

Men and Masculinity

Although aging can be challenging for both men and women, there are societal aspects that make this a different experience for men compared to women. The social construct of masculinity, or what it means to be a man in a certain time and place (Tannenbaum and Frank 2011), presents unique challenges for aging men. Even though one may argue that men enjoy many advantages in the US culture (e.g., power and prestige), these may come at a cost. The social construct of masculinity in Western culture, associated with traits of competitiveness, wealth, emotional detachment, dominance, autonomy, and physical toughness, is pervasive (Bennett 2007). Yet, adhering to the traditionally accepted masculine identity can be highly restrictive and force men to suppress and reject displays of emotion and vulnerability (Genoe and Singleton 2006; Messner 1990).

Gender role conflicts (GRS) can have a detrimental impact on men's mental health. Several GRS have been identified by O'Neil et al. (1995). One is success, power and competition, in which men focus on personal achievements and a competitive edge. Another conflict is restricted emotionality, in which men are reluctant to display expressions of emotions. Restricted affectionate behavior between men is a third GRC. All of these can create challenges for aging men as the lose career roles, have increased needs, and suffer the losses of spouses or long-term close friends. These conflicts make it difficult for men to obtain the support they might need, leaving them vulnerable to loneliness and depression (Good et al. 1995).

Furthermore, the traditional view of masculinity conflicts with many aspects of aging. For many, growing old is associated with a loss of strength, autonomy, and physical and mental resiliencies (Bennett 2007). These changes force many aging men to try to maintain a culturally accepted masculine identity and personal autonomy in the face of changing physical abilities (Spector-Mersel 2006; Smith et al. 2007). This conflict directly impacts men's choices related to health and help-seeking behaviors, including the use of health services, hence contributing to the health disparities witnessed between men and women (Smith et al. 2007; Mahalik et al. 2007).

When confronted with a health threat, many men make health care choices based on their views of traditional masculine behavior, masculine gender-role socialization, and social constructionism; often leading to a delay in seeking treatment or a lack of treatment completely (Galdas et al. 2005; Addis and Mahalik 2003; Bertakis et al. 2000). Tannenbaum (2011) has suggested that many of the tasks associated with seeking help from a health professional (e.g., relying on others, admitting a need for help, or recognizing and labeling an emotional problem), conflict with the messages men receive about the importance of self-reliance, physical toughness, and emotional control. It is not surprising, therefore, that many men avoid or delay seeking medical care and feel that addressing health concerns and seeking help is a contradiction to their views of masculinity (Tannenbaum and Frank 2011; Courtenay 2000).

For these reasons, it has been suggested that men might have a harder time adjusting to the changes that occur with aging when compared to women. As a result, many men become increasingly isolated as they age and withdraw from others as they face the challenges of growing older (Illinois Council on Long Term Care 1996). This is compounded by the challenges aging men face remaining gainfully employed. Work is often a central theme in men's lives and a crucial component of their identity. Many men suffer a loss of identity and self-esteem when they can no longer work, and as a result are at increased risk of developing depression, dependence on alcohol or drugs, or committing suicide (Illinois Council on Long Term Care 1996).

Given the increasing number of older adults and the challenges that they face, it is vitally important to identify factors related to improving quality of life in old age (Himsworth and Rock 2013). One growing area of research that could mitigate some of the negative impact of aging for men is pet ownership. It has been suggested that interactions with companion animals, and dogs in particular, have the ability to offer significant physical and psychological benefits for aging adults (McNicholas et al. 2005; Toohey and Rock 2011).

Pet Ownership

According to the 2015–2016 APPA National Pet Owners Survey, 65 % of the U.S. households own a pet, which equates to 79.7 million homes; clearly indicating that pets are an important part of the U.S. households. Many of these pet owners are 65 and older; 53 % of 65- to 69-year-olds and 34 % of those 70 and older have a pet ("Pet Population" 2014). For the majority of these owners, pets are not merely seen as animals, but as companions, as these pets share a relationship with their owners that includes codependence and mutuality (Walsh 2009). A 2013 study found that 86 % of pet owners consider their pet(s) to be part of the family, and 76 % feel they are a "pet parent" (Easterly 2013). In fact, 42.5 % of pet owners report they would not go on a vacation if they could not bring their pet, and 75 % report celebrating their pet's birthday or day of adoption ("How Do You" 2013).

People enjoy spoiling their pets; 75 % of owners report they have shared ice cream with their pet, over 99 % report their pet shares the bed with a family member, 40.3 % admit to sneaking their pet into a store or public area, and 99.4 % talk or sing to their pet ("How Do You" 2013). Another poll of more than 1000 pet owners conducted by the Associated Press reports that 35 % of owners have included their pet in a family portrait, and that 25 % of pet owners, who are married or cohabitating report that their pet is a better listener than their spouse. Other studies have found that 93 % of pet owners report they would risk their own lives for their pet and the majority of pet owners would take their pets if they had to evacuate their homes or refuse to evacuate their homes without their pets despite hazardous conditions (AAHA 2004; PR Web 2011; Knight and Herzog 2009).

Benefits of Animals and Pet Ownership

The cost of animal ownership is not cheap, however. It is estimated that small to medium-sized dogs cost between $740 and $1325 for the first year and $500–$875 annually thereafter. This equates to approximately $7240–$12,700 over the course of dog's lifetime (using an average of 14 years). Annual costs are even higher for larger breeds, but the life expectancy is shorter (8 years). The first year of owning a large or giant breed costs between $1020–$1825 and $690–$875 annually, thereafter for a total estimated lifetime cost of $5850–$7950. These are just basic figures and do not account for emergency hospitalization or treatment or cover the extra items or luxuries so many owners give to their dogs (e.g., specialty treats and food; doggie day care, spas, clothing, etc.).

Given these costs, some question the reasoning behind why people, and older people specifically, make the decision to own a pet. Many older owners cite reasons that include love for the pet, a desire for companionship, and an antidote to loneliness (Enders-Slegers 2000). The decision to own a pet is supported by a growing body of the literature that explores the many benefits pets can offer people throughout one's lifetime (Mishra 2014; Campo and Uchino 2013; McNicholas 2014). These benefits can be broadly classified into physical, psychological, and social health (Smith 2012).

Physical Health

Numerous studies have found pet ownership associated with better overall health, and in particular, cardiovascular health (Anderson et al. 1992; Bauman et al. 2001; Dembicki and Anderson 1996; Headey 1999; Raina et al. 1999; Serpell 1991). These benefits have been recognized by the National Institutes of Health, which has stated that pets should be considered as a possible protective human health factor (National Institute of Health 1988). These positive effects have been found to be especially promising for older adults, creating as trong impetus for increased research related to the potential health benefits of pet ownership for the elderly (Siegel 1993).

One of the first pivotal studies on this topic was conducted by Friedmann et al. (1980), who found that outpatients of a cardiac care unit who owned pets lived longer than non-pet owners. This seminal research influenced several other studies that subsequently supported this premise that pet ownership positively impacts physical health (Allen et al. 2001; Friedmann and Thomas 1995; Garrity et al. 1989; Koivusilta and Ojanlatva 2006; Parker et al. 2010; Parslow and Jorm 2003a, b).

Anderson et al. (1992), for example, found that pet owners have significantly lower cholesterol and blood pressure levels than non-pet owners. Another randomized control study of stockbrokers with hypertension found that pet owners experienced less stress-related increases in blood pressure when compared to non-pet owners (Allen et al. 2001). Two more recent studies support these earlier findings. Campo conducted a study that compared the cardiovascular effects of having a companion animal present during and after an emotionally stressful activity compared to having a close friend present or being alone (Campo and Uchino 2013). The results indicated that participants with their dogs experienced less unpleasant, stress-related emotions (i.e., distress, nervousness, etc.) than those who were accompanied by a friend or were alone (Campo and Uchino 2013). Conclusions of this study suggested that even when the perceived relationship quality is similar for pet dogs and close friends, dogs may provide more cardiovascular benefits during and after a stressful event (Campo and Uchino 2013). As one final example, a study by Polheber and Matchock (2014) found that the presence of a novel dog during a socially stressing event can positively impact participants' heart rate and cortisol response. Similar to results reported by Campo (2013), this study found that the presence of the dog reduced salivary cortisol levels even more than when participants were accompanied by a friend or alone (Polheber and Matchock 2014).

These studies support the premise that interaction with a dog appears to offer protective physical benefits including transitory decreases in blood pressure and heart rate (Shiloh et al. 2003). In response to these studies, the American Heart Association (AHA) published a statement on pet ownership and cardiovascular risk in which it concluded that pet ownership, *particularly dog ownership*, is probably associated with a decrease in cardiovascular risk and may actually have a causal role in reducing cardiovascular risk (Levine et al. 2013). Given the lack of social support for many older men, these findings offer exciting potential solutions in efforts to mitigate negative effects that can accompany stressful situations. This can be of significant value to men, many of whom go to great lengths to avoid appearing weak or needy. It has been suggested that even though many men may recognize they need services, they feel unable to reach out to access them (Vacha-Haase 2011). Programs that introduce social contact in a way that does not threaten their attempts at preserving their views of masculinity, such as programs designed around their pets, can offer a window of opportunity.

In addition to cardiovascular health, when compared with older adult non-pet owners, those owning a dog display slower deterioration of the ability to perform activities of daily living (Raina et al. 1999). Furthermore, other studies comparing the health of pet owners and non-pet owners suggest that pet owners are healthier, have less pharmaceutical expenditure, and are less likely to be on medication for heart problems and sleeping difficulties than non-pet owners (Siegel 1990; Headey 1999; Pachana et al. 2005; Raina et al. 1999). Pet owners also make fewer annual doctor visits. In a study of older people's utilization of general practitioner services Siegel (1990) reported that older pet owners made significantly fewer visits to their doctor than did older people who did not own pets. Greater numbers of general practitioner visits for non-pet owners were associated with greater incidence of stressful life events, whereas this association was not evident in pet owners—indicating a positive role for pets in alleviating stress in their owners and thus reducing needs for medical services. A study conducted by Headey (2007) found that pet owners in both Germany and Australia made fewer doctor visits when compared to non-pet owners. In both countries, the researchers found that pet owners make about 15 % fewer doctor visits than non-owners each year, and this effect of pet ownership remains statistically significant even after controlling for gender, age, marital status, and income (Headey and Grabka 2007).

Exercise

Physical exercise is another important component to health. As rates of obesity continue to increase in the U.S., exercise is a frequent news topic, and the search for innovative ways to help people lose weight or maintain a healthy weight is a top national priority. In 2014, the adult obesity rate in the U.S. was 27.7 % (27.9 % for men and 26.9 % for women). For those 65 and older, the rate was 27.9 %. It has been suggested that reducing obesity rates can result in numerous economic and societal benefits (McCarthy 2014). Regular physical activity can positively impact several areas of health for older adults, including, but not limited to, cognitive functioning, physical abilities, and overall quality of life (Chan et al. 2013). Yet, despite the numerous health benefits, only 35.5 % of U.S. adults 65 and older (41.1 % of men and 31.2 % of women) meet the current recommendation of 150 min of moderate-intensity physical activity per week, and only 16.1 % (18.0 % of men and 14.7 % of women) meet the current recommendations for strength training (physical activities specifically designed to strengthen muscles) at least twice per week (CDC 2014).

Due in part to the Healthy People 2020, an initiative supported by the current First Lady, Michelle Obama, the topic of health and exercise has been one of increasing the U.S. interest. Numerous suggestions are constantly offered to help people increase their activity levels, but one area that has yet to receive much attention is the effect that dog ownership can have on physical activity levels, and especially those of older adults. Several studies have found positive associations between dog ownership and physical activity of aging adults (Dembicki and Anderson 1996; Feng et al. 2014; Gretebeck et al. 2013; Toohey et al. 2013; Garcia et al. 2015; Boldt and Dellmann-Jenkins 1992; Friedmann and Thomas 1995; Cutt et al. 2008), and it has been suggested by many that dog walking may be a viable strategy to combat the frequent decline of physical activity that often accompanies the aging process (Lim and Taylor 2005; Christian et al. 2013; Cutt et al. 2008; Toohey and Rock 2011).

For example, an earlier study found that dog owners between 70 and 79 years of age were more likely to engage in any activity and non-exercise related walking when compared to non-dog owners, suggesting that the benefits of dog ownership include an increase in physical activity (Thorpe et al. 2006). A more recent study of adults aged 50 and older found that frequent dog-walkers, (defined as those who walked their dog 4 or more times per week) were more likely than non-dog owners to reach the recommendation of 150 min of moderate-intensity physical activity per week (Toohey et al. 2013). Feng (2014) found similar results: older dog owners were 12 % more active than older non-dog owners. From these results, Feng et al. (2014) suggested that dog ownership may motivate physical activity by helping older owners overcome some of the potential barriers to physical activity, including a lack of social support, bad weather, or concerns of personal safety. Further, a recent meta-analysis of 17 studies that examined the relationship between dog ownership and physical activity found that dog owners report more minutes per week of walking and overall physical activity than non-dog owners (Christian et al. 2013).

There are likely several reasons why dog ownership appears to increase physical activity (Banks and Banks 2002; Feng et al. 2014). Similar to a walking partner or workout buddy, dogs may provide external motivation for physical activity (Wells 2009). For some owners, their sense of responsibility in caring for their dogs' physical health and exercise level may serve as an impetus to walk or exercise, and may be helpful in motivating individuals to overcome barriers of minor illness or depression, lethargy, bereavement, feelings of insecurity when walking alone, and inclement weather (Cutt et al. 2007; Knight and Edwards 2008; Toohey and Rock 2011). Walking dogs can also promote socialization with people in the neighborhood, which can then incentivize additional walking (Toohey and Rock 2011; Toohey et al. 2013; Wells 2004; Wood et al. 2007). Given the number of older pet owners, even a small positive influence of pet ownership on human health could have significant public health ramifications.

Dogs not only impact exercise levels and cardiovascular health, they have also been found to impact other important health-related aspects, several of which are related to psychological and emotional well-being. For example, owning a dog has been associated with beneficial neuroendocrine changes such as increases in dopamine, oxytocin, and B-endorphin, and decreases in cortisol, even after controlling for tobacco use, body mass index, and social economic status (Odendaal 2000). Other studies have found an increase in owners' oxytocin levels when their dog looks into their eyes, suggesting that interactions with a dog can increase an owner's oxytocin levels (Nagaswa et al. 2009, 2015). Increase in oxytocin level is important in human health, as oxytocin may be a mechanism for the stress-buffering effects of social support (Heinrichs et al. 2003). It has been suggested that, similar to humans' positive relationship quality, the attachment one feels toward their pet may be a driving force behind many of the health benefits witnessed by pet owners (Crawford et al. 2006). This effect carries important implications for owners' psychological health, feelings of loneliness and isolation, and purpose in life—the topics covered in the next section.

Psychological

Many people recognize the role that animals can have in mitigating feelings of stress. One study that tried to compare retirement home residents found themselves unable to conduct the study as originally designed because 99 % of all participants chose to have the dog present. Although a comparison between groups of dog present and dog not present could not be completed, the results suggested that residents strongly preferred having a dog present during a potentially stressful event (Eshbaugh et al. 2011). In fact, the presence of dogs during therapy sessions has been demonstrated to increase willingness to disclose information by participants with a history of being reluctant to disclose (Schneider and Harley 2006), as well as show promise in helping support older adults in a variety of physical and psychosocial ways through animal-assisted therapy (Cherniack and Cherniack 2014). Part of this effect might be due to the nonjudgmental nature of animals; their presence can help facilitate feelings of safety, thereby creating an environment in which owners feel comfortable to communicate and openly express their feelings (Bryan et al. 2014).

People who seem to be particularly vulnerable to a lack of social support are individuals who have a great deal of ambivalence concerning emotional expression. Ambivalent emotional expression (AEE) results from a conflict in which one wants to express one's feelings, but is afraid of the consequences (King and Emmons 1990). Those with AEE report higher levels of psychological distress, depression, obsessive-compulsive tendencies, and fear of intimacy (Bryan et al. 2014). Owning a dog has been shown to mitigate the negative effects of AEE, suggesting that pet attachment may serve as a protective buffer for these pet owners (Bryan et al. 2014).

Additionally, pets have been found to moderate the effect of depression on mortality. For example, Friedmann et al. (2011) found pets to be beneficial for depressed patients recovering from heart attacks. In fact, older dog owners in general report fewer symptoms of depression than those without dogs (Wells 2009). Overall, pet ownership appears to have a positive effect on physical and mental health among older adults (McNicholas and Murray 2005; Baun and Johnson 2010; Siegel 2011) including the challenges of loneliness and isolation; two major issues that many elderly men face.

Loneliness and Isolation

Social support has been defined as emotional assistance from significant others; support that may either be actually received, or simply perceived to be available when needed (Thoits 2010). The disengagement theory (Cumming et al. 1961) has been used to explain the challenge men face in this area. For many men, their identity is tied to their career. When their job ends, they tend to have less involvement with others, which can lead to a downward spiral of reduced social contact. Social support has been associated with positive physical benefits, including reduced risk of developing heart disease, getting cancer or AIDS/HIV, as well as psychological benefits such as reduced risk of stress, depression, anxiety (Stanley et al. 2014; Cacioppo et al. 2002; Barth et al. 2010; Pauley and Hesse 2009; Nurullah 2012). It has been suggested that social support may reduce perceptions of stressful events, and even protect people against anxiety-related illness and enhance recovery from such serious health risks such as strokes, heart attacks, and cancer (McNicholas and Collis 2004).

Those who feel a lack of social support tend to be less healthy than those who are more connected. For example, loneliness has been linked with cardiovascular disease (Thurston and Kubzansky 2009; Udell et al. 2012), depression (Cacioppo et al. 2006) and Alzheimer's disease (Wilson et al. 2007). Loneliness negatively impacts mortality (Perissinotto et al. 2012) and has been identified as similar to other established risk factors, such as cigarette smoking, high blood pressure, obesity, low physical activity, or drinking (House et al. 1988; Holt-Lunstad et al. 2010). Loneliness is, therefore, viewed as an important public health issue, and it is critical to identify factors which can protect against or reduce vulnerability to loneliness (Pikhartoval et al. 2014). The threat of loneliness and lack of social support is especially challenging for men. One theory that can be used to help explain the challenge faced by older men when they change their roles is the selection, optimization, and compensation theory discussed by Bates (1996). Bates postulated that as men grow older, they suffer losses in social connections that not only lead to loneliness, but can create gender role-related dependency. For example, many older men rely on their wives for many areas around personal care including taking care of a house, cooking, cleaning, etc. When they no longer have this connection, they may struggle with feeling inadequate and dependent; which can conflict with their views of masculinity. To help combat these struggles it is suggested that men take an active approach to the aging process, and optimize their abilities while compensating for any declines or losses. Pets are often cited in the literature as a coping mechanism and a form of social support for older adults (Krause-Parello 2008, 2012).

People are social by nature, and it has long been recognized that the presence and support from close relationships has a powerful influence on people's well-being. Such relationships can provide a sense of well-being and the perception of feeling needed and useful—factors that are often absent in older people. The research interest in this area largely stems from the view that as people grow older, their opportunities for social interactions and for forming relationships begin to wane (McNicholas 2014). Retiring from employment, loss of older friends or family members, and a reduction in one's own health or mobility can all contribute to a reduction in a person's social network, leading to increased risk of social isolation, loneliness, and greater dependency on existing relationships. The lack of social connection and resultant loneliness is a major challenge for many older adults throughout the world. In North America, Australia, and Western Europe, approximately 40 % of adults 65 and older report severe or moderate loneliness. Countries in Central and Eastern Europe report prevalence rates of severe loneliness between 15 and 20 % (Fokkema et al. 2012).

Because of the significant number of lonely seniors, and the impact pet ownership can have on feelings of loneliness, it has been hypothesized that pet ownership may be especially beneficial to older people. Empirical research has largely supported this view. Lago and Miller (1989), for example, found that an average of 52 % of older pet owners' time is spent in the company of their pets and 29 % of their activities involve their pets, far exceeding the 2.8 % of time they spend with friends or family.

As discussed earlier, pets are not merely animals for most owners; they are often viewed as family members or friends, and owners acquire them for emotional support and companionship (Callahan 2014). For older adults, who often have limited social connections, these relationships with their pets can acquire even additional importance. McNicholas and Collis (2004), for example, found that 98 % of older adults identified pet ownership as one of their most important relationships in their lives, and found this cohort is more likely than other age groups to identify pets as a way to help alleviate emotional loneliness (McNicholas and Collis 2004).

Many older adults do not have the opportunities to establish new social contacts, but pets can provide one option for a satisfying emotional relationship (Scheibeck et al. 2011). The results of a study done by Krause-Parello (2013) support this premise by finding that attachment to a pet is significantly related to a decreased feeling of loneliness. It has been recommended that the benefits of pet relationships for older adults be examined. Programs that are geared toward helping older men's pets might be one way to address the cognitive dissonance many men feel toward accepting help (Festinger 1957).

Several studies have found that pets play an important role in the lives of older adults (Gulick and Krause-Parello 2012; Krause-Parello 2008, 2012), and especially, those living alone (Antonacopoulos and Pychy 2010; Stammbach and Turner 1999; Johnson et al. 1992; Adamelli et al. 2005). Pets can serve as a buffer against feelings of loneliness and may compensate for low (human) social connectedness (Barker and Wolen 2008; Garrity et al. 1989). For example, a recent study of older adults who presented to their primary care physician found that those owning a pet were 36 % less likely to report loneliness than older adults without pets (Stanley et al. 2014). Due in part to the results of these studies, the unique relationship older people share with their dogs as emotional companions has gained growing attention (Scheibeck et al. 2011). Contrary to some beliefs, there has been little evidence to suggest that a close relationship with a pet comes at the expense of human relationships. In fact, data appears to indicate that closeness to one's pet is mirrored, when possible, in other relationships (McConnell et al. 2011).

There are several ways in which dogs work to increase their owners' social connections and reduce isolation. Dogs may serve as a distraction from stress through games or stress-relieving activities like play or walking (Taylor et al. 2007). In addition to direct effects on loneliness, pet ownership can enhance social interactions with other people by providing an indirect effect by acting as social catalysts and helping people increase their contact with other people (McNicholas and Murray 2005). This effect has been shown to be of particular value to older adults, who often lack many other opportunities for social interactions. A case in point, Wood et al. (2007) found pet ownership positively associated with social interactions, favor exchanges, civic engagement, perceptions of neighborhood friendliness, and sense of community. It has even been suggested that pets may have a ripple effect—extending beyond their owners to non-pet owners and the broader community—and that this effect may be even more pronounced for older adult communities (Wood et al. 2007).

Purpose of Life

Another benefit of living with a companion animal is the care they require, which can have positive effects on an owner's sense of control and self-efficacy (Pachana et al. 2005). Dogs can add meaning, structure, and purpose to the lives of older adults; they give owners a reason to prepare meals, get out of bed, stay active, and keep a regular schedule (Scheibeck et al. 2011; Raina et al. 1999). Dogs depend on their owners for survival, giving their owners a sense of worth and responsibility that comes from caring for another living being (Stanley et al. 2014) This is consistent with studies of human interactions, which suggest that providing support to others, rather than receiving it, may confer greater health benefits (Brown et al. 2003).

This purpose in life, which involves having meaning and goal directedness, has been identified as a key component of psychological well-being, yet is a modifiable factor that can impact healthy aging (Yu et al. 2015; Ryff and Keyes 1995). Purpose in life is correlated with many other psychological constructs, including sense of coherence, resilience, and optimism (Nygren et al. 2005). Older adults with a greater sense of purpose are less likely to develop adverse health outcomes, including a decline in physical function (Collins et al. 2008), increased frailty (Gale et al. 2014), and disability (Boyle et al. 2010; Zaslavsky et al. 2014); Alzheimer's disease (Boyle et al. 2010) clinical strokes (Kim et al. 2013) and even mortality (Krause 2009). A recent study done by Yu (2015) found that a greater sense of purpose in life is associated with approximately a 50 % reduced likelihood of cerebral infarcts. These results are similar to those found in an earlier study in which purpose in life was found to be associated with a reduced risk of clinical strokes for people ages 53–105 (Kim et al. 2013).

Importance of Helping to Keep Pets in Home

Given the harmful effects of loneliness and social isolation on both physical and mental health, coupled with the changing demographics in the USA resulting in increasing numbers of older adults living alone, pet ownership offers many potential benefits that are often overlooked. Yet, despite the multitude of physical and psychological benefits that dog ownership can offer to older adults, and especially to older males, there are challenges in preserving this bond. Programs designed around preserving this bond, while also connecting with older male pet owners, can offer potential solutions around the challenges of cognitive dissonance many men feel toward knowing they need help but being reluctant to accept any.

The challenges that older adults face with keeping pets include the possibility that these owners 'because of fears related to their companion animals' might neglect their own health care, avoid seeking medical care, resist medical advice, or fail to leave inadequate housing conditions (McNicholas and Murray 2005; Morley and Fook 2005). For example, some older adults may avoid seeking medical care because they fear being admitted to hospital or residential care facility and have concerns about the well-being of their pet (McNicholas 2014; Raina et al. 1999). Other challenges include older adults' ability to physically and or financially care for their pet. (McNicholas 2014; Boldt and Dellmann-Jenkins 1992; McNicholas et al. 2005; Scheibeck et al. 2011).

It is not surprising therefore, that despite the health benefits for older people of owning pets, pet ownership declines with age. One recent survey conducted in the UK found that 16 % of respondents over 60 and 26 % of those over 80 who do not currently own a pet made that decision because of concerns related to becoming too frail or dying, making them unable to continue caring for a pet. These concerns were highest among those who lived alone, even though such people are the most likely to benefit from owning a pet (News and Reports 2012).

The psychological and physical benefits that can be attributed to pet ownership not only impact individuals, but can also influence the healthcare system and as a result, public expenditure for health care (Headey et al. 2002). This fact has helped fuel support for programs designed to help older adults keep their pets at home. Many of these programs are great examples of cross-sectorial partnerships that include geriatric services, animal welfare services, government agencies, recreational services, community support services, and acute and long-term care facilities. Although one such program is described in detail in the following chapter, other models include programs created by large nonprofits that have chosen to help with this issue, as well as organizations created specifically to address this need.

The Meals on Wheels Association of America is one example of a well-established nonprofit organization that created an initiative in 2006 to address this community need. Other programs share similar goals of providing needed pet supplies and services to the homebound clients (Stanley et al. 2014). An example of a program created specifically to help sick pet owners is Paws Houston, a volunteer-run program in Houston, Texas. This program helps sustain relationships between pet owners and their pets through an owner's terminal and/or chronic illness (Paws Houston 2014). The Balwyn Welfare Association in Boroondara, and the Pets of Older Persons (POOPs)' program in New South Wales (both in Australia) are two more examples of programs created to support older or disabled pet owners (Balwyn Evergreen Centre 2015; POOPS 2015). Another option to provide support in maintaining this important bond between older adults and their pets is through an intergenerational service learning course. The next chapter explores service learning and provides details on one such program—Pets Forever.

References

A Profile of Older Americans. (2013). Administration on aging and administration for community living. *U.S. Department of Health and Human Services*. Retrieved from http://www.aoa.acl.gov/Aging_Statistics/Profile/2013/docs/2013_Profile.pdf

Adamelli, S., Marinelli, L., Normando, S., & Bono, G. (2005). Owner and cat features influence the quality of life of the cat. *Applied Animal Behaviour Science, 94*, 89–98.

Addis, M. E., & Mahalik, J. R. (2003). Men, masculinity, and the contexts of help seeking. *American Psychologist, 58*, 5–14.

Allen, K., Shykoff, B. E., & Izzo, J. L, Jr. (2001). Pet ownership, but not ACE inhibitor therapy, blunts home blood pressure responses to mental stress. *Hypertension, 38*, 815–820.

American Animal Hospital Association. (2004). American animal hospital association 2004 pet owner survey. Retrieved from https://www.aahanet.org/PublicDocuments/petownersurvey2004.pdf

American Psychological Association (APA). (1998). Older adults' health and age-related changes. Retrieved from http://www.apa.org/pi/aging/resources/guides/older.aspx

Anderson, W., Reid, C., & Jennings, G. (1992). Pet ownership and risk factors for cardiovascular disease. *Medical Journal of Australia, 157*, 298–301.

Antonacopoulos, N. M. D., & Pychy, T. A. (2010). An examination of the potential role of pet ownership, human social support and pet attachment in the psychological health of individuals living alone. *Anthrozoös, 23*(1), 37–54.

Balwyn Evergreen Centre Newsletter. (2015). Retrieved from http://www.evergreen.org.au/MessageForceWebsite/Sites/206/Files/DECEMBER%202014%20AND%20JANUARY%202015.pdf

Banks, M. R., & Banks, W. A. (2002). The effects of animal-assisted therapy on loneliness in an elderly population in long-term care facilities. *Journals of Gerontology. Series A: Biological Sciences and Medical Sciences, 57*, 428–432.

Barker, S. B., & Wolen, A. R. (2008). The benefits of human companion animal interaction: A review. *Journal of Veterinary Medical Education, 35*(4), 487–495.

Barth, J., Schneider, S., & Von Kanel, R. (2010). Lack of social support in the etiology and the prognosis of coronary heart disease: A systematic review and meta analysis. *Psychosomatic Medicine, 72*(3), 229–238.

Bates, M. M. (1996). *The many faces of dependency in old age*. New York: Cambridge University Press.

Bauman, A. E., Russell, S. J., Furber, S. E., & Dobson, A. J. (2001). The epidemiology of dog walking: An unmet need for human and canine health. *Medical Journal of Australia, 175*, 632–634.

Baun, M., & Johnson, R. (2010). Human/animal interaction and successful aging. In A. H. Fine (Ed.), *The handbook on animal-assisted therapy: Theoretical foundations and guidelines for practice* (3rd ed., pp. 283–299). New York: Academic Press.

Bennett, K. M. (2007). No sissy stuff: Towards a theory of masculinity and emotional expression in older widowed men. *Journal of Ageing Studies, 21*, 347–356.

Bertakis, K. D., Azari, R., Helms, J., Callahan, E. J., & Robbins, J. A. (2000). Gender differences in the utilization of health care services. *Journal of Family Practice, 49*, 147–152.

Boldt, M. A., & Dellmann-Jenkins, M. (1992). The impact of companion animals in later life and considerations for practice. *Journal of Applied Gerontology, 11*(2), 228–239.

Boomsma, D. I., Willemsen, G., Dolan, C. V., Hawkly, L. C., & Cacioppo, J. T. (2005). Genetic and environmental contributions to loneliness in adults: The Netherlands twin register study. *Behavior Genetics, 35*, 745–752.

Bourque, P., Pushkar, D., Bonneville, L., & Beland, F. (2005). Contextual effects on life satisfaction of older men and women. *Canadian Journal on Aging, 24*, 31–44.

Boyle, P. A., Buchman, A. S., Barnes, L. L., & Bennett, D. A. (2010a). Effect of a purpose in life on risk of incident Alzheimer disease and mild cognitive impairment in community-dwelling older persons. *Archives of General Psychiatry, 67*, 304–310.

Boyle, P. A., Buchman, A. S., & Bennett, D. A. (2010b). Purpose in life is associated with a reduced risk of incident disability among community-dwelling older persons. *The American Journal of Geriatric Psychiatry, 58*, 1925–1930.

Brown, S. L., Nesse, R. M., Vinokur, A. D., & Smith, D. M. (2003). Providing social support may be more beneficial than receiving it: Results from a prospective study of mortality. *Psychological Science, 14*, 320–327.

Bryan, J. L., Quist, M. C., Young, C. M., Steers, M. N., Foster, D. W., & Lu, Q. (2014). Canine comfort: Pet affinity buffers the negative impact of ambivalence over emotional expression on perceived social support. *Personality and Individual Differences, 68*, 23–27.

Burtless, G. (2014). Changing mortality rates and income inequality among the U.S. elderly. *The Brookings Institution: Stanford Institute for Economic Policy Research*. Retrieved from http://siepr.stanford.edu/system/files/shared/events/wlc2014/Burtless-Oct-2014-Stanford-paper.pdf

Cacioppo, J. T., Cacioppo, S., Cole, W. W., Capitanio, J. P., Goossens, L., & Boomsma, D. I. (2015). Loneliness across phylogeny and a call for animal models. *Perspectives on Psychological Science, 10*, 202–212.

Cacioppo, J. T., Hawkley, L. C., Crawford, E., Ernst, J. M., Burleson, M. H., Kowalewski, R. B., et al. (2002). Loneliness and health: Potential mechanisms. *Psychosomatic Medicine, 64*, 407–417.

Cacioppo, J. T., Hughes, M. E., Waite, L. J., Hawkley, L. C., & Thisted, R. A. (2006). Loneliness as a specific risk factor for depressive symptoms: Cross-sectional and longitudinal analyses. *Psychology and Aging, 21*, 140–151.

Cacioppo, J. T., & Patrick, B. (2008). *Loneliness: Human nature and the need for social connection*. New York, NY: W.W. Norton & Company.

Callahan, A. M., & Brotherton, R. (2014). Understanding the human–animal bond: Implications for practice with community-living older adults. *International Perspectives on Aging, 9*, 253–271.

Campo, R. A., & Uchino, B. N. (2013). Humans' bonding with their companion dogs: Cardiovascular benefits during and after stress. *Journal of Sociology & Social Welfare, 40*(4), 237–259.

Centers for Disease Control and Prevention (CDCP). (2010). National center for injury prevention and control. *Web-Based Injury Statistics Query and Reporting System (WISQARS)*. Retrieved from www.cdc.gov/injury/wisqars/index.html

Chan, J. S. Y., Yan, J. H., & Payne, V. G. (2013). The impact of obesity and exercise on cognitive aging. *Front Aging Neuroscience, 5*(97). Retrieved from http://www.ncbi.nlm.nih.gov/pmc/articles/PMC3869042/pdf/fnagi-05-00097.pdf

Cherniack, E. P., & Cherniack, A. R. (2014). The benefit of pets and animal-assisted therapy to the health of older individuals. *Current Gerontology and Geriatrics Research*, Article ID: 623203.

Christian, H. E., Westgarth, C., Bauman, A., Richards, E. A., Rhodes, R., & Evenson, K. R. (2013). Dog ownership and physical activity: A review of the evidence. *Journal of Physical Activity & Health, 10*, 750–759.

Collins, A. L., Goldman, N., & Rodríguez, G. (2008). Is positive well-being protective of mobility limitations among older adults? *The Journals of Gerontology. Series B: Psychological Sciences and Social Sciences, 63*, 321–327.

Courtenay, W. H. (2000). Constructions of masculinity and their influence on men's well-being: A theory of gender and health. *Social Science and Medicine, 50*, 1385–1401.

Coyle, C. E., & Dugan, E. (2012). Social isolation, loneliness and health among older adults. *Journal of Aging and Health, 24*, 1346–1363.

Crawford, E. K., Worsham, N. L., & Swinehart, E. R. (2006). Benefits derived from companion animals, and the use of the term "attachment". *Anthrozoös, 19*, 98–112.

Cumming, E., Henry, W. E., & Damianopoulos, E. (1961). A formal statement of disengagement theory. In E. Cumming & W. E. Henry (Eds.), *Growing old: The process of disengagement*. New York: Basic Books.

Cutt, H. E., Giles-Cortia, B., Knuimana, M., & Burke, V. (2007). Dog ownership, health and physical activity: A critical review of the literature. *Health Place, 13*, 261–272.

Cutt, H. E., Knuiman, M. W., & Giles-Corti, B. (2008). Does getting a dog increase recreational walking? *International Journal of Behavioral Nutrition and Physical Activity, 5*, 17.

Dembicki, D., & Anderson, J. (1996). Pet ownership may be a factor in improved health of the elderly. *Journal of Nutrition for the Elderly, 15*(3), 15–31.

Dykstra, P. A., & De Jong Gierveld, J. (2004). Gender and marital-history differences in emotional and social loneliness among Dutch older adults. *Canadian Journal on Aging, 23*, 141–155.

Easterly, A. (2013). Techpetually speaking: How tech is transforming the pet industry. Retrieved from http://www.slideshare.net/BarkWorld/techpetually-speaking-how-tech-is-transforming-the-pet-industry-25983134?related=1

Enders-Slegers, M. (2000). The meaning of companion animals: Qualitative analysis of the life histories of elderly cat and dog owners. In A. L. Podberscek, E. S. Paul, & J. A. Serpell (Eds.), *Companion animals and us: Exploring the relationships between people and pets*. Cambridge: Cambridge University Press.

Eshbaugh, E., Somervill, J., Kotek, J., Perez, E., Nalan, K., Wilson, C., et al. (2011). Brief report: Presence of a dog, pet attachment, and loneliness among elders. *North American Journal of Psychology, 13*(1), 1–4.

Facts and Figures. (2014). American Foundation for Suicide Prevention (AFSP). Retrieved from https://www.afsp.org/understanding-suicide/facts-and-figures

Feng, Z., Dibben, C., Witham, M. D., et al. (2014). Dog ownership and physical activity in later life: A cross-sectional observational study. *Preventative Medicine, 66*, 101–106.

Festinger, L. (1957). *A theory of cognitive dissonance*. Evanston, IL: Row, Peterson.

Fokkema, T., De Jong Gierveld, J., & Dykstra, P. A. (2012). Cross-national differences in older adult loneliness. *The Journal of Psychology, 146*, 201–228.

Friedmann, E., Katcher, A. H., Lynch, J. J., & Thomas, S. A. (1980). Animal companions and one-year survival of patients after discharge from a coronary care unit. *Public Health Reports, 95*(4), 307–312.

Friedmann, E., & Thomas, S. A. (1995). Pet ownership, social support, and one-year survival after acute myocardial infarction in the cardiac arrhythmia suppression trial (CAST). *American Journal of Cardiology, 76*(17), 1213–1217.

Friedmann, E., Thomas, S. A., & Son, H. (2011). Pets, depression and long-term survival in community living patients following myocardial infarction. *Anthrozoös, 24*(3), 273–285.

Galdas, P. M., Cheater, F., & Marshall, P. (2005). Men and health help-seeking behaviour: Literature review. *Journal of Advanced Nursing, 49*, 616–623.

Gale, C. R., Cooper, C., Deary, I. J., & Aihie Sayer, A. (2014). Psychological wellbeing and incident frailty in men and women: The English longitudinal study of ageing. *Psychological Medicine, 44*, 697–706.

Garcia, D. O., Wertheim, B. C., Manson, J. E., Chlebowski, R. T., Volpe, S. L., Howard, B. V., et al. (2015). Relationships between dog ownership and physical activity in postmenopausal women. *Preventive Medicine, 70*(2015), 33–38.

Garrity, T., Stallones, L., Marx, M., & Johnson, T. (1989). Pet ownership and attachment as supportive factors in the health of the elderly. *Anthrozoos, 3*(1), 35–44.

Genoe, R. M., & Singleton, J. F. (2006). Older men's leisure experiences across their lifespan. *Topics in Geriatric Rehabilitation, 22*, 348–356.

Good, G. E., Robertson, J. M., O'Neil, J. M., Fitzgerald, L. F., Stevens, M., DeBord, K. A., et al. (1995). Male gender role conflict: Psychometric issues and relations to psychological. *Journal of Counseling Psychology, 42*, 3–10.

Grant, N., Hamer, M., & Steptoe, A. (2009). Social isolation and stress-related cardiovascular, lipid, and cortisol responses. *Annals of Behavioral Medicine, 37*, 29–37.

Gretebeck, K. A., Radius, K., Black, D. R., Gretebeck, R. J., Ziemba, R., & Glickman, L. T. (2013). Dog ownership, functional ability, and walking in community-dwelling older adults. *Journal of Physical Activity & Health, 10*, 646–655.

Gulick, E., & Krause-Parello, C. A. (2012). Factors related to type of companion pet living with older women. *Journal of Psychosocial Nursing, 50*, 30–37.

Hawkley, L. C., & Cacioppo, J. T. (2010). Loneliness matters: A theoretical and empirical review of consequences and mechanisms. *Annals of Behavioral Medicine, 40*, 218–227.

Headey, B. (1999). Health benefits and health cost savings due to pets: Preliminary estimates from an Australian national survey. *Social Indicators Research, 47*, 233–243.

Headey, B., & Grabka, M. M. (2007). Pets and human health in Germany and Australia: National longitudinal results. *Social Indicators Research, 80*, 297–311.

Headey, B., Grabka, M., Kelley, J., Reddy, P., & Tseng, Y. (2002). Pet ownership is good for your health and saves public expenditure too: Australian and German longitudinal evidence. *Australian Social Monitor, 5*, 93–99.

Heinrichs, M., Baumgartner, T., Kirschbaum, C., & Ehlert, U. (2003). Social support and oxytocin interact to suppress cortisol and subjective responses to psychosocial stress. *Biological Psychiatry, 54*(12), 1389–1398.

Himsworth, C. G., & Rock, M. (2013). Pet ownership, other domestic relationships, and satisfaction with life among seniors: Results from a Canadian national survey. *Anthrozoös, 26*(2), 295–305.

Holt-Lunstad, J., Smith, T. B., Baker, M., Harris, T., & Stephenson, D. (2015). Loneliness and social isolation as risk factors for mortality: A meta-analytic review. *Perspectives on Psychological Science, 10*(2), 227–237.

Holt-Lunstad, J., Smith, T. B., & Layton, J. B. (2010). Social relationships and mortality risk: A meta-analysis review. *PLOS Medicine, 7*, e10000316.

Holwerda, T. J., Beekman, A. T. F., Deeg, D. J. H., Stek, M. L., van Tilburg, T. G., Visser, P. J., et al. (2012). Increased risk of mortality associated with social isolation in older men: Only when feeling lonely? Results from the Amsterdam study of the elderly (AMSTEL). *Psychological Medicine, 42*, 843–853.

House, J. S., Landis, K. R., & Umberson, D. (1988). Social relationships and health. *Science, 241*, 540–544.

How Do You Spoil Your Pet? (2013). Pet360. Retrieved from http://www.pet360.com/slideshow/dog/lifestyle/how-do-you-spoil-your-pet/5/iTK9AsC8qEyZSOhBdTWJGA

Illinois Council on Long Term Care. (1996). The aging process: Unique challenges for men. Retrieved from http://www.nursinghome.org/fam/fam_007.html

NYC Coalition on Aging and Vision. (2015). Facts and Statistics. Retrieved from http://www.nycvisioncoalition.org/vision-loss-basics/facts-statistics#.VUU9o5Pe9pt

Johnson, T. P., Garrity, T. F., & Stallones, L. (1992). Psychometric evaluation of the Lexington attachment to pets scale (LAPS). *Anthrozoös, 5*, 160–175.

Kim, E. S., Sun, J. K., Park, N., & Peterson, C. (2013). Purpose in life and reduced incidence of stroke in older adults: 'The health and retirement study'. *Journal of Psychosomatic Research, 74*, 427–432.

King, L. A., & Emmons, R. A. (1990). Conflict over emotional expression: Psychological and physical correlates. *Journal of Personality and Social Psychology, 58*(5), 864–877.

Knight, S., & Edwards, V. (2008). In the company of wolves: The physical, social, and psychological benefits of dog ownership. *Journal of Aging and Health, 20*, 437–455.

Knight, S., & Herzog, H. (2009). All creatures great and small: New perspectives on psychology and human–animal interactions. *Journal of Social Issues, 65*(3), 451–461.

Koivusilta, L. K., & Ojanlatva, A. (2006). To have or not to have a pet for better health? *PLOS One*. Retrieved from http://journals.plos.org/plosone/article?id=10.1371/journal.pone.0000109

Krause, N. (2009). Meaning in life and mortality. *The Journals of Gerontology. Series B: Psychological Sciences and Social Sciences, 64*, 517–527.

Krause-Parello, C. A. (2008). The mediating effect of pet attachment support between loneliness and general health in older females living in the community. *Journal of Community Health Nursing, 25*, 1–14.

Krause-Parello, C. A. (2012). Pet ownership and older women: The relationships among loneliness, pet attachment support, human social support, and depressed mood. *Geriatric Nursing, 31*, 194–203.

Krause-Parello, C. A., & Gulick, E. E. (2013). Situational factors related to loneliness and loss over time among older pet owners. *Western Journal of Nursing Research, 35*(7), 905–919.

Lago, D., Delaney, M., Miller, M., & Grill, C. (1989). Companion animals, attitudes toward pets and health outcomes among the elderly: A long-term follow-up. *Anthrozoös, 3*, 25–34.

Levine, G. N., Allen, K., Braun, L. T., Christian, H. E., Friedmann, E., Taubert, K. A., et al. (2013). Pet ownership and cardiovascular risk: A scientific statement from the American Heart Association. *Circulation, 127*, 2353–2363.

Lim, K., & Taylor, L. (2005). Factors associated with physical activity among older people—a population-based study. *Preventative Medicine, 40*, 33–40.

Mahalik, J. R., Burns, S. M., & Syzdek, M. (2007). Masculinity and perceived normative health behaviors as predictors of men's health behaviors. *Social Science and Medicine, 64*, 2201–2209.

McCarthy, J. (2014). In U.S., adult obesity rate now at 27.7 %. *Gallup*. Retrieved from http://www.gallup.com/poll/170264/adult-obesity-rate.aspx?version=print

McConnell, A. R., Brown, C. M., Shoda, T. M., Stayton, L. E., & Martin, C. E. (2011). Friends with benefits: On the positive consequences of pet ownership. *Journal of Personality and Social Psychology, 101*(6), 1239–1252.

McNicholas, J. (2014). The role of pets in the lives of older people: A review. *Working with Older People, 18*(3), 128–133.

McNicholas, J., & Collis, G. M. (2004). The role of pets in the social networks of children, adolescents and elderly people. Retrieved from http://www.petpartners.org/document.doc?id=119

McNicholas, J., Gilbey, A., Rennie, A., Ahmedzai, S., Dono, J. A., & Ormerod, E. (2005). Pet ownership and human health: A brief review of evidence and issues. *British Medical Journal, 331*, 1252.

McNicholas, J., & Murray, A. (2005). The benefits of pets for older people: A review. In J. Dono & E. Ormerod (Eds.), *Older people and pets: A comprehensive guide 2005*. Oxford: SCAS Publications.

Messner, M. A. (1990). When bodies are weapons: Masculinity and violence in sport. *International Review for the Sociology of Sport, 25*, 203–220.

Mishra, V. (2014). Global connections, measuring the benefits of companion animals and the health of older persons. *International Federation on Aging*. Retrieved from http://www.ifa-fiv.org/wp-content/uploads/2014/09/Companion-Animals-and-Older-Persons-Full-Report-Online.pdf

Morley, C., & Fook, J. (2005). The importance of pet loss and some implications for services. *Mortality, 10*, 127–143.

Murray, J., Banerjee, S., Byng, R., Tylee, A., Bhugra, D., & McDonald, A. (2006). Primary care professionals' perceptions of depression in older people: A qualitative study. *Social Science and Medicine, 63*, 1363–1373.

Nagasawa, M., Mitsui, S., En, S., Ohtani, N., Ohta, M., Sakuma, Y., et al. (2015). Oxytocin-gaze positive loop and the coevolution of human–dog bonds. *Science, 348*(6232), 333–336.

Nagasawa, M., Mogi, K., & Kikusui, T. (2009). Attachment between humans and dogs. *Japanese Psychological Research, 51*, 209–221.

National Institute of Health. (1988). Health benefits of pets (DHHS Publication No. 1988-216-107). Washington, D.C.: U.S. Government Printing Office.

News and Reports. (2012). Survey shows declining pet ownership among older people. *Veterinary Record*. Retrieved from http://veterinaryrecord.bmj.com/content/171/21/518.2

Nurullah, A. S. (2012). Received and provided social support: A review of current evidence and future directions. *American journal of Health Studies, 27*(3), 173–188.

Nygren, B., Aléx, L., Jonsén, E., Gustafson, Y., Norberg, A., & Lundman, B. (2005). Resilience, sense of coherence, purpose in life and self-transcendence in relation to perceived physical and mental health among the oldest old. *Aging & Mental Health, 9*, 354–362.

O'Neil, J. M., Good, G. E., & Holmes, S. (1995). Fifteen years of theory and research on men's gender role conflict. In R. F. Levant & W. S. Pollack (Eds.), *The new psychology of men* (pp. 164–206). New York: Basic Books.

Odendaal, J. S. (2000). Animal-assisted therapy—magic or medicine? *Journal of Psychosomatic Research, 49*(4), 275–280.

Ortman, J. M., Velkoff, V. A., & Hogan, H. (2014). An aging nation: The older population in the United States population estimates and projections. *Current Population Reports*. Retrieved from http://www.census.gov/prod/2014pubs/p25-1140.pdf

Pachana, N. A., Ford, J. H., Andrew, B., & Dobson, A. J. (2005). Relations between companion animals and self-reported health in older women: Cause, effect or artifact? *International Journal of Behavioral Medicine, 12*(2), 102–110.
Parker, G. B., Gayed, A., Owen, C. A., Hyett, M. P., Hilton, T. M., & Heruc, G. A. (2010). Survival following an acute coronary syndrome: A pet theory put to the test. *Acta Psychiatrica Scandinavica, 121*(1), 65–70.
Parslow, R. A., & Jorm, A. F. (2003a). Pet ownership and risk factors for cardiovascular disease: Another look. *Medical Journal of Australia, 179*, 466–468.
Parslow, R. A., & Jorm, A. F. (2003b). The impact of pet ownership on health and health service use: Results from a community sample of Australians aged 40–44 years. *Anthrozoös, 16*(1), 43–56.
Paskulin, L. M. G., & Molzahn, A. (2007). Quality of life of older adults in Canada and Brazil. *Western Journal of Nursing Research, 29*, 10–26.
Pauley, P. M., & Hesse, C. (2009). The effects of social support, depression, and stress on drinking behaviors in a college student sample. *Communication Studies, 60*(5), 493–508.
Paws Houston, USA. (2014). Retrieved from www.pawshouston.org/public/pag1.aspx
Pear, R. (2008). Gap in life expectancy widens for the nation. *The New York Times*. Retrieved from http://www.nytimes.com/2008/03/23/us/23health.html?_r=0
Perissinotto, C. M., Cenzer, I. S., & Covinsky, K. E. (2012). Loneliness in older persons: A predictor of functional decline and death. *Archives of Internal Medicine, 172*, 1078–1083.
Perissinotto, C. M., & Covinsky, K. E. (2014). Living alone, socially isolated or lonely—What are we measuring? *Journal of General Internal Medicine, 11*, 1429–1431.
Pet Population and Ownership Trends in the U.S. (2014). Retrieved from www.marketresearch.com
Pikhartoval, J., Bowling, A., & Victor, C. (2014). Does owning a pet protect older people against loneliness? *BMC Geriatrics, 14*, 106–116.
Pinquart, M., & Sorensen, S. (2001). Influences on loneliness in older adults: A meta-analysis. *Basic and Applied Social Psychology, 23*(4), 245–266.
Polheber, J. P., & Matchock, R. L. (2014). The presence of a dog attenuates cortisol and heart rate in the trier social stress test compared to human friends. *Journal of Behavioral Medicine, 37*, 860–867.
POOPS (Pets of Older Persons). (2015). Retrieved from http://www.poopswa.org.au/services-provided/
PR Web. (2011). New survey reveals pet ownership at its highest level in two decades and pet owners are willing to pay when it comes to pet's health. Retrieved from http://www.prweb.com/releases/2011/4/prweb8252684.htm
Raina, P., Waltner-Toews, D., Bonnett, B., Woodward, C., & Abernathy, T. (1999). Influence of companion animals on the physical and psychological health of older people: An analysis of a one-year longitudinal study. *Journal of the American Geriatrics Society, 47*, 323–329.
Ryff, C. D., & Keyes, C. L. (1995). The structure of psychological well-being revisited. *Journal of Personality and Social Psychology, 69*, 719–727.
Scheibeck, R., Pallauf, M., Stellwag, C., & Seeberger, B. (2011). Elderly people in many respects benefit from interaction with dogs. *European Journal of Medical Research, 16*, 557–563.
Schneider, M. S., & Harley, L. P. (2006). How dogs influence the evaluation of psychotherapists. *Anthrozoös, 19*(2), 128–142.
Serpell, J. (1991). Beneficial effects of pet ownership on some aspects of human health and behaviour. *Journal of the Royal Society of Medicine, 84*, 717–720.
Shiloh, S., Sorek, G., & Terkel, J. (2003). Reduction of state-anxiety by petting animals in a controlled laboratory experiment. *Anxiety Stress Coping, 16*, 387–395.
Shor, E., Roelfs, D. J., & Yogev, T. (2013). The strength of family ties: A meta-analysis and meta-regression of self-reported social support and mortality. *Social Networks, 35*, 626–638.
Siegel, J. (1990). Stressful life events and use of physician services among the elderly: The moderating role of pet ownership. *Journal of Personality and Social Psychology, 58*(6), 1081–1086.

Siegel, J. (1993). Companion animals: In sickness and in health. *Journal of Social Issues, 49*(1), 157–167.

Siegel, J. M. (2011). Pet ownership and health. In C. Blazina, G. Boyra, & D. Shen-Miller (Eds.), *The psychology of the human–animal bond* (pp. 167–177). New York: Springer.

Smith, B. (2012). The 'pet effect' health related aspects of companion animal ownership. *Australian Family Physician, 41*(6), 439–442.

Smith, J. A., Braunack-Mayer, A., Wittert, G., & Warin, M. (2007). "I've been independent for so damn long!" Independence, masculinity and aging in a help seeking context. *Journal of Ageing Studies, 21*, 325–335.

Spector-Mersel, G. (2006). Never-aging stories: Western hegemonic masculinity scripts. *Journal of Gender Studies, 15*, 67–82.

Stammbach, K. B., & Turner, D. C. (1999). Understanding the human–cat relationship: Human social support or attachment. *Anthrozoös, 12*, 162–169.

Stanley, I. H., Conwell, Y., Bowen, C., & Van Orden, K. A. (2014). Pet ownership may attenuate loneliness among older adult primary care patients who live alone. *Aging & Mental Health, 18*(3), 394–399.

Tannenbaum, C., & Frank, B. (2011). Masculinity and health in late life men. *American Journal of Men's Health, 5*(3), 243–254.

Taylor, S. E., Welch, W. T., Kim, H. S., & Sherman, D. K. (2007). Cultural differences in the impact of social support on psychological and biological stress responses. *Psychological Science, 18*(9), 831–837.

Theeke, L. A. (2010). Sociodemographic and health-related risks for loneliness and outcome differences by loneliness status in a sample of U.S. older adults. *Research in Gerontological Nursing, 3*, 113–125.

Thoits, P. A. (2010). Stress and health: Major findings and policy implications. *Journal of Health and Social Behavior, 51*(1), 41–53.

Thoits, P. A. (2011). Mechanisms linking social ties and support to physical and mental health. *Journal of Health and Social Behavior, 52*, 145–161.

Thorpe, R. J., Kreisle, R. A., Glickman, L. T., Simonsick, E. M., Newman, A. B., & Kritchevsky, S. (2006). Physical activity and pet ownership in year 3 of the health ABC study. *Journal of Aging and Physical Activity, 14*, 154–168.

Thurston, R. C., & Kubzansky, L. D. (2009). Women, loneliness, and incident coronary heart disease. *Psychosomatic Medicine, 71*, 836–842.

Toohey, A. M., McCormack, G. R., Doyle-Baker, P. K., Adams, C. L., & Rock, M. J. (2013). Dog walking and sense of community in neighborhoods: implications for promoting regular physical activity in adults 50 years and older. *Health Place, 22*, 75–81.

Toohey, A. M., & Rock, M. J. (2011). Unleashing their potential: A critical realist scoping review of the influence of dogs on physical activity for dog-owners and non-owners. *International Journal of Behavioral Nutrition and Physical Activity, 8*, 46.

Uchino, B. N. (2006). Social support and health: A review of physiological processes potentially underlying links to disease outcomes. *Journal of Behavioral Medicine, 29*, 377–387.

Udell, J. A., Steg, P. G., Scirica, B. M., Smith, S. C., Ohman, M. E., Eagle, K. A., et al. (2012). Living alone and cardiovascular risk in outpatients at risk of or with atherothrombosis. *Archives of Internal Medicine, 172*, 1086–1095.

Vacha-Haase, T., Wester, S. R., & Fowell-Christianson, H. (2011). *Psychotherapy with older men*. New York: Routledge Taylor and Francis Group.

Van Grootheest, D. S., Beekman, A. T. F., Broese van Groenou, M. I., & Deeg, D. J. H. (1999). Sex differences in depression after widowhood. Do men suffer more? *Social Psychiatry and Psychiatric Epidemiology, 34*, 391–398.

Victor, C. R., & Yang, K. (2012). The prevalence of loneliness among adults: A case study of the United Kingdom. *The Journal of Psychology, 146*, 85–104.

Walsh, F. (2009). Human–animal bonds I: The relational significance of companion animals. *Family Process, 48*(4), 462–480.

Wells, D. L. (2004). The facilitation of social interactions by domestic dogs. *Anthrozoös, 17*, 340–352.
Wells, D. L. (2009). The effects of animals on human health and well-being. *Journal of Social Issues, 65*, 523–543.
Wilson, R. S., Krueger, K. R., Arnold, S. E., Schneider, J. A., Kelly, J. F., Barnes, L. L., et al. (2007). Loneliness and risk of Alzheimer disease. *Archives of General Psychiatry, 64*, 234–240.
Wilson, C., & Moulton, B. (2010). *Loneliness among older adults: A national survey of adults 45+*. Washington, D.C.: AARP Inc.
Wood, L. J., Giles-Corti, B., Bulsara, M. K., & Bosch, D. A. (2007). More than a furry companion: The ripple effect of companion animals on neighborhood interactions and sense of community. *Society Animals, 15*(1), 43–56.
Yu, L., Boyle, P. A., Wilson, R. S., Levine, S. R., Schneider, J. A., & Bennett, D. A. (2015). Purpose in life and cerebral infarcts in community-dwelling older people. *Stroke, 46*, 1071–1076.
Zaslavsky, O., Rillamas-Sun, E., Woods, N. F., Cochrane, B. B., Stefanick, M. L., Tindle, H., et al. (2014). Association of the selected dimensions of eudaimonic well-being with healthy survival to 85 years of age in older women. *International Psychogeriatrics, 26*, 2081–2091.

Chapter 14
Older Adults, Pets, and Intergenerational Service Learning

Lori Kogan

This chapter expands on the topic addressed in Chap. 13. The previous chapter focused on older adults, men in particular, and pet ownership. It provided the foundation for this chapter by exploring the psychological and physiological benefits of pet ownership for older adults, and how important this relationship is for many seniors. The current chapter explores one way to support this bond—intergenerational service learning. The chapter begins with helping set the stage by providing an overview of how older adults are viewed in the United States. It then moves into describing service learning, including intergenerational service learning, before moving into a description of a specific intergenerational service learning program designed to support older adults' bond with their companion animals.

Older Adults in U.S.

What defines "old age" or "older adults" is certainly relative, and the age at which people are viewed as old has changed dramatically over time. Not long ago, few people even reached the age of 65 or older ("Aging and Ageism" 2012), but life expectancy in the United States has been steadily increasing. Life expectancy in 1900 was 47 years, compared to 77 years in 2000 and over 78 years in 2010 (Arias 2010).

The demographic distribution of older adults in the U.S. is different than the rest of the population. For example, females make up 57 % of Americans aged 65 or

L. Kogan (✉)
Clinical Sciences Department, College of Veterinary Medicine and Biomedical Sciences, Colorado State University, 1601 Campus Delivery,
Fort Collins, CO 80523, USA
e-mail: Lori.kogan@colostate.edu

C. Blazina and L.R. Kogan (eds.), *Men and Their Dogs*,
DOI 10.1007/978-3-319-30097-9_14

older. Racially, 80 % are non-Latino whites (compared to 66 % in the population as a whole); 8.6 % are African American (compared to 13 % of the population); and 7.0 % are Latino (compared to 15 % of the population) (Census Data 2012). The number of Americans 65 or older as a percentage of the population is expected to continue to rise. While they comprised 4.1 % of the population in 1900, they are expected to reach 20.2 % by 2050. Labeled the "*graying of America*," this increase will have important repercussions for the elderly, as well as the individuals and support services caring for them ("Aging and Ageism" 2012).

In many countries, the elderly are valued and revered (e.g., China, India, Korea, etc.). Unfortunately, this is not the prevenient attitude in the U.S. (Hernandez and Gonzalez 2008). Several studies have documented the negative attitudes of the U.S. population toward older adults (e.g., Gugliucci and Weiner 2013; Sink 2015). Often, older adults as seen as an undesirable outside separate group, rather than viewing aging as a natural developmental process. Many see becoming old as an inevitable decline or fading away-leading to dependence, depression, and isolation. As a result of these views, many attempt to emotionally distance themselves from the elderly. Unfortunately, this only reinforces the misconceptions, because younger generations are not able to interact with elderly and have an opportunity to reshape their perceptions (Sink 2015). Given the lack of actual contact, ageism in the media only perpetuates the problem (Diamond 2013).

The reasons behind ageism are complex and multifaceted, but one theory is the U.S. culture's emphasis on individualism, independence, and the Protestant work ethic. These values result in much of a person's identity and worth tied to his/her ability to work (Martinez-Carter 2013). To compound this problem, older Americans often face age discrimination in job selection. Despite numerous studies showing that older workers offer many advantages over younger employees, ageism is common in the workplace (Reade 2013). Thus, even for older adults who are able and willing to work, finding employment can be challenging. This is especially true for technology-related jobs. Many technology companies, for example, post openings exclusively for new or recent college graduates as a way to avoid directly stating they are only interested in younger candidates. Facebook, for example, recently settled a lawsuit involving a job posting for an attorney in which they specified a specific graduating class as preferred (2007 or 2008). These issues make it challenging for many older adults to continue being gainfully employed.

In addition to difficulties maintaining or obtaining employment, other factors influence the likelihood of dependence and isolation for older Americans, including family structure and geographical location choices. More people are choosing to remain single without children as well as move more frequently and both of these factors reduce the opportunity for family support (Diamond 2013).

The issues facing many older adults create the need to explore innovative ways to help support their physical and psychological health. As discussed in the previous chapter, pet ownership is one such option. Pets offer numerous physical, psychological, and social benefits, though a significant number of older adults face challenges related to caring for a pet. To help preserve and encourage this human–animal bond, some organizations have worked to create supportive solutions. In addition to such organizations, another option worth exploring is that of service learning, which provides a way to reach beyond the scope of improving the lives of older adults and their pets to include an educational element that can positively impact another generation.

Pets Forever (PF) is an example of this type of program. The rest of this chapter will cover two major topics: the first part will explore service learning, with an emphasis on intergenerational opportunities, and the remaining part of the chapter will describe in detail PF, a program created to provide a unique opportunity to students, while helping fulfill the needs of vulnerable pet owners in the community.

Service Learning and Community Service

The willingness to give of oneself to improve one's community is universally viewed as a desirable trait and has been equated with higher levels of human development. As Maslow explained many years ago, self-actualized people have a deep feeling of empathy, sympathy, and compassion for human beings in general (Maslow 1954). Fortunately, the desire to give back to one's community is something that can be fostered and nurtured (Dharamsi et al. 2010); colleges and universities can help foster this character strength, for both men and women, through service learning.

Service learning, a form of community-based education, is a structured learning activity that balances service and learning (Bringle et al. 2004; Hood 2009). Service learning, as defined by Eyler and Giles (1999), is a teaching and learning methodology which fosters civic responsibility and applies classroom learning through meaningful service to the community. It combines formal coursework with community service in a way that promotes specific academic learning objectives, responds to community-identified needs, and is based on the premise that students can become better citizens when given opportunities to experience and understand complex social problems and apply what they learn (Eyler and Giles 1999). Bringle and Hatcher's (1995) definition of service learning focuses more on community needs: they define service learning as an educational experience in which students participate in an organized service activity that meets an identified community need, and are given the opportunity to reflect on the service as a way to encourage an enhanced sense of personal values and civic responsibility.

Examples of service learning include a communication course in which students prepare public relation materials for nonprofit organizations, education courses in which students provide after school tutoring with at-risk students, or accounting courses where students offer free tax preparation assistance to low-income clients.

Service-learning courses accomplish several goals. They provide students with experiences that allow them to gain a broader appreciation of their discipline and an enhanced sense of civic responsibility (Ash et al. 2005; Eyler et al. 2001; Pelco et al. 2014). Although studies have found that women have higher levels of participation in community service compared to men, both during school and as working adults (e.g., Trudeau and Devlin 1996; Miller 1994), it has been suggested that increased emphasis by schools on service during men's formative years might help change students' behaviors related to service after graduation (Smith 2005) and improve the chances that they will engage in more community service as working adults (Ash et al. 2005; Celio et al. 2011; Markus et al. 1993; Vogelgesang and Astin 2000). Students in dental schools help exemplify this benefit. For example, it has been suggested that dentists' willingness to treat the underserved can be influenced during dental school (Coe et al. 2014; Holtzman and Seirawan 2009; Davidson et al. 2009). More exposure and experience in providing care to the underserved, especially in community settings, has been shown to improve dental students' awareness of community needs and their willingness to provide community service to those in need (Smith et al. 2006).

In addition to positively impacting later service-related behaviors, service-learning experiences have been shown to improve students' academic performance (Zacherman and Foubert 2014). Several studies have shown that involvement in cocurricular activities can improve GPA (Carini et al. 2006; Gordon et al. 2008; Kuh et al. 2008), critical thinking skills (Pike 2004), and increase the likelihood of disadvantaged students successfully graduating (Kuh 2009). Service learning can also impact students' career decisions by increasing awareness of career options, offering practical and professional experience, and reinforcing the value of a career that serves others (Blieszner and Artale 2001; Eyler et al. 1997; Fenzel and Leary 1997).

A modification of Schwartz's model of altruistic behavior can be useful when examining relationships between service learning and the formation of students' helping behaviors and attitudes (Schwartz 1977). This model includes four steps:

Step 1 Activation—students perceive a need to respond, in the form of awareness of the need and feeling connected to the people in need.
Step 2 Obligation—students feel a moral obligation to respond to the need through a personal and situational norm and empathy.
Step 3 Defense—students reconsider costs and benefits of helping, and then reassess the situation and become serious of the need to respond.
Step 4 Response—students develop intention to engage in the community service.

With this model in mind, there are some suggested pedagogical strategies instructors can use to enhance the success of service learning courses (Roodin et al. 2013). They include the following:

Preparation: Assess the community issue to be addressed through service, evaluate the resources required for success, create relationships with community partners, and make the commitment to creating the course.
Action: Develop the course content, including specific objectives and goals; prepare students for service through training and in-class experiences. Faculty must not assume they know what students are taking with them into the service

experience, nor should they assume that students are knowledgeable about what critical reflection is, or how it is done. To that end, Stogner (2004) suggested that faculty conduct lectures on critical thinking prior to students engaging in their service experiences. Similarly, Viggiani (2004) focused on ways to prepare students with "pre-service reflection," and provided readers with a reflection assignment format and a template for how faculty might review reflective journal entries. The next step in action is to initiate the service component of the course, monitor students' engagement, and assess how well the course is meeting the needs of the community partners.

Reflection: Develop opportunities for students to process their experiences, relate them to course content, examine personal values and beliefs, and explore personal feelings and reactions.

Reward: Celebrate students' accomplishments and use campus and local media to help showcase successes of the course.

Assessment: Conduct ongoing outcomes evaluation of students, clients, and community agencies; use this data to drive changes for future development (Roodin et al. 2013).

Because of the potential benefits, more colleges are implementing and supporting service-learning courses as one way to improve comprehension of course content, develop life skills, and create a greater awareness of community, service, and civic responsibility (Kalisch et al. 2013; Astin and Sax 1998; Batchelder and Root 1994; Eyler and Giles 1999; Hamon and Way 2001; Roodin et al. 2013). One specific type of service learning that is gaining popularity is intergenerational service learning.

Intergenerational Contact

As discussed earlier, the perceptions of older adults in the U.S. involve many negative stereotypical views. The elderly are seen by many as feeble, burdensome, inflexible, and having little to offer to their communities (Cohen et al. 2004; Sauer 2006; Kimuna et al. 2005). College students tend to embrace these negative stereotypes more often than other age cohorts (Lovell 2006; Cohen et al. 2004). The views of college students toward elderly are often validated by media messages that frequently support negative stereotypes (Lovell 2006).

As suggested by social identity theory, in an effort to maintain a positive self-identity, individuals attempt to identify themselves as members of a specific group, thereby creating clear distinctions between themselves and other groups. For college students, this can result in younger adults having unfavorable or negative attitudes toward the elderly and seeing themselves as fundamentally different and better than older adults (Kalisch et al. 2013; Lovell 2006).

Yet, as the U.S. population continues to grow older, there will be an increasing need for people who want to work with older adults. For many fields, however, this presents significant challenges. For example, in the medical field, the number of physicians who specialize in the health care of older adults (geriatricians) decreased by 33 % between 1998 and 2004, and continues to decline (Gugliucci and Weiner 2013). It is estimated that by 2030 only 2.5 geriatricians will be available for every 10,000 adults age 75 and older. Since the older cohort is expected to double by 2030, a severe shortage is anticipated (American Geriatrics Society 2011). Unfortunately, many doctors do not feel comfortable caring for older adults (Gawande 2007). Only 7 % of pharmacy students, for example, describe older adults using a majority of positive terms (Sauer 2006). Lack of interest in this field will make it challenging to replace retiring geriatricians, let alone meet a growing demand. Given this backdrop, college students' career choice surrounding older adults is one of particular importance (Lovell 2006; Sauer 2006).

On a more encouraging note, there is some evidence that students who have the opportunity to interact with older adults have more positive attitudes toward them, and toward aging in general. Several studies have found that younger adults who have direct contact with older adults have fewer negative attitudes toward the elderly (O'Hanlon and Brookover 2002; Schwartz and Simmons 2001; Kite et al. 2005; Regan and Fazio 1977; Tiller and Fazio 1982). Since exposure and contact can make a difference, it is critically important that schools create opportunities to help change perceptions and foster an interest in working with older adults. It is for these reasons that intergenerational service learning has become an important component in many academic programs (Karasik 2013).

Intergenerational service learning, in which members of different age cohorts work together to achieve personal or academic goals, has been shown to be effective in reducing negative perceptions of aging populations (Kalisch et al. 2013; O'Hanlon and Brookover 2002; Vandsberger and Wakefield 2008; Knapp and Stubblefield 2000; McCrea et al. 1999). Additionally, these courses have been shown to provide "real-life" experience and knowledge about elder care and human service issues (Westacott and Hegeman 1996), dispel myths about aging and older persons (Karasik and Berke 2001; Krout et al. 2010; Whitbourne et al. 2001), increase students' understanding of the aging process (Blieszner and Artale 2001; Whitbourne et al. 2001), help students translate related theories into practice (Faria et al. 2010; Horowitz et al. 2010; Karasik and Berke 2001), and encourage students to choose careers in the field of aging (Blieszner and Artale 2001; Horowitz et al. 2010).

Studies by Dorfman et al. (2002), as well as those by Bringle and Kremer (1993), found that students who had been involved in service learning reported feeling less fearful of their own aging, were more likely to feel positive about the elderly, and had higher expectations of life in old age when compared to those who had not engaged in service learning. Roodin (2002) also found that service learning enhances students' understanding of course material and increases enthusiasm for the topic when compared to a traditional lecture course.

Other researchers have found similar positive attitude changes as a consequence of service learning (Ames and Diepstra 2006; Beling 2003; Blieszner and Artale 2001; Brown and Roodin 2001; Gutheil et al. 2006; Hegeman et al. 2002; Karasik et al. 2004; Krout et al. 2010). Hanks (2001), for example, conducted a study with gerontology and business students working with older adults in discipline-specific service-learning activities. At posttest, these students' attitudes toward older workers showed less negative stereotyping compared to pretest scores. Even more promising is the likelihood that service-learning experiences create long-term changes. One longitudinal study reported that changes identified in students who participated in a service-learning course were evident years after they graduated from college (Fenzel and Peyrot 2005).

Intergenerational service-learning courses, in addition to offering all these benefits to students, also help address community social issues by combining the strengths and resources of universities and communities to address real-world issues (Roodin et al. 2013). Intergenerational service learning creates partnerships that help communities address local issues. Many communities begin to count on these partnerships, thereby allowing them to build new programs, strengthen service delivery in older programs, improve the ratio of volunteers to older adult participants, provide relief to overburdened staff, and address underserved groups of elders or increase awareness of a community need that has heretofore gone unnoticed (Roodin et al. 2013). Pets Forever—Supporting the Life-long Bond (PF), a successful example of intergenerational service learning, operates in such a community.

PF is a seven-year-old intergenerational service-learning course offered at Colorado State University (CSU), as well as an organization working in collaboration with the nonprofit arm of the school: CSU Foundation. The goal of PF is to preserve and promote the human–animal bond by helping low-income elderly and disabled local residents keep their pets as long as possible, while improving the health and well-being of these pets and owners. The program accomplishes this by providing a variety of needed assistance and resources. PF works closely with numerous community organizations that support low-income elderly and disabled, such as CSU's Clinical Sciences Department, the CSU Veterinary Teaching Hospital, several private veterinary practitioners, local animal companies and animal groomers, as well as other nonprofit organizations that function to serve this population. As of January 2016, PF has helped over 350 clients (and currently serves approximately 155) with an average of 378 service/outreach hours each week.

PF's primary mission is the provision of direct services to clients and their pets, including companion dog walking (walking with the owner and their pet), independent dog walking, litter box scooping and cleaning, cleaning enclosures of caged pets, nail trims, bathing, brushing, feeding, yard feces removal, and transportation to/from animal-related appointments. In addition to in-home care, PF provides a full range of other health and well-being services; such services include a sponsored food program, the pick up, delivery, and administration of pet medications, and regular grooming services.

The associated service-learning course offers benefits to the University that include local and national recognition as a leader in an innovative, unique service learning, nonprofit program and helps foster positive community relationships through ongoing collaborative relationships with numerous local agencies. The community also benefits from the program through a greater awareness of the benefits that pets have for older and/or disabled individuals, a wider acceptance of older and/or disabled individuals having pets that can contribute toward the stability of these vulnerable populations as well as reducing the number of animals relinquished to local animal shelters.

PF provides students from diverse educational backgrounds with an opportunity to gain valuable real-life experience while simultaneously earning college credit. Although PF has several volunteers from the community, a major part of PF's mission is the enrichment of students' experience through the opportunity to gain community service experience. The students involved with the program include undergraduate, graduate, international, and professional veterinary students.

The course is offered as a three-credit, advanced-level undergraduate course, as well as a three-credit graduate course. Enrolled students come from all majors and departments. Approximately, 60–65 % of the students are pre-veterinary students (majoring in biology, animal sciences, etc.) who are interested in obtaining experience working directly with animals. These pre-veterinary students are able to gain valuable volunteer animal contact hours and community service, which are two critical areas assessed by veterinary school admissions committees. In fact, several previous and current PF volunteers have successfully been admitted into veterinary programs. The remaining 35–40 % of students are interested in gaining experience working with vulnerable populations and come from majors such as psychology, social work, human development and family studies, and occupational therapy.

Veterinary students are an additional group impacted by the course. These students interact with PF clients and pets as part of the program's veterinary care services. PF gives these students the opportunity to gain practical experience working with low-income elderly and disabled community pet owners—a population they otherwise have minimal exposure to. Because CSU's veterinary teaching hospital, like most teaching hospitals, is a tertiary care facility, cases tend to focus on more advanced veterinary care and many of the pet owners who visit the hospital have the funds necessary to provide advanced medical care to their pets. Yet, many students upon graduation will be employed at clinics serving clients with limited funds who are forced to make difficult choices regarding the health care of their pet. For this reason, the clients of PF are felt to be more representative of a large segment of clients these students will serve after graduation. It is viewed favorably, therefore, that PF helps these fourth year veterinary students practice practical skills including the following:

- Discussing clients' financial constraints and adjusting treatment and recommendations accordingly
- Communicating with disabled pet owners who have cognitive or physical limitations that can make clear communication more difficult
- Learning to adapt to treatment or follow up plans to match clients' physical and intellectual abilities
- Communicating through a third party (in this case, a PF volunteer) when owners are not able to communicate directly.

One additional group of students who participate with PF worth noting is international students. For these students, PF offers the opportunity to view a very different aspect of American culture than what they are exposed to while on campus. They are able to practice their English skills in a different 'real world' environment and create relationships with Americans they would not have had an opportunity to interact with otherwise. For many of these students, what often begins as a very anxiety-producing experience (e.g., calling strangers on the phone, making small talk with clients) quickly morphs into an enriched cultural experience, both for the students as well as the clients. One additional unique factor of PF is that it is one of the few classes where freshmen and graduate aged students have a chance to interact and collaborate.

Course Objectives

The course focuses on several specific objectives. Students are informed that as a result of this course, they will accomplish the following: Based on firsthand experience, students will demonstrate the ability to make a difference in the lives of others, their companion animals, and the community. Students will acquire communication techniques useful in working with vulnerable populations and the medical and animal care community, and demonstrate these skills by developing effective relationships with Pets Forever clients.

- Students will become proficient in applying needs identification strategies in real life situations to assist individual clients.
- Students will acquire critical reasoning skills by being involved with the problem solving that naturally comes from working with a dynamically changing program and clientele.
- Students will develop presentation skills and practice techniques to promote the Pets Forever program through professional work ethic and behavior.
- Students will reflect on the nature of their weekly experiences by communicating their experiences with the course instructors and classmates.

Making sure these objectives are met is accomplished in part by explicitly stating the expectations of all students. These requirements include attending the weekly 1-h class and providing 5 h of community service per week. The class period is the only set time each week; the rest of students' schedules are self-determined. With over 155 active clients to select from, students are able to select which clients they would like to work with based on client and pet characteristics, services needed, and days/times requested. Once students select their clients, they retain these clients for the semester so they are able to establish long-term relationships with both the owners and their pets.

Each class period begins with a 'check-in' process in which students share their experiences from the previous week. These might be concerns or issues about an owner or animal, or a positive experience they want to share. Since many of the clients are seen by more than one student each week, it is a great time for students to interact with other students who are providing services to the same client. There are many examples of when this type of communication is vital. For example, if a client is not home when one student goes to visit, it is important to determine the well-being of this client. Therefore, it is important to look for trends: did another student discover the client was not home? If so, this warrants further and immediate attention. Since many of the clients have limited contact with others besides PF volunteers, the program also serves as a safety net for these pet owners. PF volunteers are often the first ones to become aware of a client's changing health status (e.g., hospitalization, accidents at home, etc.). It is therefore a critical part of the program to maintain constant communication between instructors and students to help ensure rapid transmission of important information. In fact, one requirement of the course is for students to respond to all email correspondence within 24 h to ensure that important information does not fall between the cracks.

After students check-in each week, the remaining time in most class periods is filled with guest speakers from the community. Approximately, 50 % of the speakers come from local animal-related organizations (e.g., rescue shelters, humane society, pet food assistance, etc.) and the other 50 % come from organizations that service the population which PF supports. Examples include the Alzheimer's' Association, the MS Society, the Food bank, etc. In this way, students are exposed to a variety of local nonprofits designed to support vulnerable people and their pets. Feedback from students has suggested that they often have little prior access or knowledge of such programs.

In addition to their service, all students are required to complete a reflection paper that summarizes their experiences, thoughts, and insights gained from the class. Students are given the choice of either focusing their paper on one client or overall reflections related to their service work. To provide additional guidance, students are told the following:

- The reflection should be a true reflection of your experience with PF, rather than just a recap/summary of what happened.
- The reflection should be in context of the material discussed in class and the course learning objectives.
- Personal feelings are encouraged, but professional writing is expected.
- The reflection should demonstrate your ability to synthesize the experiences gained during the service-learning components of class.

The actual topic of the reflection paper can address any one or more of the following questions:

- In general, what are the most important things that you have learned through your experiences with PF?
- Discuss your experiences with one particular client and how this has changed your perceptions.
- How did your experiences affect the way you think about the issues and/or clients that PF deals with?

- What have you learned about social inequality through your service work?
- What have you learned about yourself from your service this semester?

At the end of the semester, students are asked to share their reflection papers with the class via a 5–7 min informal presentation that summarizes the key points of their paper, as well as reflections on their experience with PF. These papers and presentations provide a wonderful opportunity to assess students' perceptions of the class in addition to giving them the opportunity to personally reflect. These reflections, in addition to the informal discussions in class, help students explore their changing perceptions of the elderly and their unique experiences with each client.

Many students, through experiences with an intergenerational service learning course, began to change their previously negative perceptions of the elderly and see them in a new way (Kalisch et al. 2013; Davies et al. 2013). Similar to other research (Kalisch et al. 2013; Davies et al. 2013), we find students' reflections and experiences include descriptions of how impressed they felt by how their clients handle challenging situations, and how the experience has helped them reflect on their own personal biases and stereotypes of older people and aging. Many students talk about their own personal growth, and how they have gained a new perspective on the problems in their own lives. Often times, they come to recognize that these problems were not as big as they had originally thought they were. They meet clients who have struggled with tremendous problems and challenges, and they often report feeling a great deal of respect and inspiration. Students talk about the fact that many thought that older people would be unhappy and bitter, yet they find this is usually not the case.

Student quotes that illustrate these themes include the following:

> What really surprised me was how attached I became to all of my clients.

> This class was much more than spending time with animals; it opened my eyes to this whole other part of the community that I have unfortunately never thought much about.

> It is like having my grandmother here in Colorado instead of across the country.

Some students are able to take the experience and make significant changes in their lives related to their priorities, their concerns, and their plans for the future.

> As corny as it sounds, Pets Forever has taught me that life is fleeting and every moment and situation should not be taken advantage of, but rather cherished and appreciated.

> I absolutely love just sitting down with my clients after taking care of their animals and asking them about their week and letting them know that someone does care about what is going on in their life.

For some students, this experience has changed how they view aging; similar results were also documented by Dorfman et al. (2002) and Kalisch et al. (2013), who found that service-learning students were less fearful and more comfortable with the concept of their own aging.

Each semester, there are several students who feel anxious about calling 'strangers' on the phone and going to their home. They often have inaccurate perceptions of older or disabled adults and worry about how they will be able to communicate or relate. Inevitably, they return to class with stories about how 'normal' these people are, and how similar they are to the student in so many ways. The speed in which false impressions are dispelled each semester is always a joy to witness. One student, for example, came to class amazed that she and her client enjoy the same country western singer, and they 'celebrated' by listening to music together. Other students have reported their enjoyment in sharing television shows or talking about current events.

> I used to think that older people were so different, but I now realize how much in common I have with many of my clients.

> In reality, the way that my generation views most senior citizens (usually as frail, uptight people hopelessly stuck in the past) could not be more mistaken.

Students find they easily connect and form close relationships with their clients. Part of the reason for these types of connections is the repeated, regular contact students have with their clients over the course of the semester. Most students visited their clients at least once a week (and often more) for the entire semester.

> Not only did I get to know some of my clients on a personal basis, a lot of the time, they made my day much better than how it was going before I showed up at their houses.

> On days when I could stay longer, she would make snacks and just eat and chat with me for a long while until I needed to head home.

> It shocked me when my clients took such an interest in my life. To see them actually want to know about me and the things going on with me was unexpected.

> And this is precisely the magic of PF: While I spent time romping with canine companions, I also discovered how to become a better companion to humans.

For many students, these revelations translate into positive changes in their own personal relationships. Many students are able to engage in intimate life conversations with their clients that end up positively altering relationships with their own family, partners, and even themselves.

> Not only have my clients helped me to open up and become more comfortable with communicating, but also they have shown me how to care for others and taught me to appreciate and be thankful for all that I have.

Many students also reflect on how visits with their clients help them put things in perspective. Others discuss the reciprocal nature of the visits, recognizing that they both (student and older adult) benefit from the visits.

> Suddenly all of my daily problems seem trivial and I find myself just giving thanks.

> I have come to the realization that there are numerous people in the world less fortunate than I am, and Pets Forever has opened my eyes to how lucky I am to have the life that I have.

> This semester has taught me so much. The biggest thing I've learned is to be grateful for the life I live and how blessed I am. As well as appreciating every day I am alive, and every day I get to spend with people I love.

Although many students initally feel anxious about interacting with older adults, for most, this quickly changes to a feeling of comfort and enjoyment. As reported by (Roodin 2002), many students become excited to witness how they are able to make a difference for these clients.

> These clients are beyond appreciative of the organization's help and it feels great knowing we are making a difference.

> The amazing feeling I receive by helping make people happy is something I have never felt before and it is more rewarding than receiving a good grade or spending time with dogs and cats. It is an addictive feeling and now that I have experienced it I never want it to go away. Pets Forever has changed my life forever and made me a better person inside and out.

> When I thought of helping people, I would always think that I had to do something drastic to change their life in a positive way. Now I realize that the little things can make the biggest differences.

> I learned from this experience that as a volunteer/ helper we really do make a difference to their lives.

> Pets Forever has been a huge factor in helping me become a more patient and kind person.

> Pets Forever has definitely helped me this semester stay stress free and has taught me that giving back to the community through volunteering is probably the most important concept we should learn.

Once students have moved past their misconceptions and stereotypes, they grow increasingly able to connect on a deeper level. Students in PF change their perceptions of the elderly; such results are supported by previous research that indicates that experience with older adults can increase positive attitudes toward this population (O'Hanlon and Brookover 2002; Schwartz and Simmons 2001). Many students have reported that the experience has led them to reconsider their career path, or add a gerontology component; an increased interest in gerontology that has also been noted by Kalisch (2013).

It is not surprising that at the end of the semester, many students choose to remain involved with their clients. Many students opt to enroll in the course the following semester, largely to maintain the relationships they have created. For many, these clients have become surrogate family. As one student explained, he feels like he has several grandparents in town now, helping him make the adjustment to a new school much easier. Other students who are unable to take the course again, or are graduating, choose to stay in contact with their clients in less formal ways.

In addition to information obtained from students regarding the course, client feedback is collected regularly via personal interviews and surveys in order to assess the impacts of program. Statements from clients indicate the value and importance they feel that PF has in their lives and the lives of their pets.

The following three male clients' stories help illustrate the impact of the program.

James is a war veteran who has spent a great deal of time homeless, yet despite these challenges, he has been able to keep his 'best friend,' a small Shih Tzu, for nearly 15 years. Recently, James was able to secure housing and he and Harley are doing well in their new home. James has explained that with the help of PF, he has been able to keep Harley fed and healthy even during his most challenging times.

Daniel is a client who is blind and spends most of his time in a wheelchair. He is able to enjoy the companionship of his cat, Winston, with the help of the PF program. Through the program, volunteers help Daniel with the care and maintenance of Winston, thereby preventing Daniel from having to live alone.

Tim is one more example of the type of client that PF helps. Tim moved into an assisted living facility after suffering from congestive heart failure, whereby he inherited a 12-year-old cat, Darcy, from a previous resident. Darcy quickly became Tim's best friend and has greatly improved his quality of life. With PF's help, Tim has been able to keep Darcy, whom he credits for helping him meet the challenge of adapting from living independently to residing in an assisted living facility.

These clients benefit not only from the comfort of knowing they are able to keep and care for their pets, but also from the companionship offered by PF students. For these clients, interactions with the students are the highlight of their week, and nearly all of the clients create strong, long-lasting relationships with their students over the course of the semester.

Program Expansion and Research

From the inception of PF, the vision of the program was to expand to other communities, and plans for expansion are currently underway. It is felt that any community that has any type of college or university (including community colleges) could implement such a program. For this reason, PF has created a 'blueprint' to share with other communities in an effort to expand this program throughout the country.

Additionally, the program offers an opportunity to conduct research. For example, the positive change in mood expressed by students after they visit with clients is one area deemed worthy of exploration. One ongoing study is to assess these mood changes by having volunteers record their moods before and after their visits using a mobile application on their phone designed to monitor mood.

Additional follow up with students involved with PF is to see if they feel it has impacted their choices pertaining to altruistic behaviors during their final years at school and beyond. Studies suggest that women demonstrate higher levels of community service as adults, when compared to men (Miller 1994; Trudeau and Devlin 1996), and one suggestion to positively impact this has been for schools to offer opportunities to serve that men are interested in (Smith 2005); therefore, tracking our male students will be especially important.

In our efforts to monitor the impact of the program on the clients, PF conducts annual interviews to assess clients' thoughts and feelings related to the program. Although this data is difficult to quantify, it has helped the program identify ways in which clients feel it has benefits them beyond just caring for their pet. There are plans to continue these yearly interviews to collect data on new clients and obtain more long-term data on clients who have been with the program for several years. It is likely that the program helps older men become more open to receiving the support and care they might need, not only for their pets, but also for themselves. Assessment of this benefit would be helpful in the future.

Conclusion

The sentiments and experiences of PF students and the PF clients are not unique, as other studies have reported similar positive results. Dorfman et al. (2002) and Hegeman et al. (2002), for example, found both college students and seniors report positive companionship, social stimulation, and improved quality of life after participating in service learning. Other studies have noted an increased interest among students in working with older adults after participating in service learning with elders (Brown and Roodin 2001; Gutheil et al. 2006; Kolb 2008) as well as increased confidence in their abilities to communicate with elders, positive personal growth, increased empathy, decreased fear about their own aging, and feelings of empowerment (Ames and Diepstra 2006; Blieszner and Artale 2001; Brown and Roodin 2001; Dorfman et al. 2004). Students report a strong sense of satisfaction, often reflecting a dramatic positive shift in their attitudes toward the program from beginning to end. It is not surprising, therefore, that Dorfman et al. (2002), when comparing students who chose a service-learning option over a research project in an introductory gerontology course, found the service-learning group had more positive feelings about older adults and the possibility of working with them in the future than students who choose a research project; as many PF students have stated, service-learning involvement was their best college experience (see Brown and Roodin 2001; Dorfman et al. 2002; Hegeman et al. 2002).

Ways to enhance the college experience, especially for males, is critically important. Compared to females, fewer males are attending college, and those who attend college are graduating less often, obtaining lower grades, and pursuing advanced degrees less frequently (Weaver-Hightower 2010; Capraro 2014). While overall post-baccalaureate enrollment increased 36 % between 2000 and 2010, the number of females enrolled between 2000 and 2010 rose by 42 % compared to 28 % for males (Snyder 2014). Today, there are over 31 % more women on campus than men (Vedder 2014). Given these conditions, it has been suggested that universities have a compelling interest in making college a more viable and attractive option to a broad range of men (Weaver-Hightower 2010). Creating supportive infrastructure to help men succeed is critical. To address this issue, Weaver-Hightower (2010) has recommended schools create social opportunities that go beyond sports and other stereotypically male activities, including community service opportunities. The emphasis on community service or service learning is consistent with data related to how to best engage millennials.

Drawing from the research on millennials (people born 1980–2002), one major factor that helps these individuals be more engaged is to help give them opportunities to do things that have meaning; to make a difference. A Pew Research Center study reported that millennials place a higher priority on helping people in need (21 %) than having a high-paying career (15 %). Beyond marriage and family, 21 % of millennials say that helping people who are in need is one of the most important things in their life (Taylor and Keeter 2010). The positive feelings related to volunteering are only expected to grow, given the trends seen in the next generation. Over 77 % of Gen Z. for example, has been found to be extremely or very interested in volunteering, and over a quarter of them are currently volunteering (Schawbel 2014). These trends fit within the altruistic model proposed by Schwartz (1977) in which he indicated that altruistic behavior is influenced by the intensity of moral obligation which someone feels to take helping actions as well as their life experiences. PF might be the type of experience that helps developing young men make choices that focus more on relationships, and less on the more traditional gender roles of individualism and stoicism. Given that both the millennial and Gen Z cohorts appear to feel this obligation and desire to give back to their communities, it is likely that they will continue to exhibit high levels of giving behaviors. The impact of this type of program in these areas certainly warrants further research and exploration.

An intergenerational service learning program like PF is one way to help address this need. Caring for animals is an 'easy sell' for many male students and does not conflict with masculinity norms like some other types of volunteerism or community service might. Through this type of program, schools can increase engagement of male students, thereby positively impacting educational efforts and perhaps even patterns of social engagement upon graduation. Intergenerational service learning programs are indeed win/win proposals and should receive increasing recognition and support as ways to provide solutions for several pressing societal concerns.

> Everyone needs a hand to hold on to. Don't need to be no strong hand, don't need to be no rich hand - everyone just needs a hand to hold on to.
>
> John Mellencamp

As discussed in the previous chapter, social isolation is a challenge for many older men, and due to the masculine scripts held by many, they struggle to ask for or receive the help they need. Examples of these scripts, as defined by Mahalik et al. (2003), include the 'strong and silent,' and the 'tough-guy.' These types of scripts can limit the type of help men might be willing to accept, but can leave the door open for help related to their pet. PF offers a way to reach older men who have subscribed to the gender roles common to their generation. While in other areas of their lives they can continue to display restricted emotionality and affectionate behaviors, pets (and as an extension, caregivers of pets) create a safe outlet for otherwise unexpressed feelings and need for companionship and connection. Perhaps more than anything else, this is the real gift this program offers older men.

References

Aging and Ageism. (2012). *A primer on social problems.* Retrieved from http://2012books.lardbucket.org/books/a-primer-on-social-problems/s09-aging-and-ageism.html

American Geriatrics Society. (2011). Geriatrics Workforce Policy Study Center. Retrieved from http://www.americangeriatrics.org/files/documents/gwps/Table%201_4.pdf

Ames, N., & Diepstra, S. A. (2006). Using intergenerational oral history service-learning projects to teach human behavior concepts: A qualitative analysis. *Educational Gerontology, 32*, 721–735.

Arias, E. (2010). United States life tables, 2006. *National Vital Statistics Reports, 58*(21), 1–40.

Ash, A. L., Clayton, P. H., & Atkinson, M. P. (2005). Integrating reflection and assessment to capture and improve student learning. *Michigan Journal of Community Service Learning, 11*(2), 49–60.

Astin, A. W., & Sax, L. J. (1998). How undergraduates are affected by service participation. *Journal of College Student Development, 39*, 251–263.

Batchelder, T. H., & Root, S. (1994). Effects of an undergraduate program to integrate academic learning and service: Cognitive, prosocial cognitive, and identity outcomes. *Journal of Adolescence, 17*, 341–355.

Beling, J. (2003). Effect of service-learning on knowledge of older people and faculty teaching evaluations in a physical therapy class. *Gerontology & Geriatrics Education, 24*(1), 31–46.

Blieszner, R., & Artale, L. M. (2001). Benefits of intergenerational service-learning to human service majors. *Educational Gerontology, 27*, 71–87.

Bringle, R. C., & Hatcher, J. A. (1995). A service-learning curriculum for faculty. *Michigan Journal of Community Service Learning, 2*, 112–122.

Bringle, R. G., & Kremer, J. F. (1993). Evaluation of an intergenerational service learning project for undergraduates. *Educational Gerontology, 19*, 407–416.

Bringle, R. G., Phillips, M. A., & Hudson, M. (2004). *The measure of service learning.* Washington, DC, USA: American Psychological Association.

Brown, L. H., & Roodin, P. A. (2001). Service-learning in gerontology: An out of classroom experience. *Educational Gerontology, 27*, 89–103.

Capraro, R. (2014). *Taking male students seriously. Inside higher Ed.* Retrieved from https://www.insidehighered.com/views/2014/09/22/essay-significance-mens-studies-promoting-success-male-students

Carini, R. M., Kuh, G. D., & Klein, S. P. (2006). Student engagement and student learning: Testing the linkages. *Research in Higher Education, 47*(1), 1–32.

Celio, C. I., Durlak, J., & Dymnicki, A. (2011). A meta-analysis of the impact of service—Learning on students. *Journal of Experiential Education, 34*(2), 164–181.

Coe, J. M., Best, A. M., Warren, J. J., McQuistan, M. R., Kolker, J. L., & Isringhausen, K. T. (2014) Service-learning's impact on dental students' attitude towards community service. *European Journal of Dental Education.* Retrieved from http://onlinelibrary.wiley.com. doi:10.1111/eje.12113/pdf

Cohen, H. L., Sandel, M. H., Thomas, C. L., & Barton, T. R. (2004). Using focus groups as an educational methodology: Deconstructing stereotypes and social work practice misconceptions concerning aging and older adults. *Educational Gerontology, 30*, 329–346.

Davidson, P. L., Nakazono, T. T., Carreon, D. C., Bai, J., & Afifi, A. (2009). Practice plans of dental school graduating seniors: effects of the pipeline program. *Journal of Dental Education, 73*, 283–296.

Davies, S. M., Reitmaier, A. B., Smith, L. R., & Mangan-Danckwart, D. (2013). Capturing intergenerativity: The use of student reflective journals to identify learning within an undergraduate course in gerontological nursing. *Journal of Nursing Education, 52*(3), 139–149.

Dharamsi, S., Espinoza, N., Cramer, C., Amin, M., Bainbridge, L., & Pool, G. (2010). Social responsibility through community service-learning: Lessons learned from a pilot project. *Medical Teacher, 32*, 905–911.

Diamond, J. (2013). *How societies can grow old better. Technology, entertainment and design.* Retrieved from http://www.ted.com/talks/jared_diamond_how_societies_can_grow_old_better/transcript?language=en

Dorfman, L. T., Murty, S., Ingram, J. G., & Evans, R. J. (2002). Incorporating intergenerational service-learning into an introductory gerontology course. *Journal of Gerontological Social Work, 39*, 219–240.

Dorfman, L. T., Murty, S. A., Ingram, J. G., Evans, R. J., & Power, J. R. (2004). Intergenerational service-learning in five cohorts of students: Is attitude change robust? *Educational Gerontology, 30*, 39–55.

Eyler, J., & Giles, D. E. (1999). *Where's the service in service-learning?*. San Francisco, CA: Jossey-Bass.

Eyler, J., Giles, D. E., & Braxton, J. (1997). The impact of service-learning on college students. *Michigan Journal of Community Service-Learning, 4*, 5–15.

Eyler, J., Giles, D. E, Jr, Stenson, C. M., & Gray, C. J. (2001). *At a glance: What we know about the effects of service-learning on college students, faculty, institution and communities, 1993–2000* (3rd ed.). Nashville, TN: Vanderbilt University.

Faria, D. F., Dauenhauer, J., & Steitz, D. (2010). Fostering social work gerontological competencies: Qualitative analysis of an intergenerational service-learning course. *Gerontology and Geriatrics Education, 31*(1), 92–113.

Fenzel, L.M., & Leary, T.P. (1997, March). *Evaluating outcomes of service-learning courses at a parochial college.* Paper presented at the annual meeting of the American Educational Research Association, Chicago, IL.

Fenzel, L. M., & Peyrot, M. (2005). Comparing college community participation in future service behaviors and attitudes. *Michigan Journal of Community Service Learning, 12*(1), 15–23.

Gawande, A. (2007). Annals of medicine: The way we age now. *The New Yorker.* Retrieved from http://www.newyorker.com/reporting/2007/04/30/070430fa_fact_gawande/

Gordon, J., Ludlum, J., & Hoey, J. J. (2008). Validating NSSE against student outcomes: Are they related? *Research in Higher Education, 49*(1), 19–39.

Gugliucci, M. R., & Weiner, A. (2013). Learning by living: Life-altering medical education through nursing home-based experiential learning. *Gerontology & Geriatrics Education, 34*(1), 60–77.

Gutheil, I. A., Chernesky, R. H., & Sherratt, M. L. (2006). Influencing student attitudes toward older adults: Results of a service-learning collaboration. *Educational Gerontology, 32*, 771–784.

Hamon, R., & Way, C. (2001). Integrating intergenerational service-learning into the family science curriculum. *Journal of Teaching in Marriage and Family, 1*(3), 65–83.

Hanks, R., & Icenogle, M. (2001). Preparing for an age-diverse workforce: Intergenerational service-learning in social gerontology and business curricula. Educational Gerontology, *27*, 49–70.

Hegeman, C. R., Horowitz, B., Tepper, L., Pillemer, K., & Schultz, L. (2002). Service-learning in elder care: Ten years of growth and assessment. *Journal of Gerontological Social Work, 39*(1/2), 177–194.

Hernandez, C. R., & Gonzalez, M. Z. (2008). Effects of intergenerational interaction on aging. *Educational Gerontology, 34*, 292–305.

Holtzman, J. S., & Seirawan, H. (2009). Impact of community-based oral health experiences on dental students' attitudes towards caring for the underserved. *Journal of Dental Education, 73*, 303–310.

Hood, J. G. (2009). Service-learning in dental education: meeting needs and challenges. *Journal of Dental Education, 73*, 454–463.

Horowitz, B., Wong, S., & Dechello, K. (2010). Intergenerational service learning: To promote active aging, and occupational therapy gerontology practice. *Gerontology & Geriatrics Education, 31*, 75–91.

Kalisch, H. R., Coughlin, D. R., Ballard, S. M., & Lamson, A. (2013). Old age is a part of living: Student reflections on intergenerational service-learning. *Gerontology & Geriatrics Education, 34*(1), 99–113.
Karasik, R. J. (2013). Reflecting on reflection: Capitalizing on the learning in intergenerational service-learning. *Gerontology & Geriatrics Education, 34*(1), 78–98.
Karasik, R., & Berke, D. (2001). Classroom and community: Experiential education in family studies and gerontology. *Journal of Teaching in Marriage and Family: Innovations in Family Science Education, 1*(4), 13–38.
Karasik, R., Maddox, M., & Wallingford, M. (2004). Intergenerational service-learning across levels and disciplines: "One size (does not) fit all". *Gerontology & Geriatrics Education, 25*(1), 1–17.
Kimuna, S. R., Knox, D., & Zusman, M. (2005). College students' perceptions about older people and aging. *Educational Gerontology, 31*, 563–572.
Kite, M., Stockdale, G., Whitley, B, Jr, & Johnson, B. (2005). Attitudes toward younger and older adults: An updated meta-analytic review. *Journal of Social Issues, 61*, 241–266.
Knapp, J. L., & Stubblefield, P. (2000). Changing students' perceptions of aging: The impact of an intergenerational service-learning course. *Educational Gerontology, 26*, 611–621.
Kolb, P. (2008). Interest of racially and ethnically diverse social work students in gerontological social work. *Educational Gerontology, 34*, 907–922.
Krout, J., Bergman, E., Bianconi, P., Caldwell, K., Dorsey, J., Durnford, S., et al. (2010). Intergenerational service learning with elders: Multidisciplinary activities and outcomes. *Gerontology & Geriatrics Education, 31*, 55–74.
Kuh, G. D. (2009). What student affairs professionals need to know about student engagement. *Journal of College Student Development, 50*(6), 683–706.
Kuh, G. D., Cruce, T. M., Shoup, R., Kinzie, J., & Gonyea, R. M. (2008). Unmasking the effects of student engagement on first year college grades and persistence. *The Journal of Higher Education, 79*(5), 540–563.
Lovell, M. (2006). Caring for the elderly: Changing perceptions and attitudes. *Journal of Vascular Nursing, 24*, 22–26.
Mahalik, J. R., Good, G. E., & Englar-Carlson, M. (2003). Masculinity scripts, presenting concerns and help seeking: implications for practice and training. *Professional Psychology: Research and Practice, 34*(2), 123–131.
Markus, G. B., Howard, J. P. F., & King, D. C. (1993). Integrating community service and classroom instruction enhances learning: Results from an experiment. *Educational Evaluation and Policy Analysis, 15*, 410–419.
Martinez-Carter, K. (2013). How the elderly are treated around the world. *The Week*. Retrieved from http://theweek.com/articles/462230/how-elderly-are-treated-around-world
Maslow, A. H. (1954). *Motivation and personality*. New York: Harper & Bros.
McCrea, J. M., Nichols, A., & Newman, S. (Eds.). (1999). *Intergenerational service learning in gerontology: A compendium* (Vol. II). Pittsburgh, PA: University of Pittsburgh Press.
Miller, F. (1994). Gender differences in adolescents' attitudes toward mandatory community service. *Journal of Adolescence, 17*(4), 381–393.
O'Hanlon, A. M., & Brookover, B. C. (2002). Assessing changes in attitudes about aging: Personal reflections and a standardized measure. *Educational Gerontology, 28*, 711–725.
Pelco, L. E., Ball, C. T., & Lockeman, K. S. (2014). Student growth from service-learning: A comparison of first-generation and non-first-generation college students. *Journal of Higher Education Outreach and Engagement, 18*(2), 49.
Pike, G. R. (2004). The influence of fraternity or sorority membership on students' college experiences and cognitive development. *Research in Higher Education, 41*(1), 117–139.
Reade, N. (2013). The surprising truth about older workers. *AARP The Magazine*. Retrieved from http://www.aarp.org/work/job-hunting/info-07-2013/older-workers-more-valuable.html
Regan, D. T., & Fazio, R. (1977). On the consistency between attitudes and behavior: Look to the method of attitude formation. *Educational Gerontology, 13*, 28–45.

Roodin, P. (2002). *Questions and answers about service-learning*. Paper presented at the Intergenerational service.
Roodin, P., Brown, L. H., & Shedlock, D. (2013). Intergenerational service-learning: A review of recent literature and directions for the future. *Gerontology & Geriatrics Education, 34*(1), 3–25.
Sauer, B. L. (2006). Student-directed learning in a community geriatrics advanced pharmacy practice experience. *American Journal of Pharmaceutical Education, 70*(3), 1–7.
Schawbel, D. (2014). *51 of the most interesting facts about Generation Z*. Retrieved from http://danschawbel.com/blog/39-of-the-most-interesting-facts-about-generation-z/
Schwartz, S. H. (1977). Normative influences on altruism. *Advances in Experimental Social Psychology, 10*, 221–279.
Schwartz, L. K., & Simmons, J. P. (2001). Contact quality and attitudes toward the elderly. *Educational Gerontology, 27*, 127–137.
Sink, V. (2015) *Are we speaking the same language when it comes to aging? A New Report from Expert Collaborative Hopes to Get Us Closer*. Retrieved from http://www.ncoa.org/press-room/press-release/Gauging-Aging-Report.html
Smith, TJ. (2005). Ethnic and gender differences in community service participation among working adults. *Journal of Extension, 43*(2). Retrieved from http://www.joe.org/joe/2005april/rb1.php
Smith, C. S., Ester, T. V., & Inglehart, M. R. (2006). Dental education and care for underserved patients: an analysis of students' intentions and alumni behavior. *Journal of Dental Education, 70*, 398–408.
Snyder, Thomas D. (2014). Mobile Digest of Education Statistics, 2013 (NCES 2014-085). National Center for Education Statistics, Institute of Educational Sciences, U.S. Department of Education. Washington, DC
Stogner, C. D. (2004). Priming students for the benefits of service-learning: The benefits of supplemental lectures on critical thinking, reflection, and journaling. In J. McCrea, M. Weissman, D. Stepp, & B. Ciha (Eds.), *Intergenerational servicelearning in gerontology: a compendium, volume IV—Reflection in servicelearning: Practical guidance from multiple perspectives* (pp. 9–15). Washington, DC and Pittsburgh, PA: Association for Gerontology in Higher Education & Generations Together.
Taylor, P., & Keeter, S. (2010). Millennials: A portrait of generation next. *Pew Research Center*. Retrieved from http://www.pewsocialtrends.org/files/2010/10/millennials-confident-connected-open-to-change.pdf
Tiller, M. G., & Fazio, R. (1982). The relation between attitudes and later behavior following dissonance-produced attitude change. *Personality and Social Psychology Bulletin, 8*, 280–285.
Trudeau, K. J., & Devlin, A. S. (1996). College students and community service: Who, with whom, and why? *Journal of Applied Social Psychology, 26*(21), 1867–1888.
U.S. Census Bureau, Population Division. (2012). Table 2. *Projections of the population by selected age groups and sex for the United States: 2015 to 2060*. Retrieved from http://www.census.gov/population/projections/data/national/2012/summarytables.html
Vandsberger, E., & Wakefield, M. (2008). Service learning with rural older adults. *Journal of Intergenerational Relationships, 3*(4), 83–97.
Vedder, R. (2014). the disappearing male on college campuses. *Forbes*. Retrieved from http://www.forbes.com/sites/ccap/2014/12/29/the-disappearing-male-on-college-campuses/
Viggiani, K. (2004). Pre-service reflection. In J. McCrea, M. Weissman, D. Stepp, & B. Ciha (Eds.), *Intergenerational service-learning in gerontology: A compendium, volume IV—Reflection in service-learning: Practical guidance from multiple perspectives* (pp. 33–35). Washington, DC and Pittsburgh, PA: Association for Gerontology in Higher Education & Generations Together.
Vogelgesang, L. J., & Astin, L. W. (2000). Comparing the effects of community service and service learning. *Michigan Journal of Community Service Learning, 7*, 25–34.

Weaver-Hightower, M. B. (2010). Where the guys are: Males in higher education. *Change*. Retrieved from http://www.changemag.org/archives/back%20issues/may-june%202010/where-guys-full.html

Westacott, B., & Hegeman, C. (Eds.). (1996). *Service learning in elder care: A resource manual*. Albany, NY: Foundation for Long Term Care.

Whitbourne, S., Collins, K., & Skultety, K. (2001). Formative reflections on service learning in a course on the psychology of aging. *Educational Gerontology, 27*, 105–115.

Zacherman, A., & Foubert, J. (2014). The relationship between engagement in cocurricular activities and academic performance: Exploring gender differences. *Journal of Student Affairs Research and Practice, 51*(2), 157–169.

Chapter 15
Continuing Bonds Research with Animal Companions: Implications for Men Grieving the Loss of a Dog

Wendy Packman, Cori Bussolari, Rachel Katz and Betty J. Carmack

Introduction

It is evident that animal companions have a deep capacity for acceptance, adoration, attention, forgiveness, and unconditional love, thus, satisfying some of our greatest human needs. Pets also help humans to overcome or prevent a sense of isolation that is frequently experienced due to life struggles (Levinson 1969). Because our emotional health is continuously impacted by important relationships, pets have become significant attachment figures who benefit our general social, physical and psychological well-being (Sable 1995). Our connection with animals goes as far back as recorded history, and as Oyama and Serpell (2013) put it, "…humans have always suspected an ability of animals to improve the human condition" (p. 374). In 2012 (Humane Society 2014), in the U.S. alone, 47 % of households owned at least one dog, and over half of U.S. households owned some other species of pet. At the

W. Packman (✉)
2578 16th Avenue, San Francisco, CA 94116, USA
e-mail: wpackman@paloaltou.edu

C. Bussolari
1921 Grove Street, San Francisco, CA 94117, USA
e-mail: bussolari@usfca.edu

R. Katz
208 Douglass Street, San Francisco, CA 94114, USA
e-mail: rachelkatzsf@gmail.com

B.J. Carmack
1400 Geary Blvd. Apt 1402, San Francisco, CA 94109, USA
URL:http://www.bettyjcarmack.com

C. Blazina and L.R. Kogan (eds.), *Men and Their Dogs*,
DOI 10.1007/978-3-319-30097-9_15

same time, an all time high of almost 60 billion dollars will be spent this year on our animal companions, up from 21 billion from 1996 (Manning 2014).

Research has demonstrated that for humans, pets provide companionship, protection, non-judgmental acceptance (Labrecque and Walsh 2011), increased quality of life (Peacock et al. 2012), reduction of mental distress (Aydin et al. 2012), accelerated adaption to traumatic events (Wolfe 1977; Aydin et al. 2012) as well as love and nurturance (Garrity et al. 1989; Zasloff and Kidd 1994). It has been suggested that transitional objects help children feel confident and protected without their primary attachment figure or parents, thus empowering them to transfer their affections from parents to others (Barba 1991). Robin and ten Bensel (1985) noted that as transitional objects, pets help children feel safe, whether or not their parents are around. During adolescence, pets can "be a confidant, an object of love, a protector, a social facilitator or a status symbol" (Robin and ten Bense 1985, p. 66). Levinson (1969) has also noted that pets fulfill the need for touch or physical contact without most of the fear that accompanies human contact. In the same vein, there is evidence to indicate that positive feelings and interactions with an animal transfers to improved interactions with other humans (Moneymaker and Strimple 1991; Ruth 1992; Mallon 1992; Thompson 2009; Barba 1991; Ryder 1973; Savishinsky 1983). Animal companions have been additionally described as social lubricants (Messent 1983) or bridges to social interactions (Lockwood 1983), indicating that pets tend to facilitate positive human interactions. Aydin et al. (2012) found that for people who experienced social exclusion, just the presence of a dog reduced emotional distress.

Similar to humans, pets carry the potential to provide an emotional attachment bond that promotes a sense of security and well-being (Sable 1995). The attachment relationship between humans and pets is reinforced by the fact that pets are often viewed as part of the family (Raupp 1999; Raupp et al. 1997). Indeed, over 99 % of pet owners consider his or her pet to be family member (Stutts 1994). People become emotionally close and committed to pets, accept responsibility for pets, share activities with pets and grieve when their pet dies. Thus, it seems evident that the human–pet attachment bond is similar to that between humans, suggesting that one of the most important things a pet can provide is someone to love (Arehart-Treichel 1982) and unconditional love and acceptance.

In this chapter, we examine the human animal bond and the implications for men when their pets die. This will specifically include a discussion about attachment, human–canine bond, gender, grief, and continuing bonds (CB). Continuing Bonds expressions (CBE) (e.g., dreams, fond memories, rituals, memorials) have been found in the literature to be an adaptive means of coping following the loss of a beloved relationship with an attachment figure, including pets. In our research and clinical practice, we have consistently found that men have difficulties expressing their emotions and accessing support following a death. Because of the strong relationship between men and their dogs, a death can be especially devastating. Thus, using CBE may be helpful in affect regulation.

Attachment to Animal Companions

The need for attachment is common to both humans and animals. Humans have a tendency to develop attachment bonds with animals due to anthropomorphism, neoteny, and alleomemetic behaviors (Lagoni et al. 1994). Anthropomorphism is the attribution of humanlike traits to nonhumans, neoteny signifies the presence of infant-like characteristics, and alleomemetic behaviors are human behaviors that are mimicked by animals. Attachment theorists have outlined specific behaviors that are essential to the attachment between human beings and other animals such as the amount of time spent together, physical closeness, care-giving and care-soliciting behavior, sharing of emotional experiences, dependency, cooperative behavior, tactile and visual stimulation, and feelings of happiness evoked by behaviors of the attached figure (Voith 1985; Triebenbacher 1998). Bowlby (1969) noted two important and similar attachment behaviors observed in birds and mammals such as maintaining proximity to and taking care of another animal, as well as specificity and discrimination in the relationship, such as the connection between a parent and child. From a biological perspective, Nagasawa et al. (2009) highlighted the distinct relationship that humans have with dogs, due in particularly, to recent "evolved social cognitive abilities in close symbiosis with humans" (p. 217). Animal behaviorists acknowledge that the love and attentiveness humans give to animal companions is reciprocal and beneficial to both (Rynearson 1978; Ory and Goldberg 1983; Garrity et al. 1989).

Attachment theory has often been used to explain the human/animal bond as well and animal companions are considered to be attachment figures. Animal companions appear to provide an alternative opportunity for humans to experience bonding. Recent research (Nagasawa et al. 2009), assessing the biological aspects of the human–dog relationship using physiological and neuroendocrinological approaches, revealed that dogs can discriminate between humans and are the only animals with the ability to use and respond to human-like social cues. Specifically, when a dog "gazes" at their owners (a factor that contributes greatly to social bonding), their oxytocin levels increase. Oxytocin is a "neuropeptide produced in the hypothalamus linked to feelings of trust and bonding, especially between a breast-feeding mother and her newborn child, oxytocin is best known as the mammalian hormone of love" (Frankel 2014, p. 61). Nagasawa et al. (2009), hypothesized that humans and dogs may have similar attachment styles and that these are the elements that could possibly form cross species empathy, thereby creating powerful bonds between men and their dogs. In a similar study, researchers looked at oxytocin levels within humans and dogs and found that after spending quality time together, both humans and dogs had an increase in oxytocin (Handlin et al. 2011), suggesting a reciprocal or similar bonding experience.

This capacity to make an emotional connection beyond typical human relationships is important. Bowlby (1980) investigated the attachment feelings and behaviors beyond childhood and postulated "working models" or an inner psychological organization of the self and attachment figures. Similarly, Sable (1995) proposed that family pets have the potential to provide an emotional bond of attachment that promotes a sense of well-being and security. According to Levinson (1997), how individuals feel about themselves reflects in the ways they treat their animals and how people treat their animals also tends to mirror the way in which they relate to other people.

The formation of an emotional attachment to animal companions is especially relevant for men. In order to look at the interconnections between our relationship with humans and pets, Cohen (2002) assessed family relationships and pet attachment and found that men reported fewer feelings of psychological kinship and intimacy with both pets and people. At the same time, Williams et al. (2009) assessed children age 9–13 regarding attachment, attitude, and empathy towards their pets. Their findings suggested that regardless of gender, children have strong attachments with their pets. For children, Williams et al. (2009) noted that having a pet is valuable for their overall development and may also increase empathy through the practice of nurturance. Kurdek (2009) studied the extent to which adult owners turn to their dogs in times of emotional duress and found that dog owners scored strongest in the area of proximity maintenance, highlighting how much they enjoyed spending time with their dogs. He also found that "men were more likely than women to prefer dogs to mothers, sisters, best friends and children, but not to partners", underscoring the notion that dogs are "man's best friend" (p. 445).

Human–Canine Bond and Gender

Research continues to demonstrate a strong bond between humans and dogs (Cain 1985; Serpell 1996). Dogs provide unconditional and non-judgmental love (Cusack 1988), lowered blood pressure (Anderson et al. 1992), fewer health and mental health problems (Serpell 1996), decreases in isolation and loneliness (Duncan 1995) and support for stress (Allen et al. 1991). Much of the research specifically regarding the human–dog bond and attachment has been limited and sometimes contradictory. In one study, gender was not found to be a factor in how much people cared for their pet dogs (Ramirez 2006). In another study, compared to men, women were found to have a stronger attachment with their dogs (Margolies 1999). In contrast, Prato-Previde et al. (2006) observed 25 owner-dog pairs in various scenarios to assess gender differences in the interactions of owners and their pet dogs in an adapted version of the 'strange situation procedure' (Ainsworth and Bell 1970). Results suggested no gender differences in play or providing physical comfort. There were no significant differences in the strength of reported attachment. However, women were more likely to interact verbally with their dog and their verbal communication closely resembled infant directed speech. Prato-Previde et al. (2006) concluded that "the behavior of modern pet owners towards their dogs is parental behavior directed towards individuals of another species" (p. 71). The more primitive behaviors of caregiving, such as physical touch and comfort, could be less affected by gender than the modern (primarily female) use of speech, and most importantly, males and females have equally strong bonds (Prato-Previde et al. 2006). These contradictory outcomes regarding gender and the human–canine bond mirror the complicated and inconclusive findings arising from gender research, in general. This may be due to the suggestion that compared to within gender variations, gender differences are small across cultures (Costa et al. 2001).

Frankel (2014) elucidates the strength of the male-canine bond in her book entitled *War Dogs*. She writes about her observations of military dogs and their handlers, noting Any handler who has brought a dog with him or her to war will say it made all the difference in the world. They will say that the dog by their side provided them with something more than just a living, breathing piece of home—the dog acted as a talisman, insulating them from whatever horrors unfolded, bringing them peace in turbulence, offering companionship in times of loneliness. "The dog's presence made the path through war bearable, the unendurable somehow endurable, and many will say they came through the other side more stable." (p. 23)

Pet Attachment and Grief

The loss of a loved one is devastating and nothing but the return of the lost attachment object can truly relieve the emotional pain (Bowlby 1980). Although Bowlby was referring to the loss of a human loved one, research has shown that the loss of a pet rivals or exceeds the pain of the loss of a human in terms of psychological and social difficulties (Quackenbush 1985). Bowlby's (1980) framework underscores the specific phases of mourning: numbing, yearning and searching, disorganization and despair, and the phase of greater or lesser disorganization and despair. Bowlby (1980) states that these four phases occur in a sequence, although the actual way people move in and out of these phases are often not linear.

These phases, as outlined by Bowlby (1980) are equally applicable in pet loss. Unfortunately, our research and clinical practice repeatedly show that the loss of a pet is often unvalidated. According to Sable (2013), clients who come for emotional support after the death of their pet are often most distressed due to lack of sympathy from those around them. Because there are numerous people who do not consider a pet to be an important attachment figure, they also do not acknowledge other people's grief when their animal companion dies (Wrobel and Dye 2003). As a result, bereaved pet owners may hide their feelings and suffer in silence. Doka (1989) uses the term disenfranchised grief to describe a grief that is not socially sanctioned or readily acknowledged. Doka (1989) states that disenfranchised grief occurs when: the relationship with the deceased is unrecognized; the loss itself is unrecognized; or the griever is unrecognized. As the majority of society still fails to recognize the depth of relationships people can have with their pets, most, if not all, of these criteria are met in the loss of a pet (Clements et al. 2003).

Gosse (1988) found a positive relationship between pet attachment and the grief response to the loss of a pet, with more grief symptoms reported if a stronger attachment was found. In a similar study, Gerwolls and Labbott (1994) assessed whether the loss of a close human companion was different from the loss of a pet. The authors found that at two and eight weeks post-loss, the grief scores of those who had lost a pet were similar to those who had lost a human companion, suggesting that the loss of a pet was very similar to the loss of a human. In addition, those reporting deeper connections with their animal companions had more difficulties adjusting to the loss.

Planchon and Templer (1996) found that well-adjusted individuals faired psychologically better in the grieving process than less adjusted individuals. Similarly, in a later study, Planchon et al. (2002) found that greater grief following the death of a pet was associated with general depression, depression following bereavement, as well as strong attachments to pets. In another study Adams et al. (2000) found that 30 % of participants reported severe grief and that the most prominent predictors were strength of attachment, the incidence of euthanasia, societal attitudes toward pet death, and professional support from the veterinary team. In fact, higher strength of attachment was once again associated with a higher incidence of severe grief.

At present, there is only a small body of literature that specifically looks at gender and pet loss, with several findings suggesting that females, rather than males, exhibit more distress following the loss of an animal companion (Brown et al. 1996; McCutcheon and Fleming 2002; Planchon and Templer 1996; Gage and Holcomb 1991; Gosse 1994; Reynolds 1999). In a study conducted by Wrobel and Dye (2003) using adult participants, results suggested that the strength of attachment to a pet predicted severity of negative emotional symptoms such as guilt, depression, anger, loneliness, and length of grieving process. In addition, for each of these symptoms, the rate of endorsement was higher for females than for males. McCutcheon and Fleming (2002) found similar results, with females also showing more distress. Wrobel and Dye (2003) note, however, that these data reflect the percent of occurrences of symptoms, and not the intensity of experience. It could be hypothesized that these gender specific disparities are due to socialization and cultural differences (Reynolds 1999) rather than the potency of the loss. It is possible that males might express fewer emotions on questionnaires or interviews (Brown et al. 1996; McCutcheon and Fleming 2002). In fact, in a comprehensive literature review looking at gender differences and bereavement, Rothaupt and Becker (2007) concluded that there were no gender differences in the level of grief, but rather men and women demonstrate their grief in very specific and different ways.

In a comprehensive analysis of gender and human–animal attachment, Herzog (2007) noted that most of the studies he evaluated did not use effect sizes; thus, the comparison of gender responses were inadequately documented. He cautioned not to look at gender differences in human–animal attachment as static, but rather, as a result of "the interaction of factors that operate at multiple levels and it is unlikely that any single factor can account for the array of differences in human–animal relationships that have been documented over different behaviors and cultures" (p. 17). It is evident that we attach to our animal companions similarly to how we attach to other humans, sometimes even to a more intense degree.

Continuing Bonds and Pet Loss

It is clear that losing a pet is similar to losing a valued human attachment relationship. This is especially salient for bereaved men as they may find it harder to express their emotions, access support, or engage in positive coping skills (Brown et al. 1996; Wroebel and Dye 2003).

In recent bereavement literature the concept of CB has received growing attention, especially its function in relation to coping following a death. (Field and Friedrichs 2004; Field et al. 2005; Stroebe et al. 1992; Klass et al. 1996). Despite the permanence of physical separation, the bereaved can be emotionally sustained through a continuing bond to the deceased (Field et al. 1999). Examples of CB include reminiscing about the loved one, memorials and rituals, dreams, and holding onto special possessions as remembrances. Thus, resolving grief does not involve ending a relationship with the deceased, but rather includes a renegotiation and transformation of the meaning of the loss over time (Field 2008; Klass et al. 1996).

Until 2010, the concept of "continuing bonds" (CB) had not been described in the pet bereavement literature (Packman et al. 2011). Earlier writers described phenomena that were experienced as CBs but not labeled as such (Carmack 2003; Cowles 1985; Podrazik et al. 2000; Weisman 1990/1991). Packman et al. (2011) examined and quantified CB expressions (CBE) experienced by bereaved pet owners. Participants who had lost a dog or cat within the past year completed a set of measures that assessed psychosocial adjustment, (grief, symptoms, growth), and CBE. The measures consisted of the Inventory of Complicated Grief, the Brief Symptom Inventory the Post-Traumatic Growth Inventory and projective drawings.

The Continuing Bonds Interview (CBI) of Field et al. (2007) was used to evaluate the degree of connection that the bereaved maintains with the deceased pet and how that bond affects functioning. This interview-based CB measure is designed to investigate the different facets of CB and goes well beyond simply assessing extent of CB usage to distinguish whether the CBE are indicative of poor versus successful adaptation to the loss (Field 2008). If the participant endorsed CBE, they were asked to describe and rate if the experience was comforting, distressing, or both and the degree to which this occurred (see Table 15.1).

Table 15.1 Continuing bonds expressions endorsement

CB Expression	Pet loss ($N = 33$)			Spousal loss ($N = 24$)		
	Percent	Comfort MN	Distress SD	Percent	Comfort MN	Distress SD
Continuing connection Sense of deceased's presence	48	3.56* (1.32)	1.94 (1.12)	46	3.89*** (.93)	1.11 (.33)
Belongings Use of deceased's belongings for comfort	79	3.42*** (1.21)	1.73 (1.15)	75	3.05*** (1.13)	1.74 (0.99)
Associated Places Drawn to places associated with deceased	48	3.12* (1.31)	2.12 (1.36)	42	2.80 (1.23)	2.50 (1.65)
Fond Memories Focus on fond memories of deceased	85	3.54** (1.07)	2.32 (1.52)	92	3.23*** (1.07)	1.45 (0.86)
Dreams Dreams involving deceased	52	2.71 (1.16)	2.18 (1.38)	54	2.62 (1.56)	1.62 (1.04)
Reunited with Deceased Thoughts of being reunited with deceased	58	3.74*** (1.44)	1.58 (1.17)	54	2.92* (1.61)	1.54 (.66)
Living up to Ideals or Wishes of Deceased Aware of wanting to be more like or live up to ideals of deceased	39	3.54*** (1.19)	1.54 (.776)	38	3.00 (1.73)	1.56 (1.01)
Everyday Decisions Making everyday decisions based on deceased's preferences	18	3.17* (1.16)	1.17 (0.408)	8	3.50 (2.12)	1.00 (0.00)
Reminisce Reminisce with others about deceased	79	3.46** (1.27)	1.88 (1.31)	96	3.39*** (1.08)	1.43 (1.08)
Memorials Organize special events to commemorate deceased	39	3.77*** (1.09)	1.85 (1.21)	33	3.38** (1.19)	1.63 (1.06)

(continued)

Table 15.1 (continued)

CB Expression	Pet loss ($N = 33$)			Spousal loss ($N = 24$)		
	Percent	Comfort MN	Distress SD	Percent	Comfort MN	Distress SD
Intrusion Mistaking other sounds or sights for deceased	39	3.15 (1.52)	1.62 (.768)	29	1.57 (1.51)	3.00 (1.29)
Lessons Learned/ Positive Influence Positive lasting influence of deceased	76	3.64*** (1.11)	1.56 (1.15)	63	3.33*** (1.18)	1.60 (1.18)

*$p < 0.05$, **$p < 0.01$, ***$p < 0.001$

Presence and Prevalence of Continuing Bonds

The most frequently endorsed CBE about the pet were recalling fond memories (85 %), holding onto or using belongings (79 %), reminiscing with others (79 %), and lessons learned/positive influences (76 %) (Packman et al. 2011). To investigate the similarities in the use of CBE in pet loss, the authors compared their sample with a spousal loss sample (Field 2010). Importantly, both groups were similar in terms of relative frequency of endorsement of each CBE. For example, both samples have high endorsement of reminiscing with others, focusing on fond memories and use of deceased's belongings. A mean score was derived for the extent of comfort and distress in the use of CBE. Both the pet loss and spousal loss groups showed an overall tendency to experience a CB as more comforting than distressing (see Table 15.1).

Packman et al. (2011) assessed whether the comfort and distress mean score ratings moderated the relationship between the Continuing Bond Ongoing Connection Factor (comprised of five of the CBE) and the psychosocial adjustment measures. Analyses revealed that the comfort variable moderated the relationship between the ongoing bond on the one hand and grief, as well as other symptoms on the other hand. Significant trends were found for the moderating role of comfort on the relationship between ongoing connection and post-traumatic growth and drawing measures. Importantly, the research suggests that the relationship between CBE and both grief and symptoms is contingent on comfort: those who use more CBE and derive comfort from them experience less grief and fewer symptoms. In addition, those who use CBE and derive comfort from them experience growth. On the other hand, these relationships do not hold for the distress variable, i.e., individuals who report using many CBE accompanied by distress experience more grief and symptoms.

In a later and ongoing cross-cultural study, Packman et al. (2014) use qualitative and quantitative methodology to compare, analyze, and report responses of U.S. and French Canadian participants to the last open-ended question on an online pet loss survey.

Now that you have answered our questions are there any other feelings or thoughts about your experience of grieving for your pet that you would like to share with us? Feel free to write as much or as little as you like.

The survey provided respondents with a place and a means to describe their experiences. Four major themes emerged: intensity of loss; lack of validation and support; nature of the human pet relationship; and CB. In this part of the chapter, we include representative quotes from some of the men respondents who participated in the cross-cultural survey.

Intensity of Loss

It was not unusual to have grievers speak about intensity of loss. Men wrote of their symptoms of grief, some expressing them on a physical level while others described them in terms of emotional pain often reflected in behavioral ways. Intensity was expressed by statements such as, "I am missing her terribly and feel a piece of my heart is gone and it won't ever heal. I'm trying to adjust to the emptiness and loss, but it's a struggle." A police officer stated: "I was emotionally immobilized for almost two weeks and couldn't perform my duties. This could have jeopardized mine or other people's lives." Still another stated, "I thought I was a tough guy, but can't believe how weak I am with her being gone."

Another man talked about his grief as follows: Since Tracy died, I get waves of tremendous sadness. She died two weeks ago and fortunately these feelings are starting to decrease in number but not in intensity as of yet. Although I have lost 2 parents, losing my dog is even worse in some respects—in a special kind of way. I was not expecting this. Although I love my wife and my kids tremendously, the love I had for my dog was somehow just as strong; I did not expect to feel the grief that I've been feeling.

Another respondent said: My dog Clancy was my soulmate. When I'd had a bad day, I could always look forward to coming home, being greeted by Mr. Clancy as I walked in the door…. He was my "go to" thing in life… He was the one who slept right by my side…. I was his primary caregiver who fed, walked, bathed, groomed, and medically cared for him…. Now that he is gone after suffering a brain tumor, I am lost on a sea alone in the world, and the world seems more lonely and meaner than before when he was by my side. How will I go on without him? Additionally, it was not unusual to have grievers speak of their intensity in terms of suicidal ideation.

I miss my dog. I cry too easy. I don't want to feel this way all the time. I'm very sad. My dog was one of the only things in my life which was perfect and pure. I sometimes thought about killing myself but wondered who would feed my dog. And that kept me alive. Now, I don't have a good reason to live. My wife will be fine without me but my dog needed me.

Disenfranchised Grief: Lack of Validation and Support

In spite of the intensity of loss, respondents had limited places for expression of their grief as well as minimal support for their loss, i.e., their grief was disenfranchised. One man expressing his lack of validation and support wrote:

> People seem to somehow trivialize the loss of a pet as if it is the loss of agricultural livestock; they think there is no way that sane, well socially integrated people can become so emotionally attached or dependant on a 'dumb animal'. Well, I can tell you that's not the case. After a decade and a half of living together, Randy was my best friend and my little boy, and he knew me and my little habits and idiosyncrasies just like I knew his, and we lived together perfectly as a result.

The Nature of the Human–Pet Relationship

The intensity and strength of men's relationships with their animal companion cannot be underestimated. Several examples illuminate the depth of their connection:

> I am always uncomfortable letting people know how much I love my dog, and how much I grieve for him. Many people will never understand how much a part of my life my dog is. I love my wife more than anything in the world, but I have always had a special relationship with dogs. I can't imagine being happy without a dog. A dog is like a familiar spirit; they are an attachment to the soul, they give me something that no person can. I trust people, but I trust dogs more. When a dog meets me, it's as if they are meeting another dog instead of a person. I like to think that I have a heart and soul good enough for a dog.

Another man described his connection with his beloved dog Moby, as follows: Moby and I were inseparable… I could take him to work with me daily, and after that he and I would walk for two hours… I was definitely clinging to him as my marriage fell apart. He got me through my divorce. Even the dog people realized we had a very great bond and were a little pack of our own. Although I was obviously overly attached to him I didn't care and both of us were really only happy if the other one was nearby.

Coping with Loss/Continuing Bonds (CB)

In terms of CB, resolving grief does not involve ending a relationship (detachment), but instead involves a reorganization of the relationship with the deceased (Field 2008). In earlier work, Packman et al. (2012) described both the comforting and distressing aspects of CB. The qualitative data from the cross-cultural sample also supported both the adaptive nature of CB as well as their distressing nature.

One participant described both aspects when he wrote, “It was my wife’s idea to give away or destroy all objects which would remind us of our boy. The sole exception is the wooden box which houses his ashes. It now sits next to the one that houses his brother who died nearly ten years ago.”

Two other men talked about the hope of being reunited with their dog:

> I am missing her terribly and feel a piece of my heart is gone and it won’t ever heal. I’m trying to adjust to the emptiness and loss, but it’s a struggle. I want to honor her and what she meant to a lot of people, but find myself dwelling on the events of the loss and not the joy of her life.... I loved her so much and know I will struggle with her being gone until I see her again. Each time I look out of the window I expect to see the little white tail go trotting past with such purpose as he surveys his garden, but of course I won’t. He’s exploring the great garden in the sky, waiting until we meet again.

Clinical Implications

Within our research, (Packman et al. 2014) men have frequently reported that they grieve more for their animal companion than they did for some humans. This finding is corroborated by our clinical experience and underscores the strong connection between men and their dogs.

With respect to gender, our experience suggests that therapeutic interventions with men will understandably vary, depending upon a number of person specific factors (e.g., strength of attachment, ethnic identity and practices, age, style of grieving, prior experience of loss and grief, perceived degree of social support, and safety in expression of emotions). Professional literature describes many men from an early age being socialized into not expressing emotions. Men grieve deeply, but the ways in which they grieve can be very different from the way females grieve (Doka and Martin 2010). At the same time, our clinical experience suggests that all men do not grieve the same way.

Additionally, a client’s ability to access various clinical options must be considered. For example, some men attend pet loss support groups, participate in online pet loss chat rooms and pet loss hotlines, or see an individual counselor. Other men choose to be more private within their own world and life. Still, other men do not know how to recognize their feelings, access help, or move through their grief, especially if the death of their dog is their first experience of significant grief.

Because CBE can be an adaptive means of coping following the loss of an attachment relationship, clinicians need to address CBE and pet loss. Both research and clinical practice emphasize that male pet owners do maintain ongoing, meaningful ties with their pet, e.g., creating rituals and memorials, looking at photographs and reminiscing, having thoughts of being reunited with their pets after their own death, or holding onto a pet’s possessions (Packman et al. 2012). Therefore, clinicians are encouraged to assess whether clients experience CBE and if the CBE are a source of comfort, distress, or both. In fact, in many cases they are mixed (Packman et al. 2012). Clinical experience suggests that those men who find comfort or more comfort than distress from these CBE are more likely to integrate them into their loss experience. In contrast, if CBE are too distressing, it is also adaptive to not engage in them. For those men who do not know about CBE, clinicians can educate about their nature and potential benefits of CBE as a coping strategy for loss as well as a means to maintain a meaningful connection to their dog.

Counselors must not trivialize pet loss and grief, as too often, clients' experience is disenfranchised and minimized (Packman et al. 2014). Clients have reported clinicians looking to uncover the "real reason" for the grief, either within their family or within areas of dysfunction in personal or professional relationships. Such an approach discounts that the loss of a loved animal companion can, in fact, be the cause of intense grief. Along the same lines, some clinicians determine that such intense grief for a dog implies that their clients' have difficulties in relationships with people. When the clients' loss for their beloved animal companions is disenfranchised and minimized, they may experience social constraint when talking to others about their loss (Kiel et al. 2015). For a man, the impact of having his story heard and his grief legitimized must not be underestimated. They expect to hurt, but they are often unprepared for how much or how long. Thus, validation and normalization of feelings are essential therapeutic interventions.

Providing non-verbal ways to access and express client grief can also be useful, e.g., journaling, expressive arts such as drawing or sketching, and music. In our pet loss support group (CB and BC), several men have shared poetry they have written or art they have created. One male participant's stated, "I write her (his dog) a little more each night in a letter I'm writing her." This reflects and models another way of grief expression. In a related vein, Jimmy Greene, a saxophonist, in an interview on NPR November 25, 2014, described the creation of his album, "*Beautiful Life*" as a memorial to his daughter, Ana, who was killed in the 2012 Sandy Hook Elementary School shootings. He said, "when there's not an accurate way to express my emotion or my struggle or my trauma, there's music. It's helpful in that way. It's akin to talking it out with someone." It is important to let men know there is no one right way to grieve and to help them find the strategy or strategies most appropriate for them.

Providing men with resource lists such as on-line chat rooms, pet loss support groups and pet loss hot lines, in addition to books, pamphlets and articles can be helpful. Clients can take these resource lists and consider them in the privacy of their home. Articles and books authored by men about their relationships with their dogs and their resulting grief can also be particularly helpful. Reading descriptions by men about the intensity of their grief for their dogs allows other men to recognize that the intensity of their grief is not that unusual, serving again to validate and normalize the experience.

In conclusion, there exists a continuum of male grief following the loss of a deeply loved attachment relationship, his dog. This continuum reflects both intensity and duration of grief. In this section we have presented a framework for recognition, care and treatment of male client grief following the death of a dog. Our framework, consisting of the component parts of recognition and validation of the grief experience, openness to a variety of clinical modalities, and integration of CBE, provides a useful guide to professionals for whom pet loss is a new or unfamiliar clinical experience.

Future Directions

Recent research has demonstrated that there is no difference between the intensity of grief between males and females (Rothaupt and Becker 2007; Wrobel and Dye 2003); rather, they cope differently with their emotions. A clear interface exists between research and clinical practice in relation to CBE and pet loss. Research findings reflect the comfort men often receive from their ongoing bond with their pets (Packman et al. 2011). We know that both men and women use CBE, but there is little information regarding frequency, duration, type of CBE, and most importantly, the extent to which men derive comfort from the use of CBE. In our ongoing cross-cultural pet loss research (Kiel et al. 2015) we assessed the specific process or predictor variables associated with pet loss, including gender. Preliminary results indicated that women reported higher levels of social constraint, that is, negative social responses to expressing grief, than men. It is possible that women talk more openly about their loss with others. Thus, they may be more likely to receive negative social responses (high social constraint) than men. These preliminary results support further investigation and analyses of the relationship between social constraints, gender, attachment, loss and CBE.

In addition, future research should use a longitudinal research design and repeated measures of CBE and other constructs in order to see how CBE change over time. It would then be possible to clarify the developmental course of various CBE for men in pet loss.

Future research should also include an in depth exploration of contextual factors related to pet loss. Specifically, we recommend examining the situational factors related to euthanasia and their impact on grief. Of interest would be the relationship between the euthanasia decision-making process and the subsequent intensity and duration of grief, in addition to the impact on CBE. Clinicians and researchers are in need of knowing how CBE are experienced similarly or differently, if they are, in various groups, e.g., within and between gender variables, children, adults and elders. Specifically, we should identify and explore the person specific factors which contribute to a client's ability or willingness to utilize CBE as an adaptive coping strategy. Knowledge about multi-cultural and different spiritual experiences of pet owners is also lacking. Because of this, our ongoing international cross-cultural research related to CBE and pet loss is significant for clinical practice.

References

Adams, C. L., Bonnett, B. N., & Meek, A. H. (2000). Predictors of owner response to companion animal death in 177 clients from 14 practices in Ontario. *Journal of the American Veterinary Medical Association, 9*, 1303–1309.

Ainsworth, M. D. S., & Bell, S. M. (1970). Attachment, exploration and separation: Illustrated by the behavior of one year olds in a strange situation. *Child Development, 41*, 49–67.

Allen, K. M., Blascovich, J., Tomaka, J., & Kelsey, R. M. (1991). Presence of human friends and pet dogs as moderators of autonomic responses to stress in women. *Journal of Personality and Social Psychology, 61*, 582–589.
Anderson, W., Reid, C., & Jennings, G. (1992). Pet ownership and risk factors for cardiovascular disease. *Medical Journal of Australia, 157*(5), 298–301.
Arehart-Treichel, J. (1982). Pets: The health benefits. *Science News, 220–223.*
Aydin, N., Krueger, J. I., Fischer, J., Hahn, D., & Kastenmüller, A. (2012). "Man's best friend": How the presence of a dog reduces mental distress after social exclusion. *Journal of Experimental Social Psychology, 48*, 446–449.
Barba, B. (1991). The human companion animal relationship: Philosophical inquiry (Doctoral dissertation, New York University, 1991). Dissertation Abstracts International.
Bowlby, J. (1969). *Attachment and loss* (Vol. I). Attachment. New York: Basic Books.
Bowlby, J. (1980). *Attachment and Loss, Vol. 3: Loss* (2nd ed.). New York: Basic Books.
Brown, B. H., Richards, H. C., & Wilson, C. A. (1996). Pet bonding and pet bereavement among adolescents. *Journal of Counseling and Development, 74*(5), 505.
Cain, A. O. (1985). Pets as family members. *Marriage and Family Review, 8*, 5–10.
Carmack, B. J. (2003). *Grieving the death of a pet*. Minneapolis: Augsburg Books.
Clements, P. T., Benasutti, K. M., & Carmone, A. (2003). Support for bereaved owners of pets. *Perspectives in Psychiatric Care, 39*(2), 49–54.
Cohen, S. P. (2002). Can pets function as family members? *Western Journal of Nursing Research, 24*(6), 621–638.
Costa, P. J., Terracciano, A., & McCrae, R. R. (2001). Gender differences in personality traits across cultures: Robust and surprising findings. *Journal of Personality and Social Psychology, 8*(12), 322–331.
Cowles, K. V. (1985). The death of a pet: Human responses to the breaking of the bond. *Marriage & Family Review, 8*(3–4), 135–148.
Cusack, O. (1988). *Pets and mental health*. New York: Haworth Press.
Doka, K. J. (1989). *Disenfranchised grief: Recognizing hidden sorrow*. Lexington, MA: Lexington Books.
Doka, K. J., & Martin, T. L. (2010). *Grieving beyond gender: Understanding the ways men and women mourn*. New York: Routledge.
Duncan, S. L. (1995). Loneliness: A health hazard of modern times. *Interactions, 13*(1), 5–9.
Field, N. P. (2008). Whether to relinquish or maintain a bond with the deceased. In M. S. Stroebe, R. O. Hansson, H. Schut, & W. Stroebe (Eds.), *Handbook of bereavement research and practice: Advances in theory and intervention* (pp. 113–132). Washington, DC: American Psychological Association.
Field, N. P. (2010). Continuing bonds in coping with the loss of a husband (Unpublished raw data).
Field, N. P., & Friedrichs, M. (2004). Continuing bonds in coping with the death of a husband. *Death Studies, 28*(7), 597–620.
Field, N. P., Gao, B., & Paderna, L. (2005). Continuing bonds in bereavement: An attachment theory based perspective. *Death Studies, 29*, 277–299.
Field, N. P., Nichols, C., Holen, A., & Horowitz, M. (1999). The relation of continuing attachment to adjustment in conjugal bereavement. *Journal of Consulting and Clinical Psychology, 67*, 212–218.
Field, N. P., Packman, W., & Carmack, B. J. (2007). Continuing bonds interview (Unpublished instrument).
Frankel, R. (2014). *War dogs: Tales of canine heroism, history, and love*. New York: Palgrave Macmillan.
Gage, M., & Holcomb, R. (1991). Couples' perception of stressfulness of death of the family pet. *Family Relations, 40*(1), 103–105.
Garrity, T. F., Stallones, L., Marx, M. B., & Johnson, T. P. (1989). Pet ownership and attachment as supportive factors in the health of the elderly. *Anthrozoös, 3*, 35–44.

Gerwolls, M. K., & Labott, S. M. (1994). Adjustments to the death of a companion animal. *Anthrozoös, VII*(3), 172–187.
Gosse, G. H. (1994). Human grief resulting from the death of a pet. *Journal of the Delta Society, 7*(2), 103–112.
Gosse, G. (1988). Factors associated with the human grief experience as a result of the death of a pet. Doctoral dissertation available from ProQuest Dissertations and Theses (AAT No. 8825153).
Handlin, L., Hydbring-Sandberg, E., Nilsson, A., Ejdebäck, M., Jansson, A., & Uvnäs-Moberg, K. (2011). Short-Term Interaction between Dogs and Their Owners: Effects on Oxytocin, Cortisol, Insulin and Heart Rate—An Exploratory Study. *Anthrozoos: A Multidisciplinary Journal of The Interactions of People & Animals, 24*(3), 301–315.
Herzog, H. A. (2007). Gender differences in human-animal interactions: A review. *Anthrozoös, 20*(1), 7–21.
Kiel, K., Makhoulian, S., Habarth, J., Packman, W., & Field, N. (2015, August). *Gender and pet loss: Social constraints as a mediator of physical and mental health outcomes*. Poster accepted and to be presented at the annual meeting of the American Psychological Association, Toronto, Canada.
Klass, D., Silverman, P., & Nickman, S. L. (Eds.). (1996). *Continuing bonds—New understanding of grief*. Philadelphia: Taylor & Francis.
Kurdek, L. (2009). Pet dogs as attachment figures for adult owners. *Journal of Family Psychology, 23*(4), 439–446.
Labrecque, J., & Walsh, C. A. (2011). Homeless women's voices on incorporating companion animals into shelter services. *Anthrozoös, 24*(1), 79–95.
Lagoni, L., Butler, C., & Hetts, S. (1994). *The human-animal bond and grief*. New York: W.B. Saunders Company.
Levinson, B. (1969). *Pet oriented child psychotherapy*. Springfield, Illinios: Charles C. Thomas.
Levinson, B. (1997). *Pet oriented child psychotherapy* (2nd ed.). Springfield, IL: Charles C. Thomas.
Lockwood, R. (1983). The influence of animals on social perception. In A. H. Katcher & A. M. Beck (Eds.), *New perspectives on our lives with companion animals* (pp. 64–71). Philadelphia: University of Pennsylvania Press.
Mallon, G. P. (1992). Utilization of animals as therapeutic adjuncts with children and youth: A review of the literature. *Child & Youth Care Forum, 21*(1), 53–67.
Manning, S. (2014, March 13). *US trade group: spending on pets at all-time high*. Retrieved from http://bigstory.ap.org/article/ap-exclusive-americans-spend-56-billion-pets.
Margolies, L. (1999). The long good-bye: Women, companion animals, and maternal loss. *Clinical Social Work Journal, 27*(3), 289–304.
McCutcheon, K. A., & Fleming, S. J. (2002). Grief resulting from euthanasia and natural death of companion animals. *OMEGA, 44*(2), 169–188.
Messent, P. R. (1983). Social facilitation of contact with other people by pet dogs. In A. H. Katcher & A. M. Beck (Eds.), *New perspectives on our lives with companion animals* (pp. 37–46). Philadelphia: University of Pennsylvania Press.
Moneymaker, J. M., & Strimple, E. O. (1991). Animals and inmates: A sharing companionship behind bars. *Journal of Offender Rehabilitation, 16*, 133–152.
Nagasawa, M., Mogi, K., & Kikusui, T. (2009). Attachment between humans and dogs. *Japanese Psychological Research, 51*(3), 209–221.
Ory, M. G., & Goldberg, E. L. (1983). Pet possession and life satisfaction in elderly women. A.H. Katcher, & A. M. Beck (Eds.), *New perspectives on our lives with companion animals* (pp. 303–317). Philadelphia: University of Pennsylvania Press.
Oyama, M. A., & Serpell, J. A. (2013). General commentary: Rethinking the role of animals in human well-being. *Frontiers in Psychology for Clinical Settings, 4*, 374.
Packman, W., Carmack, B. J., Katz, R., Carlos, F., Field, N. P., & Landers, C. (2014). Online survey as empathic bridging for the disenfranchised grief of pet loss. *Omega, 69*(4), 333–356.
Packman, W., Carmack, B. J., & Ronen, R. (2012). Therapeutic implications of continuing bonds expressions following the death of a pet. *Omega, 64*(4), 335–356.

Packman, W., Field, N. P., Carmack, B. J., & Ronen, R. (2011). Continuing bonds and psychosocial adjustment in pet loss. *Journal of Loss and Trauma,16:4,* 341–357. doi:10.1080/15325024.2011.572046

Peacock, J., Chur-Hansen, Al, & Winefield, H. (2012). Mental health implications of human attachment to companion animals. *Journal of Clinical Psychology, 68*(3), 292–303.

Planchon, L. A., & Templer, D. L. (1996). The correlates of grief after death of pet. *Anthrozoos, 9*(2–3), 107–113.

Planchon, L. A., Templer, D. I., Stokes, S., & Keller, J. (2002). Death of a companion cat or dog and human bereavement: Psychosocial variables. *Society & Animals: Journal of Human-Animal Studies, 10*(1), 93–105.

Podrazik, D., Shackford, S., Becker, L., & Heckert, T. (2000). The death of a pet: Implications for loss and bereavement across the lifespan. *Journal of Personal and Interpersonal Loss, 3*, 361–395.

Prato-Previde, E., Fallani, G., & Valsecchi, P. (2006). Gender differences in owners interacting with pet dogs: An observational study. *Ethnology, 112*(1), 64–73.

Quackenbush, J. E. (1985). The death of a pet: How it can affect owners. *The Veterinary Clinics of North America. Small Animal Practice, 15*, 395–402.

Ramirez, M. (2006). My dog's just like me: Dog ownership as a gender display. *Symbolic Interaction, 29*(3), 373–391.

Raupp, D. C. (1999). Treasuring, trashing or terrorizing: Adult outcomes of childhood socialization about companion animals. *Society & Animals, 7*(2), 141–159.

Raupp, D. C., Barlow, M., & Oliver, J. (1997). Perceptions of family violence: Are companion animals in the picture? *Society and Animals, 5*(3), 219–237.

Reynolds, T. E. (1999). *Pet bonding and pet bereavement as a function of culture and gender differences among adolescents* (Doctoral dissertation). Retrieved from ProQuest Dissertations and Theses (Accession Order No. AA19935416).

Robin, M., & ten Bensel, R. (1985). Pets and the socialization of children. In M. B. Sussman (Ed.), *Pets and the family* (pp. 63–78). New York: The Haworth Press.

Rothaupt, J. W., & Becker, K. (2007). A literature review of western bereavement theory: From decathecting to continuing bonds. *The Family Journal: Counseling and Therapy for Couples and Families, 15*(1), 6–15.

Ruth, R. (1992). Animals are helping children overcome physical and emotional challenges. *Interactions, 10*, 16–18.

Ryder, R. D. (1973). Pets in man's search for sanity. *Journal of Small Animal Practice, 14*, 657–668.

Rynearson, E. K. (1978). Humans and pets and attachment. *British Journal of Psychiatry, 133*, 550–555.

Sable, P. (1995). Pets, attachment, and well-being across the life-cycle. *Social Work, 40*(3), 334–341.

Sable, P. (2013). The pet connection: An attachment perspective. *Clinical Social Work Journal, 41*(1), 93–99.

Savishinsky, J. S. (1983). Pet ideas; The domestication of animals, human behavior, and human emotions. In A. H. Katcher & A. M. Beck (Eds.), *New perspectives on our lives with companion animals* (pp. 112–131). Philadelphia: University of Pennsylvania Press.

Serpell, J. A. (1996). Evidence for an association between pet behavior and owner attachment levels. *Applied Animal Behaviour Science, 47*(1–2), 49–60.

Stroebe, M., Gergen, M. M., Gergen, K. J., & Stroebe, W. (1992). Broken hearts or broken bonds: Love and death in historical perspective. *American Psychologist, 47*, 1205–1212.

Stutts, J. C. (1994). *Pet bereavement counseling: Factors related to pet owner depression in a local veterinary hospital versus a veterinary teaching hospital.* Doctoral Dissertation, Walden University, Minneapolis, MN.

The Humane Society. (2014, January 30). *Pets by the numbers.* Retrieved from http://www.humanesociety.org/issues/pet_overpopulation/facts/pet_ownership_statistics.html

Thompson, M. J. (2009). Animal-assisted play therapy: Canines as co-therapists. Compelling counseling interventions. *VISTAS, 2009*, 199–209.

Triebenbacher, S. L. (1998). The relationship between attachment to companion animals and self esteem: A developmental perspective. In C. Wilson & D. Turner (Eds.), *Companion animals in human health* (pp. 135–148). Thousand Oakes, CA: Sage Publications.

Voith, V. (1985). Attachment of people to companion animals. *Veterinary Clinics of North America: Small Animal Practice, 15*(2), 289–295.

Weisman, A. D. (1990). Bereavement and companion animals. *Omega, 22*(4), 241–248. 1991.

Williams, J. M., Muldoon, J., & Lawrence, A. (2009). Children and their pets: Exploring the relationships between pet ownership, pet attitudes, attachment to pets and empathy. *Education and Health, 28*(1), 12–15.

Wolfe, J. (1977). The use of pets as transitional objects in adolescent interpersonal functioning. *Dissertation Abstracts International, 28*(5), 2391.

Wrobel, T. A., & Dye, A. L. (2003). Grieving pet death: Normative, gender, and attachment issues. *OMEGA: Journal of Death and Dying, 47*(4), 385–393.

Zasloff, R. L., & Kidd, A. H. (1994). Loneliness and pet ownership among single women. *Psychological Reports, 75*, 747–752.

Index

Note: Page numbers followed by *f* and *t* indicate figures and tables, respectively

C. Blazina and L.R. Kogan (eds.), *Men and Their Dogs*,
DOI 10.1007/978-3-319-30097-9

MIX
Papier aus verantwortungsvollen Quellen
Paper from responsible sources
FSC® C105338

If you have any concerns about our products,
you can contact us on
ProductSafety@springernature.com

In case Publisher is established outside the EU,
the EU authorized representative is:
Springer Nature Customer Service Center GmbH
Europaplatz 3, 69115 Heidelberg, Germany

Printed by Libri Plureos GmbH
in Hamburg, Germany